中医经典译丛
Chinese-English Translation of Traditional Chinese Medicine Classics

救荒本草
Materia Medica for Famine Relief
（汉英对照）

原　著　朱　橚
主　译　范延妮
副主译　李　琳
译　者　王芳芳　张　洁
　　　　李　琳　范延妮

本书为山东中医药大学"中医英译及中医文化对外传播研究"科研创新团队项目资助成果、山东中医药大学英语专业学科建设资助成果。

苏州大学出版社

图书在版编目(CIP)数据

救荒本草 = Materia Medica for Famine Relief：汉英对照 /(明)朱橚原著；范延妮主译. — 苏州：苏州大学出版社，2019.9
(中医经典译丛)
ISBN 978-7-5672-2757-6

Ⅰ.①救… Ⅱ.①朱… ②范… Ⅲ.①食物本草-研究-汉、英 Ⅳ.①R281.5

中国版本图书馆 CIP 数据核字(2019)第 142532 号

| 书　　名：救荒本草 JIU HUANG BEN CAO |
| Materia Medica for Famine Relief |
| （汉英对照） |

原　　著：朱　橚
主　　译：范延妮
责任编辑：汤定军
策划编辑：汤定军
装帧设计：刘　俊

出版发行：苏州大学出版社(Soochow University Press)
社　　址：苏州市十梓街1号　邮编：215006
印　　装：虎彩印艺股份有限公司
网　　址：www.sudapress.com
邮　　箱：sdcbs@suda.edu.cn
邮购热线：0512-67480030
销售热线：0512-67481020
开　　本：700mm×1 000mm　1/16　印张：25　字数：398 千
版　　次：2019 年 9 月第 1 版
印　　次：2019 年 9 月第 1 次印刷
书　　号：ISBN 978-7-5672-2757-6
定　　价：88.00 元

凡购本社图书发现印装错误，请与本社联系调换。服务热线：0512-67481020

《救荒本草》序

植物之生于天地间，莫不各有所用，苟不见诸载籍，虽老农老圃亦不能尽识，而可亨可茹者，皆躏藉于牛羊鹿豕而已。自神农氏品尝草木，辨其寒温甘苦之性，作为医药，以济人之夭札，后世赖以延生。而《本草》书中所载，多伐病之物，而于可茹以充腹者，则未之及也。

敬惟周王殿下，体仁遵义，孳孳为善，凡可以济人利物之事，无不留意。尝读孟子书，至于五谷不熟，不如荑稗，因念林林总总之民，不幸罹于旱涝，五谷不熟，则可以疗饥者，恐不止荑稗而已也。苟能知悉而载诸方册，俾不得已而求食者，不惑甘苦于荼荠，取昌阳，弃乌喙，因得以裨五谷之缺，则岂不为救荒之一助哉。于是购田夫野老，得甲坼勾萌者四百余种，植于一圃，躬自阅视。俟其滋长成熟，乃召画工绘之为图，仍疏其花、实、根、干、皮、叶之可食者，汇次为书一帙，名曰《救荒本草》。命臣同为之序。

臣惟人情于饱食暖衣之际，多不以冻馁为虞，一旦遇患难，则莫知所措，惟付之于无可奈何，故治己治人鲜不失所。今殿下处富贵之尊，保有邦域，于无可虞度之时，乃能念生民万一或有之患，深得古圣贤安不忘危之旨，不亦善乎。神农品尝草木，以疗斯民之疾，殿下区别草木，欲济斯民之饥，同一仁心之用也。虽然，今天下方乐雍熙泰和之治，禾麦产瑞，家给人足，不必论及于荒政，而殿下亦岂忍睹斯民仰食于草木哉？是编之作，盖欲辨载嘉植，不没其用，期与《图经本草》并传于后世，庶几萍实有征，而凡可以亨茹者，得不躏藉于牛羊鹿豕；苟或见用于荒岁，其及人之功利，又非药石所可拟也。尚虑四方所产之多，不能尽录，补其未备，则有俟于后日云。

永乐四年岁次丙戌秋八月奉议大夫周府左长史臣卞同拜手谨序。

卞同
1406 年 8 月

重刻《救荒本草》序

《淮南子》曰："神农尝百草之滋味，一日而七十毒。"由是《本草》兴焉。陶隐居、徐之才、陈藏器、日华子、唐慎微之徒，代有演述，皆为疗病也。嗣后孟诜有《食疗本草》，陈士良有《食性本草》，皆因饮馔以调摄人，非为救荒也。《救荒本草》二卷，乃永乐间周藩集录而刻之者，今亡其板。濂家食时，访求善本，自汴携来。晋台按察使石冈蔡公，见而嘉之，以告于巡抚都御使蒙斋毕公。公曰："是有裨荒政者。"乃下令刊布，命濂序之。

按，《周礼·大司徒》以荒政十二聚万民，五曰舍禁。夫舍禁者，谓舍其虞泽之厉禁，纵民采取，以济饥也。若沿江濒湖诸郡邑，皆有鱼虾螺蚬、菱芡茭藻之饶，饥者犹有赖焉。齐梁秦晋之墟，平原坦野，弥望千里，一遇大侵，而鹄形鸟面之孚，枕藉丁道路。呼，可悲已！后汉永兴二年，诏令郡国种芜菁以助食。然五方之风气异宜，而物产之形质异状，名汇既繁，真赝难别，使不图列而详说之，鲜有不以虺床当蘼芜，荠苨乱人参者，其弊至于杀人，此《救荒本草》之所以作也。是书有图有说，图以肖其形，说以著其用。首言产生之壤、同异之名，次言寒热之性、甘苦之味，终言淘浸烹煮、蒸晒调和之法。草木野菜，凡四百一十四种，见旧《本草》者一百三十八种，新增者二百七十六种云。或遇荒岁，按图而求之，随地皆有，无艰得者。苟如法采食，可以活命。是书也，有功于生民大矣。昔李文靖为相，每奏对，常以四方水旱为言。范文正为江淮宣抚使，见民以野草煮食，即奏而献之。毕、蔡二公刊布之盛心，其类是夫。

嘉靖四年岁次乙酉春二月之吉，赐进士出身奉政大夫山西等处提刑按察司金事奉敕提督屯政大梁李濂撰。

李濂

1525 年 2 月

翻译说明

1. 本次所译的《救荒本草》以中华书局1959年影印本为底本,以文渊阁《四库全书》为校本,并参考了多个通行本。

2. 为了更准确地展现和传递《救荒本草》的基本信息,本书的本草采用中文原文、中文注释、英文译文、英文注释予以编排。

3. 本草名称的翻译采取"四保险"的翻译方法,即每个本草名称均按拼音、汉字、英文和拉丁文的方式进行翻译,如"荠菜"译为 Jicai [荠菜,shepherd's purse, Capsellae Bursa-Pastoris (L.) Medic.]。

4. 本草名称如果是三个字及以下,其音译合并在一起;如果是四个字及以上,根据文义将其音译分开,便于阅读。

5. 古籍名称采用音译的方法翻译,括号中附以中文和英文翻译,音译中的每个字独立音译。例如,《图经本草》译为 Tu Jing Ben Cao [《图经本草》,Illustrated Classic of Materia Medica]。

6. 《救荒本草》中部分中药名称经多方考证,至今仍无法确定为何种中药,在翻译成英文的时候,采取音译加 medicinal 的方法;翻译成拉丁文的时候,采取 materia medica 加音译的方法。

7. 书中出现的繁体字、异体字根据现行出版规范改为简体字、通行字。书中涉及的剂量单位采用音译方法,基本形式和释义如下:

传统剂量单位	公制剂量单位	音译形式
尺	0.3333333 米	Chi
寸	0.0333333 米	Cun
丈	3.3333333 米	Zhang

Preface of *Materia Medica for Famine Relief*

All of the plants on the earth have their own values and functions. If not recorded in books, they would not be identified and familiarized even by experienced farmers. Especially those edible ones are treaded and eaten by such livestock as cows, sheep, deer and pigs instead of being taken by people. Thanks to Agriculture God's efforts to taste all kinds of plants and herbs and distinguish their different properties of cold, warm, sweet and bitter, these plants and herbs can be applied as medicinal to save and protect people from dying early and prolong people's life-span. However, those plants recorded in the *Shen Nong Ben Cao Jing*[《神农本草经》, *Agriculture God's Canon of Materia Medica*] are mainly to treat disease, there is almost no record found about the edible ones to relieve famine.

Our respected King Zhou, virtuous and moral, was devoted in carrying out benefactions and focused on anything beneficial to the people and society. He once read the writings of Mencius and knew that the five cereals were far less helpful than the weeds like Baizi [稗子, barnyard grass, Echinochloa crusgalli (L.) Beauv] if crop failure happened. This reminded him of the fact that besides Baizi, there probably existed more weeds and wild plants edible to relieve famine in case of natural disasters like flood, drought and crop failures. It would be a good method to relieve famine and cover shortage of food by recognizing and recording these edible plants, with the purpose to help people clarify different tastes of the plants like Tucai [荼菜, Tucai Medicinal, Materia Medica Tucai] and Jicai [荠菜, shepherd's purse, Capsellae Bursa-Pastoris (L.) Medic.], select edible plants like Changpu [菖蒲, acorus, Acori Tatarinowii Rhizoma] and discard toxic ones like Wutou [乌头, aconite,

Aconitum carmichaelii Debx.]. Based on these thoughts, King Zhou collected and paid for about 400 kinds of edible young plants and planted them in a nursery garden. He observed and cared for these plants till they grew to full maturity. Then he asked painters to draw their pictures, classified and recorded their edible parts like flowers, fruits, roots, stems, peels and leaves, arranged and compiled them into a book named *Jiu Huang Ben Cao* [《救荒本草》, *Materia Medica for Famine Relief*], for which I was asked to write a preface.

It is believed that people would not worry about such things as cold and hunger when in abundance. So they feel overwhelmed and helpless once in famine with no way out. This often happens not only to the common people but also to the rulers. Presently King Zhou, with his own state and glorious life, is concerned about people's life in unexpected disaster and can be regarded as a good practitioner for the ancient saint's principle of "being prepared for danger in times of safety". Both of the Agriculture God and King Zhou are kind and benevolent, with the former tasting plants to treat disease and the latter identifying them to relieve famine. Of course, there is no need to discuss famine and take these plants as food in this peaceful and prosperous age. The purpose of this book is to identify, record and spread different kinds of edible plants and hand them down to later generations together with *Tu Jing Ben Cao* [《图经本草》, *Illustrated Classic of Materia Medica*]. This book would help people when searching for and using edible plants instead of letting them destroyed by cows, sheep, deer and pigs. Its function and benefit to the common people would be especially felt in the year of famine due to crop failures, far greater than medicinal. It is impossible for a book to include all the species of plants for their great variety from different regions, so future work is needed for further supplement.

Bian Tong

August, 1406

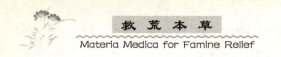

Preface to the Republication of *Materia Medica for Famine Relief*

According to *Huai-nan Tzu*, "Shennong has tasted hundreds of herbs and ever encountered seventy toxic plants in one day". From then on, this kind of monograph on materia medica has developed. Tao Hongjing, Xu Zhicai, Chen Zangqi, Ri Huazi, Tang Shenwei and others have performed deductives from generation to generation. Their purpose in writing *Materia Medica* is to cure diseases. Later the intention of *Shi Liao Ben Cao* [《食疗本草》, *Materia Medica for Dietotherapy*] written by Meng Shen and *Shi Xing Ben Cao* [《食性本草》, *Materia Medica for Therapeutic efficacy*] by Chen Shiliang were not for famine relief but for dietary health maintenance. The two volumes of *Jiu Huang Ben Cao* [《救荒本草》, *Materia Medica for Famine Relief*] were recorded in the collection of Zhou Dingwang in the Yongle Period. Now the original version has lost. When I was at home, I searched the rare version of the book and brought it back from Zhangzhou. After the inspection in Shanxi, the Shigang officer Cai Tianyou was very appreciative after seeing it, so he told the governor Bi of Mengzhai. Bi said, "This is a book that is good for the famine." So the order was issued to ask me to preface the book.

According to *Zhouli · Dasitu* [《周礼·大司徒》, *The Rites of Zhou · Grand Minister of Education*], there are 12 policies for famine relief to convene the public with the fifth policy named Shejin. The so-called Shejin refers to lift the previous ban of lakes and rivers, and permit the common people to fish and pick at will and overcome the famines. The prefectures and towns, which are along watersides, are rich in fishes, shrimps, clams and snails. The famine refugees still can survive by relying on them. While in the areas of Qi, Liang, Qin and Jin prefecture which is featured with flatlands, the

Preface to the Republication of *Materia Medica for Famine Relief*

common people would starve at the roadsides in big famine due to crop failures. What a terrible thing! In the second year of Yongxing of the Eastern Han Dynasty (154), Emperor Sui of the Sui Dynasty ordered the country to plant turnips to help solve the shortage of food. However, the suitable terroir and climate in different places are different. The physical appearance of the products is also different. The names are complicated and difficult to distinguish. If you do not draw them and explain the characteristics of these plants in detail, most people will take Huichuang [虺床, cnidium monnieri, Cnidium monnieri (L.) Cuss.] as Miwu [蘪芜, Sichuan lovage rhizome, Ligusticum Chuanxiong Hort.] and confuse Jini [荠苨, adenophora trachelioides, Adenophora trachelioides Maxim.] with Renshen [人参, ginseng, Panax ginseng C. A. Mey.]. Thus it will do harm to people and even lead to death. This is the reason why the book was written. The pictures describe the plant images and the plant applications can be clarified by the relevant texts. The book elaborates on producing areas, the names and alternative names, characteristics and properties of the plants. The processing methods such as rinsing, soaking, boiling, steaming and drying, and the compatibilities are also elucidated. There are 414 herbaceous and woody plants with 138 listed in the original *Bencao* [《重修政和经史证类备急本草》, *Revised Zhenghe Classified Materia Medica from Historical Classics for Emergency*] and 276 new supplements. In the famine years, it is easy to find the plants everywhere according to the pictures recorded in this book. And people can survive by the methods of collecting and cooking plants for food listed in the book. This book would be great beneficial for the common people. The Prime Minister Li Hang used to report the floods and droughts across the country to the emperor, Fan Zhongyan ever respectfully reported and presented wild herbs eaten by common people to the emperor when he served as the officer of Xuan Fushi in Jianghuai region. Bi Zhao and Cai Tianyou also have the same intentions to inscribe and publish this book.

Li Lian

February, 1525

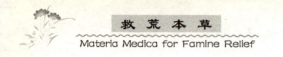

Translation Specification

1. The translation of *Materia Medica for Famine Relief* takes its Chinese photocopy published by Chung Wha Book Company in 1959 as the master copy, the *Complete Library in the Four Branches of Literature* stored in Imperial Library as the checked copy, and also refers to many current versions.

2. For a better presentation and transmission of the content of *Materia Medica for Famine Relief*, this book is arranged in the order like the following: Chinese text, Chinese notes, English translation and English notes.

3. As to the translation of herbal names, the "Four Assurance Method" is adopted, namely, every herbal name is translated in the way that its four forms are listed in the sequence of Pinyin, Chinese character, English and Latin. For instance, "荠菜" is translated as Jicai [荠菜, shepherd's purse, Capsellae Bursa-Pastoris (L.) Medic.].

4. If a herbal name has three Chinese characters, its transliteration of Pinyin is put together; if a herbal name has four or more than four Chinese characters, its transliteration of Pinyin is divided into two parts according to its literal meaning for the convenience of easy reading.

5. The names of ancient books are transliterated with its Chinese names and English versions in brackets, every Chinese character being transliterated separately. For instance,《图经本草》is translated as *Tu Jing Ben Cao* [《图经本草》, *Illustrated Classic of Materia Medica*].

6. There are some herbal names from *Materia Medica for Famine Relief*, even after textual research, hard to be exactly clarified and confirmed till now, so they are translated into English with Pinyin plus "medicinal" and into Latin

with "materia medica" plus Pinyin.

7. The traditional Chinese characters and variant Chinese characters in this book are changed into the simplified and current Chinese characters according to the current publishing standards. Dose unit involved in this book is translated with Pinyin. Refer to the table below:

Traditional dose unit	Metric dose unit	Pinyin
尺	0.3333333 meter	Chi
寸	0.0333333 meter	Cun
丈	3.3333333 meter	Zhang

目录

卷上 上之前

草 部

叶可食

《本草》原有

1. 刺蓟菜 ………………………… 1
2. 大蓟 …………………………… 3
3. 山苋菜 ………………………… 4
4. 款冬花 ………………………… 5
5. 萹蓄 …………………………… 7
6. 大蓝 …………………………… 8
7. 石竹子 ………………………… 9
8. 红花菜 ………………………… 10
9. 萱草花 ………………………… 11
10. 车轮菜 ……………………… 12
11. 白水荭苗 …………………… 13
12. 黄耆 ………………………… 14
13. 威灵仙 ……………………… 15
14. 马兜零 ……………………… 17
15. 旋覆花 ……………………… 18
16. 防风 ………………………… 19
17. 郁臭苗 ……………………… 20
18. 泽漆 ………………………… 21
19. 酸浆草 ……………………… 22
20. 蛇床子 ……………………… 23
21. 桔梗 ………………………… 24
22. 茴香 ………………………… 26
23. 夏枯草 ……………………… 27
24. 藁本 ………………………… 28
25. 柴胡 ………………………… 29
26. 漏芦 ………………………… 30
27. 龙胆草 ……………………… 31
28. 鼠菊 ………………………… 32
29. 前胡 ………………………… 33
30. 猪牙菜 ……………………… 34
31. 地榆 ………………………… 35
32. 川芎 ………………………… 36
33. 葛勒子秧 …………………… 38
34. 连翘 ………………………… 39
35. 仙灵脾 ……………………… 40
36. 青杞 ………………………… 41
37. 野生姜 ……………………… 42
38. 马兰头 ……………………… 43
39. 豨莶 ………………………… 44
40. 泽泻 ………………………… 45

新增

41. 竹节菜 ……………………… 46
42. 独扫苗 ……………………… 47
43. 歪头菜 ……………………… 48
44. 兔儿酸 ……………………… 48
45. 碱蓬 ………………………… 49

46. 茼蒿 ……	50	79. 青荚儿菜 ……	71
47. 水莴苣 ……	50	80. 八角菜 ……	72
48. 金盏菜 ……	51	81. 耐惊菜 ……	72
49. 水辣菜 ……	51	82. 地棠菜 ……	73
50. 紫云菜 ……	52	83. 鸡儿肠 ……	73
51. 鸦葱 ……	53	84. 雨点儿菜 ……	74
52. 匙头菜 ……	53	85. 白屈菜 ……	75
53. 鸡冠菜 ……	54	86. 扯根菜 ……	76
54. 水蔓菁 ……	55	87. 草零陵香 ……	77
55. 野园荽 ……	55	88. 水落藜 ……	77
56. 牛尾菜 ……	56	89. 凉蒿菜 ……	78
57. 山萮菜 ……	57	90. 粘鱼须 ……	79
58. 绵丝菜 ……	57	91. 节节菜 ……	80
59. 米蒿 ……	58	92. 野艾蒿 ……	80
60. 山芥菜 ……	59	93. 堇堇菜 ……	81
61. 舌头菜 ……	59	94. 婆婆纳 ……	82
62. 紫香蒿 ……	60	95. 野茴香 ……	82
63. 金盏儿花 ……	60	96. 蝎子花菜 ……	83
64. 六月菊 ……	61	97. 白蒿 ……	84
65. 费菜 ……	62	98. 野茼蒿 ……	84
66. 千屈菜 ……	62	99. 野粉团儿 ……	85
67. 柳叶菜 ……	63	100. 蚵蚾菜 ……	86
68. 婆婆指甲菜 ……	64	101. 狗掉尾苗 ……	87
69. 铁杆蒿 ……	64	102. 石芥 ……	88
70. 山甜菜 ……	65	103. 獾耳菜 ……	88
71. 剪刀股 ……	65	104. 回回蒜 ……	89
72. 水苏子 ……	66	105. 地槐菜 ……	90
73. 风花菜 ……	67	106. 螺黡儿 ……	90
74. 鹅儿肠 ……	67	107. 泥胡菜 ……	91
75. 粉条儿菜 ……	68	108. 兔儿丝 ……	92
76. 辣辣菜 ……	69	109. 老鹳筋 ……	93
77. 毛连菜 ……	69	110. 绞股蓝 ……	93
78. 小桃红 ……	70	111. 山梗菜 ……	94

112. 㸬娘蒿	95		140. 地花菜	118
113. 鸡肠菜	95		141. 杓儿菜	119
114. 水葫芦苗	96		142. 佛指甲	119
115. 胡苍耳	97		143. 虎尾草	120
116. 水棘针苗	98		144. 野蜀葵	121
117. 沙蓬	99		145. 蛇葡萄	121
118. 麦蓝菜	100		146. 星宿菜	122
119. 女娄菜	100		147. 水蓑衣	123
120. 委陵菜	101		148. 牛奶菜	124
121. 独行菜	102		149. 小虫儿卧单	124
122. 山蓼	103		150. 兔儿尾苗	125

卷上　上之后
草部
叶可食
新增

			151. 地锦苗	126
			152. 野西瓜苗	126
123. 花蒿	105		153. 香茶菜	127
124. 葛公菜	106		154. 蔷蘼	128
125. 鲫鱼鳞	106		155. 毛女儿菜	129
126. 尖刀儿苗	107		156. 牻牛儿苗	129
127. 珍珠菜	108		157. 铁扫帚	130
128. 杜当归	109		158. 山小菜	131
129. 风轮菜	110		159. 羊角苗	131
130. 拖白练苗	110		160. 耧斗菜	132
131. 透骨草	111		161. 瓯菜	133
132. 酸桶笋	112		162. 变豆菜	134
133. 鹿蕨菜	113		163. 和尚菜	134
134. 山芹菜	113		**根可食**	
135. 金刚刺	114		*《本草》原有*	
136. 柳叶青	115		164. 萎蕤	136
137. 大蓬蒿	116		165. 百合	137
138. 狗筋蔓	116		166. 天门冬	139
139. 兔儿伞	117		167. 章柳根	141
			168. 沙参	142
			169. 麦门冬	144
			170. 苇根	145

171. 苍术 …………………… 146
172. 菖蒲 …………………… 148
新增
173. 菖子根 ………………… 149
174. 萩蒮根 ………………… 150
175. 野胡萝卜 ……………… 151
176. 绵枣儿 ………………… 152
177. 土圞儿 ………………… 153
178. 野山药 ………………… 153
179. 金瓜儿 ………………… 154
180. 细叶沙参 ……………… 155
181. 鸡腿儿 ………………… 156
182. 山蔓菁 ………………… 157
183. 老鸦蒜 ………………… 158
184. 山萝卜 ………………… 158
185. 地参 …………………… 159
186. 獐牙菜 ………………… 160
187. 鸡儿头苗 ……………… 160

实可食
《本草》原有
188. 雀麦 …………………… 161
189. 回回米 ………………… 162
190. 蒺藜子 ………………… 163
191. 苘子 …………………… 164
新增
192. 稗子 …………………… 165
193. 穄子 …………………… 166
194. 川谷 …………………… 167
195. 莠草子 ………………… 168
196. 野黍 …………………… 168
197. 鸡眼草 ………………… 169
198. 燕麦 …………………… 170
199. 泼盘 …………………… 170

200. 丝瓜苗 ………………… 171
201. 地角儿苗 ……………… 172
202. 马㼎儿 ………………… 173
203. 山黧豆 ………………… 173
204. 龙芽草 ………………… 174
205. 地稍瓜 ………………… 175
206. 锦荔枝 ………………… 176
207. 鸡冠果 ………………… 176

叶及实皆可食
《本草》原有
208. 羊蹄苗 ………………… 177
209. 苍耳 …………………… 178
210. 姑娘菜 ………………… 180
211. 土茜苗 ………………… 181
212. 王不留行 ……………… 182
213. 白薇 …………………… 183
新增
214. 蓬子菜 ………………… 185
215. 胡枝子 ………………… 185
216. 米布袋 ………………… 186
217. 天茄儿苗 ……………… 187
218. 苦马豆 ………………… 188
219. 猪尾把苗 ……………… 189

根叶可食
《本草》原有
220. 黄精苗 ………………… 190
221. 地黄苗 ………………… 192
222. 牛蒡子 ………………… 193
223. 远志 …………………… 194
224. 杏叶沙参 ……………… 196
225. 藤长苗 ………………… 197
226. 牛皮消 ………………… 198
227. 菹草 …………………… 199

228. 水豆儿 …………………… 199
229. 草三奈 …………………… 200
230. 水葱 ……………………… 201

根笋可食
《本草》原有

231. 蒲笋 ……………………… 202
232. 芦笋 ……………………… 203
233. 茅芽根 …………………… 204

根及花皆可食
《本草》原有

234. 葛根 ……………………… 205
235. 何首乌 …………………… 206

根及实皆可食
《本草》原有

236. 瓜楼根 …………………… 208

新增

237. 砖子苗 …………………… 210

花叶皆可食
《本草》原有

238. 菊花 ……………………… 211
239. 金银花 …………………… 212

新增

240. 望江南 …………………… 213
241. 大蓼 ……………………… 214

茎可食
《本草》原有

242. 黑三棱 …………………… 215

新增

243. 荇丝菜 …………………… 216
244. 水慈菰 …………………… 217

笋及实皆可食
《本草》原有

245. 茭笋 ……………………… 217

卷下 下之前
木 部
叶可食
《本草》原有

246. 茶树 ……………………… 219
247. 夜合树 …………………… 220
248. 木槿树 …………………… 221
249. 白杨树 …………………… 222
250. 黄栌 ……………………… 223
251. 椿树芽 …………………… 223
252. 椒树 ……………………… 225
253. 椋子树 …………………… 226

新增

254. 云桑 ……………………… 227
255. 黄楝树 …………………… 227
256. 冻青树 …………………… 228
257. 穞芽树 …………………… 229
258. 月芽树 …………………… 229
259. 女儿茶 …………………… 230
260. 省沽油 …………………… 231
261. 白槿树 …………………… 231
262. 回回醋 …………………… 232
263. 槭树芽 …………………… 233
264. 老叶儿树 ………………… 233
265. 青杨树 …………………… 234
266. 龙柏芽 …………………… 234
267. 兜栌树 …………………… 235
268. 青冈树 …………………… 236
269. 檀树芽 …………………… 236
270. 山茶科 …………………… 237
271. 木葛 ……………………… 238

272. 花楸树 …… 238	302. 野木瓜 …… 259
273. 白辛树 …… 239	303. 土栾树 …… 260
274. 木栾树 …… 239	304. 驴驼布袋 …… 260
275. 乌棱树 …… 240	305. 婆婆枕头 …… 261
276. 刺楸树 …… 241	306. 吉利子树 …… 262

叶及实皆可食

《本草》原有

277. 黄丝藤 …… 241	307. 枸杞 …… 262
278. 山格剌树 …… 242	308. 柏树 …… 264
279. 筕树 …… 242	309. 皂荚树 …… 265
280. 报马树 …… 243	310. 楮桃树 …… 266
281. 椴树 …… 244	311. 柘树 …… 267

新增

282. 臭萩 …… 244	312. 木羊角科 …… 268
283. 坚荚树 …… 245	313. 青檀树 …… 269
284. 臭竹树 …… 246	314. 山茼树 …… 269

花可食

新增

285. 马鱼儿条 …… 246	315. 藤花菜 …… 270
286. 老婆布毡 …… 247	316. 把齿花 …… 271

实可食

《本草》原有

287. 蕤核树 …… 248	317. 楸树 …… 272
288. 酸枣树 …… 249	318. 腊梅花 …… 272
289. 橡子树 …… 249	319. 马棘 …… 273
290. 荆子 …… 250	
291. 实枣儿树 …… 251	
292. 孩儿拳头 …… 252	

花叶皆可食

《本草》原有

	320. 槐树芽 …… 274

新增

花叶实皆可食

新增

293. 山菜儿 …… 254	
294. 山里果儿 …… 254	321. 棠梨树 …… 275
295. 无花果 …… 255	322. 文冠花 …… 276
296. 青舍子条 …… 255	
297. 白棠子树 …… 256	
298. 拐枣 …… 257	

叶皮及实皆可食

《本草》原有

299. 木桃儿树 …… 257	
300. 石冈橡 …… 258	323. 桑椹树 …… 277
301. 水茶臼 …… 259	

324. 榆钱树 ………………………… 279

笋可食
《本草》原有
325. 竹笋 ……………………………… 280

米谷部
实可食
新增
326. 野豌豆 …………………………… 282
327. 䉎豆 ……………………………… 283
328. 山扁豆 …………………………… 283
329. 回回豆 …………………………… 284
330. 胡豆 ……………………………… 285
331. 蚕豆 ……………………………… 286
332. 山绿豆 …………………………… 286

卷下 下之后
米谷部
叶及实皆可食
《本草》原有
333. 荞麦苗 …………………………… 288
334. 御米花 …………………………… 289
335. 赤小豆 …………………………… 290
336. 山丝苗 …………………………… 291
337. 油子苗 …………………………… 293

新增
338. 黄豆苗 …………………………… 294
339. 刀豆苗 …………………………… 294
340. 眉儿豆苗 ………………………… 295
341. 紫豇豆苗 ………………………… 296
342. 苏子苗 …………………………… 297
343. 豇豆苗 …………………………… 297
344. 山黑豆 …………………………… 298
345. 舜芒谷 …………………………… 299

果部
实可食
《本草》原有
346. 樱桃树 …………………………… 300
347. 胡桃树 …………………………… 301
348. 柿树 ……………………………… 302
349. 梨树 ……………………………… 303
350. 葡萄 ……………………………… 304
351. 李子树 …………………………… 305
352. 木瓜 ……………………………… 306
353. 樝子树 …………………………… 307
354. 郁李子 …………………………… 308
355. 菱角 ……………………………… 309

新增
356. 软枣 ……………………………… 310
357. 野葡萄 …………………………… 311
358. 梅杏树 …………………………… 312
359. 野樱桃 …………………………… 312

叶及实皆可食
《本草》原有
360. 石榴 ……………………………… 313
361. 杏树 ……………………………… 314
362. 枣树 ……………………………… 316
363. 桃树 ……………………………… 318

新增
364. 沙果子树 ………………………… 319

根可食
《本草》原有
365. 芋苗 ……………………………… 320
366. 铁葧脐 …………………………… 321

根及实皆可食
《本草》原有
367. 莲藕 ……………………………… 323

368. 鸡头实 …………………… 324

菜 部

叶可食

《本草》原有

369. 芸薹菜 …………………… 326
370. 苋菜 ………………………… 327
371. 苦苣菜 ……………………… 328
372. 马齿苋菜 …………………… 329
373. 苦荬菜 ……………………… 329
374. 莙荙菜 ……………………… 330
375. 邪蒿 ………………………… 331
376. 茼蒿 ………………………… 332
377. 冬葵菜 ……………………… 333
378. 蓼芽菜 ……………………… 334
379. 苜蓿 ………………………… 335
380. 薄荷 ………………………… 335
381. 荆芥 ………………………… 337
382. 水蘄 ………………………… 338

新增

383. 香菜 ………………………… 339
384. 银条菜 ……………………… 340
385. 后庭花 ……………………… 340
386. 火焰菜 ……………………… 341
387. 山葱 ………………………… 342
388. 背韭 ………………………… 342
389. 水芥菜 ……………………… 343
390. 遏蓝菜 ……………………… 343
391. 牛耳朵菜 …………………… 344
392. 山白菜 ……………………… 345
393. 山宜菜 ……………………… 345
394. 山苦荬 ……………………… 346

395. 南芥菜 ……………………… 347
396. 山萮苣 ……………………… 347
397. 黄鹌菜 ……………………… 348
398. 燕儿菜 ……………………… 349
399. 孛孛丁菜 …………………… 349
400. 柴韭 ………………………… 350
401. 野韭 ………………………… 350

根可食

新增

402. 甘露儿 ……………………… 351
403. 地瓜儿苗 …………………… 352

根叶皆可食

《本草》原有

404. 泽蒜 ………………………… 353

新增

405. 楼子葱 ……………………… 353
406. 薤韭 ………………………… 354
407. 水萝卜 ……………………… 355
408. 野蔓菁 ……………………… 356

叶及实皆可食

《本草》原有

409. 荠菜 ………………………… 357
410. 紫苏 ………………………… 358
411. 茬子 ………………………… 359

新增

412. 灰菜 ………………………… 360
413. 丁香茄儿 …………………… 361

根及实皆可食

《本草》原有

414. 山药 ………………………… 362

Contents

Volume 1　The First Half

Herbaceous Plant

- **Leaf Edible**

Original Ones

1. Cijicai ［刺蓟菜, field thistle herb, Cirsium arvense (L.) Scop. var. integrifolium Wimm. et Grab.］
　/ 2

2. Daji ［大蓟, Japanese thistle herb, Carduus crispus L.］　/ 3

3. Shanxiancai ［山苋菜, twotoothed achyranthes root, Achyranthes bidentata Blume］　/ 4

4. Kuandonghua ［款冬花, common coltsfoot flower, Tussilago farfara L.］　/ 6

5. Bianxu ［萹蓄, common knotgrass herb, Polygonum aviculare L.］　/ 8

6. Dalan ［大蓝, leaf and stem of true indigo, Isatis tinctoria L.］　/ 9

7. Shizhuzi ［石竹子, Chinese pink, Dianthus chinensis L.］　/ 10

8. Honghuacai ［红花菜, safflower, Carthamus tinctorius L.］　/ 11

9. Xuancaohua ［萱草花, day lily, Hemerocallis fulva L.］　/ 12

10. Cheluncai ［车轮菜, plantago seed, Plantago asiatica L.］　/ 13

11. Baishuihong Miao ［白水荭苗, oriental smartweed, Polygonum lapathifolium L.］　/ 14

12. Huangqi ［黄耆, milkvetch root, Astragalus membranaceus (Fisch.) Bunge］　/ 15

13. Weilingxian ［威灵仙, clematis root, Eupatorium fortune Turca］　/ 16

14. Madouling ［马兜零, dutohmanspipe fruit, Aristolochia debilis Sieb. et Zucc.］　/ 17

15. Xuanfuhua ［旋覆花, inula flower, Inula Britannica L.］　/ 18

16. Fangfeng ［防风, divaricate saposhnikovia root, Saposhnikovia divaricata (Turcz.) Schischk.］　/ 19

17. Yuchoumiao ［郁臭苗, motherwort fruit, Lagopsis supine (Steph. ex Willd.) Ik. -Gal. ex Knorr.］　/ 21

18. Zeqi ［泽漆, sun spurge, Apocynum venetum L.］　/ 22

19. Suanjiangcao ［酸浆草, creeping wood sorrel, Oxalis corniculata L.］　/ 23

20. Shechuangzi［蛇床子, chidium fruit, Cnidium monnieri (L.) Cuss.］	/ 24
21. Jiegeng［桔梗, platycodon root, Platycodon grandiflorus (Jacq.) A. DC.］	/ 25
22. Huixiang［茴香, fennel, Foeniculum vulgare Mill.］	/ 26
23. Xiakucao［夏枯草, common selfheal fruit-spike, Prunella vulgaris L.］	/ 27
24. Gaoben［藁本, Chinese lovage, Ligusticum sinense Oliv.］	/ 28
25. Chaihu［柴胡, Chinese thorowax root, Bupleurum chinense DC.］	/ 29
26. Loulu［漏芦, uniflower swissentaury, Rhaponticum uniflorum (L.) DC.］	/ 30
27. Longdancao［龙胆草, Chinese Gentian, Gentiana manshurica Kitag.］	/ 31
28. Shuju［鼠菊, European verbena herb, Verbena officinalis L.］	/ 33
29. Qianhu［前胡, hogfennel root, Peucedanum praeruptorum Dunn］	/ 34
30. Zhuyacai［猪牙菜, Chinese incarvillea, Incarvillea sinensis Lam.］	/ 35
31. Diyu［地榆, garden burnet root, Sanguisorba officinalis L.］	/ 36
32. Chuanxiong［川芎, Sichuan lovage rhizome, Ligusticum chuanxiong S. H. Qiu et al.］	/ 37
33. Gelezi Yang［葛勒子秧, Japanese hop, Humulus scandens (Lour.) Merr.］	/ 38
34. Lianqiao［连翘, forsythia, Forsythia suspense (Thunb.) Vahl］	/ 39
35. Xianlingpi［仙灵脾, epimedium, Epimedium brevicornu Maxim.］	/ 40
36. Qingqi［青杞, climbing nightshade, Solanum septemlobum Bunge］	/ 42
37. Yeshengjiang［野生姜, anomalous artemisia, Siphonostegia chinensis Benth.］	/ 43
38. Malantou［马兰头, kalimeris, Aster indicus L.］	/ 44
39. Xixian［豨莶, siegesbeckia, Sigesbeckia orientalis L.］	/ 45
40. Zexie［泽泻, alisma, Alisma orientale (Sam.) Juz.］	/ 46

New Supplements

41. Zhujiecai［竹节菜, dayflower, Commelina communis L.］	/ 46
42. Dusaomiao［独扫苗, kochia shoot, Kochia scoparia (L.) Schrad.］	/ 47
43. Waitoucai［歪头菜, vicia unijuga, Vicia unijuga A. Br.］	/ 48
44. Tu'ersuan［兔儿酸, amphibious polygonum, Polygonum amphibium L.］	/ 48
45. Jianpeng［碱蓬, suaeda, Suaeda glauca (Bunge) Bunge］	/ 49
46. Lvhao［蓾蒿, common mugwort, Artemisia selengensis Turcz. ex Bess.］	/ 50
47. Shuiwoju［水莴苣, water speedwell, Veronica undulate Wall. ex Jack］	/ 50
48. Jinzhancai［金盏菜, Tripolium, Tripolium pannonicum (Jacq.) Dobrocz.］	/ 51
49. Shuilacai［水辣菜, Japanese artemisia, Artemisia Japonica Thunb.］	/ 52
50. Ziyuncai［紫云菜, peruvian groundcherry herb, Clinopodium chinense (Benth.) Kuntze］	/ 52
51. Yacong［鸦葱, scorzonera root, Scorzonera sinensis (Lipsch. et Krasch) Nakai］	/ 53
52. Shitoucai［匙头菜, violet, Viola collina Bess.］	/ 54
53. Jiguancai［鸡冠菜, feather cockscomb, Celosia argentea L.］	/ 54

Contents

54. Shuimanjing［水蔓菁, kochia, Pseudolysimachion linariifolia Pall. ex Link subsp. dilatata (Nakai et Kitag.) Hong］ / 55
55. Yeyuansui［野园荽, wild coriander, Umbelliferae］ / 56
56. Niuweicai［牛尾菜, riparian greenbrier root and rhizome, Smilax riparia A. DC.］ / 56
57. Shanyucai［山蒢菜, Eutrema yunnanense, Eutrema yunnanense Franch.］ / 57
58. Miansicai［绵丝菜, silk floss, Pseudognaphalium luteoalbum (L.) Hilliard & B. L. Burtt］ / 58
59. Mihao［米蒿, artemisia, Descurainia Sophia (L.) Webb ex Prantl］ / 58
60. Shanjiecai［山芥菜, wild mustard leaf, Cruciferae］ / 59
61. Shetoucai［舌头菜, Kirilow Groundsel Herb, Tephroseris kirilowii］ / 59
62. Zixianghao［紫香蒿, Annuae Sweet Wormwood Herb, Artemisia］ / 60
63. Jinzhan'er Hua［金盏儿花, Calendula, Calendula officinalis L.］ / 61
64. Liuyueju［六月菊, tatarian aster root, Compositae］ / 61
65. Feicai［费菜, phedimus aizoon, Sedum aizoon L.］ / 62
66. Qianqucai［千屈菜, lythrum, Lythrum salicaria L.］ / 63
67. Liuyecai［柳叶菜, swamp willow herb, Epilobium hirsutum L.］ / 63
68. Popo Zhijiacai［婆婆指甲菜, grasswort, Cerastium fontanum subsp. Vulgare (Hartm.) Greuter et Burdet］ / 64
69. Tieganhao［铁杆蒿, Artemisia vestita, Aster］ / 64
70. Shantiancai［山甜菜, climbing nightshade, Solanum lyratum Thunb.］ / 65
71. Jiandaogu［剪刀股, lactuca debilis maxim, Ixeris japonica (N. L. Burman) Nakai］ / 66
72. Shuisuzi［水苏子, bur beggarticks herb, Bidens tripartita L.］ / 66
73. Fenghuacai［风花菜, Indian rorippa herb, Rorippa globosa (Turca. ex Fisch. et C. A. Mey.) Hayek］ / 67
74. E'erchang［鹅儿肠, malachium, Myosoton aquaticum (L.) Moench］ / 68
75. Fentiao'er Cai［粉条儿菜, root of Austrian serpentroot, Scorzonera albicaulis Bge.］ / 68
76. Lalacai［辣辣菜, garden cress, Lepidium apetalum Willd.］ / 69
77. Maoliancai［毛连菜, picris, Picris hieracioides L.］ / 70
78. Xiaotaohong［小桃红, garden balsam flower, Impatiens balsamina L.］ / 70
79. Qingjia'er Cai［青荚儿菜, heterophyllous patrinia, Patrinia heterophylla Bunge］ / 71
80. Bajiaocai［八角菜, umbelliferous vegetables, Umbelliferae］ / 72
81. Naijingcai［耐惊菜, eclipta prostrata, Eclipta prostrata (L.) L.］ / 72
82. Ditangcai［地棠菜, figwort root, Scrophularia ningpoensis Hemsl.］ / 73
83. Ji'erchang［鸡儿肠, Indian Kalimeris Herb, Kalimeris indica (L.) Sch. -Bip.］ / 74
84. Yudian'er Cai［雨点儿菜, willowleaf rhizome, Cynanchum stauntonii (Decne.) Schltr. ex Levl.］ / 74

85. Baiqucai〔白屈菜, celandine, Chelidonium majus L.〕 / 75
86. Chegencai〔扯根菜, Chinese penthorum, Penthorum chinense Pursh〕 / 76
87. Caoling Lingxiang〔草零陵香, sweet clover, Melilotus officinalis (L.) Pall.〕 / 77
88. Shuiluoli〔水落藜, chenopodium serotinum, Chenopodium serotinum L.〕 / 78
89. Lianghaocai〔凉蒿菜, wild chrysanthemum, Dendranthema indicum (L.) Des Moul.〕 / 78
90. Nianyuxu〔粘鱼须, Glabrous Greenbrier Rhizome, Smilax glabra Roxb〕 / 79
91. Jiejiecai〔节节菜, Rotala indica, Rotala indica (Willd.) Koehne〕 / 80
92. Yeaihao〔野艾蒿, artemisia lavandulaefolia, Artemisia lavandulaefolia DC.〕 / 80
93. Jinjincai〔堇堇菜, Tokyo violet herb, Viola philippica Cavanilles〕 / 81
94. Popona〔婆婆纳, speedwell, Veronica didyma Tenore〕 / 82
95. Yehuixiang〔野茴香, wild fennel, Foeniculum vulgare Mill.〕 / 83
96. Xiezi Huacai〔蝎子花菜, limonium bicolor, Limonium bicolor (Bag.) Kuntze〕 / 83
97. Baihao〔白蒿, virgate wormwood herb, Artemisia capillaris Thunb.〕 / 84
98. Yetonghao〔野茼蒿, artemisia scoparia, Artemisia scoparia Waldst. et Kit.〕 / 85
99. Yefen Tuan'er〔野粉团儿, kalimeris integrifolia, Kalimeris integrifolia Turcz. ex DC.〕 / 85
100. Hebocai〔蚵蚾菜, common carpesium root and leaf, Carpesium abrotanoides L.〕 / 86
101. Goudiaowei Miao〔狗掉尾苗, herba solani, Solanum lyratum Thunb.〕 / 87
102. Shijie〔石芥, cardamine leucantha, Cardamine leucantha (Tausch) O. E. Schulz〕 / 88
103. Huan'ercai〔獾耳菜, lithospermum arvense, Lithospermum arvense L.〕 / 88
104. Huihuisuan〔回回蒜, Chinese buttercup herb, Ranunculus chinensis Bunge〕 / 89
105. Dihuaicai〔地槐菜, herba phyllanthi urinariae, Phyllanthus urinaria L.〕 / 90
106. Luoyan'er〔螺黡儿, copperleaf herb, Acalypha australis L.〕 / 91
107. Nihucai〔泥胡菜, hemistepta lyrata, Hemisteptia lyrata (Bunge) Fischer & C. A. Meyer〕 / 92
108. Tu'ersi〔兔儿丝, lysimachia christinae, Lysimachia christinae Hance〕 / 92
109. Laoguanjin〔老鹳筋, potentilla supina, Potentilla supina L.〕 / 93
110. Jiaogulan〔绞股蓝, Japanese cayratia herb, Cayratia japonica (Thunb.) Gagnep.〕 / 94
111. Shangengcai〔山梗菜, lobelia sessilifolia, Lobelia sessilifolia Lamb.〕 / 94
112. Bunianghao〔㧯娘蒿, descurainia sophia, Descurainia sophia (L.) Webb ex Prantl〕 / 95
113. Jichangcai〔鸡肠菜, salvia umbratica, Salvia umbratica Hance〕 / 96
114. Shuihulu Miao〔水葫芦苗, halerpestes cymbalaris, Halerpestes sarmentosa var. multisecta (S. H. Li & Y. H. Huang) W. T. Wang〕 / 97
115. Hucang'er〔胡苍耳, gycyrrhiza pallidilora, Glycyrrhiza pallidiflora Maxim.〕 / 97
116. Shuijizhen Miao〔水棘针苗, amethystea coerulea, Amethystea caerulea L.〕 / 98
117. Shapeng〔沙蓬, corispermum puberulum, Corispermum puberulum Iljin〕 / 99
118. Mailancai〔麦蓝菜, vaccaria pyramidata, Vaccaria segetalis〕 / 100

Contents

119. Nvloucai［女娄菜, sunward melandrium herb, Silene firma Sieb. et Zucc. var. pubescens (Makino) S. Y. He］ / 101
120. Weilingcai［委陵菜, Chinese cinquefoil, Potentilla chinensis Ser.］ / 102
121. Duxingcai［独行菜, garden cress, Lepidium apetalum Willd.］ / 103
122. Shanliao［山蓼, cematis flammula, Clematis hexapetala Pall.］ / 103

Volume 1　The Second Half

Herbaceous Plant

- Leaf Edible

New Supplements

123. Huahao［花蒿, scorzonera austriaca wild, Scorzonera austriaca Willd.］ / 105
124. Gegongcai［葛公菜, danshen root, Salvia miltiorrhiza Bunge］ / 106
125. Jiyulin［鲫鱼鳞, caryopteris terniflora, Caryopteris terniflora Maxim.］ / 107
126. Jiandao'er Miao［尖刀儿苗, paniculate swallowwort root, Cynanchum paniculatum (Bunge) Kitag.］ / 107
127. Zhenzhucai［珍珠菜, lysimachia clethroide duby, Lysimachia clethroides Duby］ / 108
128. Dudanggui［杜当归, aralia cordata, Aralia continentalis Kitagawa］ / 109
129. Fengluncai［风轮菜, Clinopodium chinense, Clinopodium chinense (Benth.) O. Ktze.］ / 110
130. Tuobailian Miao［拖白练苗, sedum polytrichoides, Sedum polytrichoides Hemsl.］ / 111
131. Tougucao［透骨草, motherwort herb, Leonurus artemisia (Laur.) S. Y. Hu］ / 111
132. Suantongsun［酸桶笋, giant knotweed rhizome, Reynoutria japonica Houtt.］ / 112
133. Lujuecai［鹿蕨菜, fern, Pteridium aquilinum (L.) Kuhn var. latiusculum (Desv.) Underw. ex Heller］ / 113
134. Shanqincai［山芹菜, sanicle, Sanicula chinensis Bunge］ / 114
135. Jingangci［金刚刺, smilax scobinicaulis, Smilax scobinicaulis C. H. Wright］ / 114
136. Liuyeqing［柳叶青, anaphalis margaritacea, Anaphalis margaritacea (L.) Benth. et Hook. f.］ / 115
137. Dapenghao［大蓬蒿, senecio argunensis, Senecio argunensis Turcz.］ / 116
138. Goujinman［狗筋蔓, baccifera, Cucubalus baccifer L.］ / 117
139. Tu'ersan［兔儿伞, aconiteleaf syndeilesis herb, Syneilesis aconitifolia (Bge.) Maxim.］ / 117
140. Dihuacai［地花菜, atrina glass, Patrinia rupestris (Pall.) Juss. Subsp. scabra (Bunge) H. J. Wang］ / 118
141. Shao'ercai［杓儿菜, carpesium cernuum, Carpesium cernuum L.］ / 119
142. Fozhijia［佛指甲, hypericum ascyron, Hypericum ascyron L.］ / 120

143. Huweicao［虎尾草, lysimachia barystachys, Lysimachia barystachys Bunge］　/ 120

144. Yeshukui［野蜀葵, Japanese Cryptotaenia, Cryptotaenia japonica Hassk.］　/ 121

145. Sheputao［蛇葡萄, ampelopsis aconitifolia, Ampelopsis aconitifolia Bunge］　/ 122

146. Xingxiucai［星宿菜, lysimachia fortunei, Lysimachia fortunei Maxim.］　/ 123

147. Shuisuoyi［水蓑衣, veronica peregrina, Veronica peregrina L.］　/ 123

148. Niunaicai［牛奶菜, marsdenia sinensis, Marsdenia sinensis Hemsl.］　/ 124

149. Xiaochong'er Wodan［小虫儿卧单, euphorbia humifusa, Euphorbia humifusa Willd. ex Schlecht.］　/ 125

150. Tu'erwei Miao［兔儿尾苗, longifolia, Veronica longifolia L.］　/ 125

151. Dijinmiao［地锦苗, Herb of Common Corydalis, Corydalis edulis Maxim.］　/ 126

152. Yexigua Miao［野西瓜苗, hibiscus trionum, Hibiscus trionum Linn.］　/ 127

153. Xiangchacai［香茶菜, rabdosia rubescens, Rabdosia rubescens (Hemsl.) Hara］　/ 127

154. Qiangmi［蔷蘼, multiflora rose, Rosa multiflora Thunb.］　/ 128

155. Maonv'er Cai［毛女儿菜, gnaphalium japonicum, Gnaphalium japonicum Thunb.］　/ 129

156. Mangniu'er Miao［牻牛儿苗, erodium stephanianum, Erodium stephanianum Willd.］　/ 130

157. Tiesaozhou［铁扫帚, lespedeza cuneata, Lespedeza cuneata (Dum.-Cours.) G. Don］　/ 130

158. Shanxiaocai［山小菜, spotted bellflower, Campanula puncatata Lam.］　/ 131

159. Yangjiaomiao［羊角苗, cynanchum chinense, Cynanchum chinense R. Br.］　/ 132

160. Loudoucai［耧斗菜, aquilegia yabeana, Aquilegia yabeana Kitag.］　/ 133

161. Oucai［瓯菜, black nightshade, Solanum nigrum L.］　/ 133

162. Biandoucai［变豆菜, sanicle, Sanicula chinensis Bunge］　/ 134

163. Heshangcai［和尚菜, adenocaulon himalaicum, Adenocaulon himalaicum Edgew.］　/ 135

- **Root Edible**

Original Ones

164. Weirui［萎蕤, fragrant solomonseal rhizome, Polygonatum odoratum (Mill.) Druce］　/ 136

165. Baihe［百合, lily bulb, Lilium brownii Lilium brownii F. E. Brown var. viridulum Baker］　/ 138

166. Tianmendong［天门冬, radix asparagi, Asparagus cochinchinensis (Lour.) Merr.］　/ 139

167. Zhangliugen［章柳根, pokeberry root, Phytolacca acinosa Roxb.］　/ 141

168. Shashen［沙参, the root of straight ladybell, Adenophora stricta Miq.］　/ 143

169. Maimendong［麦门冬, radix ophiopogonis, Ophiopogon japonicus (L. f.) Ker-Gawl］　/ 144

170. Zhugen［苎根, ramie, Boehmeria nivea (L.) Gaudich.］　/ 146

171. Cangzhu［苍术, atractylodes rhizome, Atractylodes Lancea (Thunb.) DC.］　/ 147

172. Changpu［菖蒲, calamus, Acorus calamus］　/ 148

Contents

New Supplements

173. Fuzigen［菖子根, calystegia hederacea, Calystegia hederacea Wall. ex. Roxb.］ / 150

174. Maosaogen［荗葀根, water gladiole, Butomus umbellatus Linn.］ / 151

175. Ye Huluobo［野胡萝卜, wild carrot, Daucus carota L.］ / 151

176. Mianzao'er［绵枣儿, common squill bulb, Scilla scilloides（Lindl.）Druce］ / 152

177. Tuluan'er［土圞儿, root of Fortune Apios, Apios fortunei Maxim.］ / 153

178. Yeshanyao［野山药, wild yam rhizome, Dioscorea opposita Thunb.］ / 154

179. Jingua'er［金瓜儿, thladiantha dubia, Thladiantha dubia Bunge］ / 155

180. Xiye Shashen［细叶沙参, adenophora paniculata, Adenophora paniculata Nannf.］ / 156

181. Jitui'er［鸡腿儿, potentilla discolor, Potentilla discolor Bge.］ / 156

182. Shanmanjing［山蔓菁, adenophora trachelioides, Adenophora trachelioides Maxim.］ / 157

183. Laoyasuan［老鸦蒜, lycoris, Lycoris radiata（L'Her.）Herb.］ / 158

184. Shanluobo［山萝卜, scabiosa japonica, Scabiosa japonica Miq.］ / 158

185. Dishen［地参, adenophora wawreana, Adenophora wawreana Zahlbr.］ / 159

186. Zhangyacai［獐牙菜, oriental waterplantain rhizome, Alisma plantago-aquatica Linn.］ / 160

187. Ji'ertou Miao［鸡儿头苗, potentilla reptans, Potentilla reptans L. var. sericophylla Franch.］ / 161

- **Fruit Edible**

Original Ones

188. Quemai［雀麦, Japanese bromegrass, Bromus japonicus Thunb. ex Murr.］ / 162

189. Huihuimi［回回米, the seed of job's tears, Coix chinensis Tod.］ / 163

190. Jilizi［蒺藜子, puncturevine caltrop fruit, Tribulus terrester L.］ / 164

191. Qingzi［苘子, abutilon, Abutilon theophrasti Medicus］ / 165

New Supplements

192. Baizi［稗子, barnyard millet, Echinochloa crusgalli（L.）Beauv.］ / 166

193. Canzi［穇子, barnyard millet, Echinochloa crusgalli（L.）Beauv. var. crusgalli］ / 166

194. Chuangu［川谷, adlay, Coix lacryma-jobi L.］ / 167

195. Youcaozi［莠草子, green bristlegrass, Setaria viridis（L.）Beauv.］ / 168

196. Yeshu［野黍, wild broom corn millet, Panicum miliaceum L.］ / 169

197. Jiyancao［鸡眼草, Japan clover herb, Kummerowia striata（Thunb.）Schindl.］ / 169

198. Yanmai［燕麦, roegneria kamoji, Roegneria kamoji Ohwi］ / 170

199. Popan［泼盘, Japanese Raspberry Herb, Rubus parvifolius L.］ / 171

200. Siguamiao［丝瓜苗, luffa, Luffa cylindrica（L.）Roem.］ / 172

201. Dijiao'er Miao［地角儿苗, oxytropis bicolor, Oxytropis bicolor Bunge］ / 172

202. Mabao'er［马㼆儿, zehneria indica, Zehneria indica（Lour.）Keraudren］ / 173

203. Shanlidou［山黧豆, lathyrus quinquenervius, Lathyrus quinquenervius (Miq.) Litv.］/ 174

204. Longyacao［龙芽草, agrimony, Agrimonia pilosa Ldb.］/ 174

205. Dishaogua［地稍瓜, cynanchum thesioides, Cynanchum thesioides K. Schum.］/ 175

206. Jinlizhi［锦荔枝, balsam pear, Momordica charantia L.］/ 176

207. Jiguanguo［鸡冠果, Indian mock strawberry, Duchesnea indica (Andr.) Focke］/ 177

- **Leaf and Fruit Edible**

Original Ones

208. Yangtimiao［羊蹄苗, curly dock, Rumex crispus L.］/ 178

209. Cang'er［苍耳, xanthium sibiricum, Xanthium sibiricum Patrin ex Widder］/ 179

210. Guniangcai［姑娘菜, winter cherry, Physalis alkekengi L.］/ 180

211. Tuqianmiao［土茜苗, madder, Rubia cordifolia L.］/ 181

212. Wangbuliu Xing［王不留行, cowherb seed, Silene aprica Turcz. ex Fisch. et C. A. Mey.］/ 183

213. Baiwei［白薇, blackend swallowwort root, Cynanchum atratum Bunge］/ 184

New Supplements

214. Pengzicai［蓬子菜, true galium, Galium verum L.］/ 185

215. Huzhizi［胡枝子, bicolor lespedeza stem and leaf, Lespedeza bicolor Tricz］/ 186

216. Mibudai［米布袋, Gueldenstaedtia verna, Gueldenstaedtia verna (Georgi) Boriss.］/ 187

217. Tianqie'er Miao［天茄儿苗, solanum nigrum, Solanum nigrum L.］/ 187

218. Kumadou［苦马豆, Sphaerophysa salsula, Sphaerophysa salsula (Pall) DC.］/ 188

219. Zhuweiba Miao［猪尾把苗, Lysimachia, Lysimachia］/ 189

- **Root and Leaf Edible**

Original Ones

220. Huangjingmiao［黄精苗, yellow essence, Polygonatum sibiricum Redouté］/ 191

221. Dihuangmiao［地黄苗, ehmannia, Rehmannia glutinosa (Gaert.) Libosch. ex Fisch et Mey.］/ 192

222. Niubangzi［牛蒡子, arctium, Arctium lappa L.］/ 193

223. Yuanzhi［远志, polygala, Polygala sibirica L.］/ 195

224. Xingye Shashen［杏叶沙参, adenophora hunanensis, Adenophora petiolata Pax et Hoffm. subsp. hunanensis (Nannf.) D. Y. Hong et S. Ge］/ 196

225. Tengchangmiao［藤长苗, calystegia pellita, Calystegia pellita (Ledeb.) G. Don］/ 197

226. Niupixiao［牛皮消, cynanchum auriculatum, Cynanchum auriculatum Royle ex Wight］/ 198

227. Zucao［菹草, algae, Potamogeton crispus］/ 199

228. Shuidou'er［水豆儿, utricularia, Utricularia vulgaris L.］/ 200

229. Caosannai［草三奈, belamcanda chinensis, Belamcanda chinensis (L.) Redouté］/ 200

230. Shuicong [水葱, robust bullrush, Scirpi Validi Caulis] / 201

- **Root and Shoot Edible**

  Original Ones

  231. Pusun [蒲笋, typha, Typha orientalis Presl.] / 202

  232. Lusun [芦笋, phragmites shoot, Phragmititis Surculus] / 203

  233. Maoyagen [茅芽根, imperata, Imperatae Cylindrica (L.) Beauv.] / 204

- **Root and Flower Edible**

  Original Ones

  234. Gegen [葛根, pueraria, Puerariae montana (Lour.) Merr.] / 205

  235. Heshouwu [何首乌, flowery knotweed, Polygonum multiflorum Thunb.] / 207

- **Root and Fruit Edible**

  Original Ones

  236. Gualonggen [瓜楼根, trichosanthes root, Trichosanthes kirlowii Maxim.] / 209

  New Supplements

  237. Zhuanzimiao [砖子苗, compact mariscus, Marisci Compacti Herba] / 210

- **Flower and Leaf Edible**

  Original Ones

  238. Juhua [菊花, chrysanthemum, Chrysanthemum morifolium Ramat] / 211

  239. Jinyinhua [金银花, lonicera, Lonicera japonica Thunb] / 212

  New Supplements

  240. Wangjiangnan [望江南, coffee senna, Senna occidentalis (L.) Link] / 213

  241. Daliao [大蓼, flowering clematis, Clematidis Floridae Herba] / 214

- **Stem Edible**

  Original Ones

  242. Heisanleng [黑三棱, sparganium, Sparganium stoloniferum (Buch.-Ham. ex Graebn) Buch.-Ham. ex Juz] / 215

  New Supplements

  243. Xingsicai [荇丝菜, Nymphoides peltata (S.G. Gmelin) Kuntze] / 216

  244. Shuicigu [水慈菰, savory, Clinopodii Herba] / 217

- **Shoot and Fruit Edible**

  Original Ones

  245. Jiaosun [茭笋, infested ear of wild rice, Zizaniae Spica Infestata] / 218

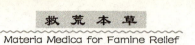

Volume 2 The First Half

Woody Plant

- **Leaf Edible**

Original Ones

246. Chashu［茶树, tea tree, Camellia sinensis（L.）Ktze］ / 220

247. Yeheshu［夜合树, Maackia amurensis, Albizia julibrissin Durazz./ Albizia kalkora Prain］ / 221

248. Mujinshu［木槿树, hibiscus syriacus, Hibiscus syriacus L.］ / 222

249. Baiyangshu［白杨树, white poplar, Populus alba L.］ / 222

250. Huanglu［黄栌, cotinus coggygria Cotinus coggygria Scop.］ / 223

251. Chunshuya［椿树芽, cedrela sinensis, Toona sinensis（A. Juss.）Roem.］ / 224

252. Jiaoshu［椒树, Sichuan pepper, Zanthoxylum simulans Hance］ / 225

253. Liangzishu［椋子树, cornus, Cornus macrophylla Wall.］ / 226

New Supplements

254. Yunsang［云桑, Acer ginnala, Acer tataricum L. subsp. ginnala（Maxim.）Wesmael］ / 227

255. Huanglianshu［黄楝树, pistacia chinensis bunge, Pistacia chinensis Bunge］ / 228

256. Dongqingshu［冻青树, ligustrum lucidum, Ligustrum lucidum Ait.］ / 228

257. Rongyashu［稱芽树, hoary willow, Fontanesia phillyreoides Labill. subsp. fortunei（Carrière）Yalt.］ / 229

258. Yueyashu［月芽树, hoary willow, Fontanesia phillyreoides Labill. subsp. fortunei（Carrière）Yalt.］ / 230

259. Nv'ercha［女儿茶, Rhamnus davurica, Rhamnus davurica Pall.］ / 230

260. Shengguyou［省沽油, Staphylea bumalda, Staphylea bumalda DC.］ / 231

261. Baijinshu［白槿树, fraxinus chinensis Fraxinus chinensis Roxb.］ / 232

262. Huihuicu［回回醋, rhus chinensis, Rhus chinensis Mill.］ / 232

263. Seshuya［械树芽, Acer mono, Acer pictum Thunb］ / 233

264. Laoye'er Shu［老叶儿树, Quercus variabilis, Quercus variabilis Bl.］ / 234

265. Qingyangshu［青杨树, Cathay poplar, Populus cathayana Rehd.］ / 234

266. Longboya［龙柏芽, Exochorda giraldii, Exochorda giraldii Hesse.］ / 235

267. Doulushu［兜栌树, Platycarya strobilacea Sieb., Platycarya strobilacea Sieb. et Zucc.］ / 235

268. Qinggangshu［青冈树, Quercus serrata, Quercus serrata Murray］ / 236

269. Tanshuya［檀树芽, Dalbergia hupeana Dalbergia hupeana Hance］ / 237

270. Shanchake［山茶科, Rhamnus bungeana J. Vass.］ / 237

271. Muge［木葛, pawpaw, Chaenomeles sinensis（Thouin）Koehne］ / 238

Contents

272. Huaqiushu［花楸树, Sorbus pohuashanensis, Sorbus pohuashanensis（Hance）Hedl.］ / 238
273. Baixinshu［白辛树, Pterostyrax psilophyllus, Pterostyrax psilophyllus Diels ex Perk.］ / 239
274. Muluanshu［木栾树, Koelreuteria paniculata, Koelreuteria paniculata Laxm.］ / 240
275. Wulengshu［乌棱树, lindera glauca, Lindera glauca（Sieb. et Zucc.）Bl.］ / 240
276. Ciqiushu［刺楸树, Kalopanax septemlobus, Kalopanax septemlobus（Thunb.）Koidz.］ / 241
277. Huangsiteng［黄丝藤, Dodder seed, Semen Cuscutae］ / 241
278. Shangela Shu［山格剌树, Celastrus gemmatus, Celastrus gemmatus Loes.］ / 242
279. Hangshu［箲树, Euonymus verrucosoides, Euonymus verrucosoides Loes.］ / 243
280. Baomashu［报马树, Celtis koraiensis, Celtis koraiensis Nakai］ / 243
281. Duanshu［椴树, linden, Tilia mongolica Maxim］ / 244
282. Chouhong［臭蓣, Eleutherococcus nodiflorus, Eleutherococcus nodiflorus（Dunn）S. Y. Hu］ / 245
283. Jianjiashu［坚荚树, Viburnum schensianum Maxim］ / 245
284. Chouzhushu［臭竹树, Clerodendrum trichotomum, Clerodendrum trichotomum Thunb.］ / 246
285. Mayu'er Tiao［马鱼儿条, Gleditsia microphylla, Gleditsia microphylla D. A. Gordon ex Isely］ / 247
286. Laopo Butie［老婆布帖, Celastrus angulatus, Celastrus angulatus Maxim］ / 247
287. Ruiheshu［蕤核树, Prinsepia uniflora Batal, Prinsepia uniflora Batal］ / 248
288. Suanzaoshu［酸枣树, crataegus, Ziziphus jujuba var. spinosa（Bunge）Hu ex H. F. Chow］ / 249
289. Xiangzishu［橡子树, acorn, Quercus acutissima Carr.］ / 250
290. Jingzi［荆子, negundo vitex, Vitex negundo L.］ / 250
291. Shizao'er Shu［实枣儿树, cornus, Cornus officinalis Sieb. et Zucc］ / 251
292. Hai'er Quantou［孩儿拳头, Viburnum dilatatum, Grewia biloba G. Don var. parviflora（Bge.）Hand.-Mazz.］ / 253

New Supplements

293. Shanli'er［山蓠儿, Smilax china, Smilax china L.］ / 254
294. Shanli Guo'er［山里果儿, Crataegus pinnatifida Bunge, Crataegus pinnatifida Bunge var. pinnatifida］ / 254
295. Wuhuaguo［无花果, fig, Ficus carica L.］ / 255
296. Qingshe Zitiao［青舍子条, Berchemia floribunda, Berchemia floribunda（Wall.）Brongn］ / 256
297. Baitang Zishu［白棠子树, Elaeagnus multiflora, Elaeagnus multiflora Thunb.］ / 256
298. Guaizao［拐枣, honey raisin tree, Hovenia dulcis Thunb.］ / 257
299. Mutao'er Shu［木桃儿树, Celtis bungeana, Celtis bungeana Bl.］ / 258
300. Shigangxiang［石冈橡, Quercus baronii, Quercus baronii Skan］ / 258
301. Shuichajiu［水茶臼, Rosaceae, Rosaceae］ / 259

302. Yemugua［野木瓜, trifoliate akebia, Akebia quinata（Houtt.）Decne］　　　　/ 259

303. Tuluanshu［土栾树, Viburnum schensianum, Viburnum schensianum Maxim］　　/ 260

304. Lvtuo Budai［驴驼布袋, Lonicera fragrantissima, Lonicera fragrantissima Lindl. et Paxt.］　/ 261

305. Popo Zhentou［婆婆枕头, Bilobed Grewia, Grewia biloba G. Don］　　/ 261

- **Leaf and Fruit Edible**

Original Ones

306. Jilizi Shu［吉利子树, Root of Bilobed Grewia, Grewia biloba G. Don var. parviflora
　　　（Bge.）Hand.-Mazz.］　　　　　　　　　　　　　　　　　　　　　　　/ 262

307. Gouqi［枸杞, medlar, Lycium chinense Mill.］　　　　　　　　　　　　　　/ 263

308. Baishu［柏树, cypress tree, Platycladus orientalis（L.）Franco］　　　　　　　/ 264

309. Zaojiashu［皂荚树, soap-bark tree, Gleditsia sinensis Lam.］　　　　　　　　/ 265

310. Chutaoshu［楮桃树, paper mulberry, Broussonetia papyrifera（L.）L'Hér. ex Vent.］/ 266

311. Zheshu［柘树, cudrania, Cudraniae Lignum］　　　　　　　　　　　　　/ 267

New Supplements

312. MuyangJiao Ke［木羊角科, periploca, Periploca sepium Bunge］　　　　　/ 268

313. Qingtanshu［青檀树, celtis, Celtis bungeana Bl.］　　　　　　　　　　　/ 269

314. Shanqingshu［山苘树, alangium platanifolium, Alangium platanifolium（Sieb. et Zucc.）
　　　Harms, var. trilobum（Miq.）Ohwi］　　　　　　　　　　　　　　　　　/ 270

- **Flower Edible**

New Supplements

315. Tenghuacai［藤花菜, wisteria villosa, Wisteria villosa Rehd.］　　　　　　　/ 271

316. Bachihua［把齿花, caragana, Caragana sinica（Buc'hoz）Rehd.］　　　　　　/ 271

317. Qiushu［楸树, catalpa bungei, Catalpa bungei C. A. Mey.］　　　　　　　/ 272

318. Lameihua［腊梅花, Winter sweet, Chimonanthus praecox（L.）Link］　　　/ 273

319. Maji［马棘, sophora davidii, Sophora davidii（Franch.）Skeels］　　　　　/ 273

- **Flower and Leaf Edible**

Original Ones

320. Huaishuya［槐树芽, sophora japonica, Sophora japonica L.］　　　　　　　/ 274

- **Flower, Leaf and Fruit Edible**

New Supplements

321. Tanglishu［棠梨树, pyrus betulifolia, Pyrus betulifolia Bunge］　　　　　　/ 276

322. Wenguanhua［文冠花, Xanthoceras sorbifolium, Xanthoceras sorbifolium Bunge］/ 276

- **Leaf, Peel and Fruit Edible**

Original Ones

323. Sangshenshu [桑椹树, mulberry, Morus alba L.] / 278

324. Yuqianshu [榆钱树, ulmus pumila, Ulmus pumila L.] / 279

- **Shoot Edible**

Original Ones

325. Zhusun [竹笋, bamboo shoot, Bambusoideae] / 281

Herbaceous Cereal

- **Fruit Edible**

New Supplements

326. Yewandou [野豌豆, vicia sepium, Vicia sativa L.] / 282

327. Laodou [捞豆, wild soybean, Glycine soja Sieb. et Zucc.] / 283

328. Shanbiandou [山扁豆, senna, Senna nomame (Makino) T. C. Chen] / 284

329. Huihuidou [回回豆, chickpea, Cicer arietinum L.] / 285

330. Hudou [胡豆, indigofera decora, Indigofera decora Lindl.] / 285

331. Candou [蚕豆, broad bean, Vicia faba L.] / 287

332. Shanlvdou [山绿豆, indigofera kirilowii Maxim. ex Palibin, Indigofera kirilowii Maxim. ex Palibin] / 286

Volume 2   The Second Half

Herbaceous Cereal

- **Leaf and Fruit Edible**

Original Ones

333. Qiaomaimiao [荞麦苗, fagopyrum esculentum, Fagopyrum esculentum] / 288

334. Yumihua [御米花, papaver somniferum, Papaver somniferum L.] / 289

335. Chixiaodou [赤小豆, azuki Bean, Vigna angularis (Willd.) Ohwi et Ohashi] / 290

336. Shansimiao [山丝苗, cannabis sativa, Cannabis sativa L.] / 292

337. Youzimiao [油子苗, sesamum indicum, Sesamum indicum Linn.] / 293

New Supplements

338. Huangdoumiao [黄豆苗, soybean, Glycine max (L.) Merr.] / 294

339. Daodoumiao [刀豆苗, sword bean, Canavalia gladiata Dc. Merr.] / 295

340. Mei'erdou Miao [眉儿豆苗, lablab purpureus, Lablab purpureus (L.) sweet] / 295

341. Zijiangdou Miao [紫豇豆苗, cowpea, Vigna unguiculata (Linn.) Walp.] / 296

342. Suzimiao [苏子苗, perilla frutescens, Perilla frutescens (L.) Britt.] / 297

343. Jiangdoumiao [豇豆苗, cowpea, Vigna unguiculata (Linn.) Walp.] / 298

344. Shanheidou [山黑豆, wild black soybean, Glycine soja Sieb. et Zucc.] / 298

345. Shunmanggu［舜芒谷, chenopodium giganteum, Chenopodium giganteum D. Don.］ / 299

Herbaceous Fruit

- **Fruit Edible**

Original Ones

346. Yingtaoshu［樱桃树, cherry tree, Cerasus pseudocerasus (Lindl.) G. Don］ / 300

347. Hutaoshu［胡桃树, walnut tree, Juglans regia L.］ / 301

348. Shishu［柿树, persimmon tree, Diospyros kaki Thunb.］ / 302

349. Lishu［梨树, pear tree, Pyrus pyrifolia (Burm.) Nakai］ / 304

350. Putao［葡萄, grape, Vitis vinifera L.］ / 304

351. Lizishu［李子树, plum tree, Prunus salicina Lindl.］ / 306

352. Mugua［木瓜, pawpaw, Chaenomeles sinensis (Thouin) Koehne］ / 307

353. Zhazishu［楂子树, cydonia oblonga, Cydonia oblonga Mill.］ / 308

354. Yulizi［郁李子, cerasus japonica, Cerasus japonica (Thunb.) Lois.］ / 309

355. Lingjiao［菱角, water chestnut, Trapa natans L.］ / 310

New Supplements

356. Ruanzao［软枣, diospyros lotus, Diospyros lotus L.］ / 311

357. Yeputao［野葡萄, wild grape, Vitis bryoniifolia Bunge］ / 311

358. Meixingshu［梅杏树, plum apricot tree, Armeniaca limeixing J. Y. Zhang et Z. M. Wang］ / 312

359. Yeyingtao［野樱桃, nanking cherry, Cerasus tomentosa (Thunb.) Wall.］ / 313

- **Leaf and Fruit Edible**

Original Ones

360. Shiliu［石榴, pomegranate, Punica granatum L.］ / 314

361. Xingshu［杏树, apricot tree, Armeniaca vulgaris Lam］ / 315

362. Zaoshu［枣树, jujube tree, Ziziphus jujuba Mill.］ / 316

363. Taoshu［桃树, peach tree, Amygdalus persica L.］ / 318

New Supplements

364. Shaguozi Shu［沙果子树, crab apple, Malus asiatica Nakai］ / 320

- **Root Edible**

Original Ones

365. Yumiao［芋苗, taro roots, Colocasia esculenta (L.) Schoot］ / 321

366. Tieboqi［铁荸荠, water-chestnuts, Bolboschoenus yagara (Ohwi) Y. C. Yang et M. Zhan］ / 322

- **Root and Fruit Edible**

Original Ones

367. Lian'ou［莲藕, lotus root, Nelumbo nucifera Gaertn.］ / 323

368. Jitoushi［鸡头实, euryale ferox, Euryale ferox Salisb.］ / 325

Herbaceous Vegetable

- **Leaf Edible**

Original Ones

369. Yuntaicai［芸薹菜, brassica campestris, Brassica campestris L. var. campestris］ / 326

370. Xiancai［苋菜, amaranth, Amaranthus tricolor］ / 327

371. Kujucai［苦苣菜, common sowthistle herb, Sonchus wightianus DC.］ / 328

372. Machixian Cai［马齿苋菜, purslane herb, Portulaca oleracea L.］ / 329

373. Kumaicai［苦荬菜, field sowthistle herb, Ixeridium sonchifolium（Maxim.）Shih］ / 330

374. Jundacai［莙荙菜, spinach beet, Beta vulgaris L. var. Cicla L.］ / 331

375. Xiehao［邪蒿, artemisia carvifolia, Artemisia carvifolia var. schochii（Mattf.）Pamp.］ / 331

376. Tonghao［茼蒿, garland chrysanthemum, Glebionis coronaria（L.）Cass. Ex Spach］ / 332

377. Dongkuicai［冬葵菜, malva verticillata, Malva verticillata L. var. Crispa L.］ / 333

378. Liaoyacai［蓼芽菜, polygonum hydropiper, Polygonum hydropiper L.］ / 334

379. Muxu［苜蓿, medicago sativa, Medicago sativa L.］ / 335

380. Bohe［薄荷, field-mint, Mentha canadensis L.］ / 336

381. Jingjie［荆芥, schizonepeta herba, Nepeta tenuifolia Benth.］ / 337

382. Shuiqin［水蕲, cress, Oenanthe javanica（Blume）DC.］ / 338

New Supplements

383. Xiangcai［香菜, coriander herb with root, Ocimum basilicum L.］ / 339

384. Yintiaocai［银条菜, rorippa globosa, Rorippa globosa（Turcz.）Hayek］ / 340

385. Houtinghua［后庭花, amaranthus, Amaranthus tricolor L.］ / 341

386. Huoyancai［火焰菜, beta vulgaris, Beta vulgaris L.］ / 341

387. Shancong［山葱, scallion, Allium victorialis L.］ / 342

388. Beijiu［背韭, allium paepalanthoides, Allium paepalanthoides Airy-Shaw］ / 342

389. Shuijiecai［水芥菜, rorippa palustris, Rorippa palustris（L.）Bess.］ / 343

390. Elancai［遏蓝菜, boor's mustard herb, Thlaspi arvense L.］ / 344

391. Niu'erduo Cai［牛耳朵菜, chirita eburnea, Brassica rapa L. var. Olefera DC.］ / 344

392. Shanbaicai［山白菜, aster, Aster tataricus L., f.］ / 345

393. Shanyicai［山宜菜, lactuca raddeana, Lactuca raddeana Maxim.］ / 346

394. Shankumai［山苦荬, field sowthistle herb, Paraixeris denticulata（Houtt.）Nakai］ / 346

395. Nanjiecai［南芥菜, nanjiecai medicinal, Cruciferae］ / 347

396. Shanwoju［山莴苣, herb of Indian Lettuce, Lactuca indica L.］ / 347

397. Huang'ancai [黄鹌菜, herb of Japanese Youngia, Youngia japonica (L.) DC.] / 348

398. Yan'ercai [燕儿菜, herb of Hygrometric Boea, Boea hygrometrica (Bunge) R. Brown] / 349

399. Beibeiding Cai [孛孛丁菜, dandelion, Taraxacum mongolicum Hand. -Mazz.] / 349

400. Chaijiu [柴韭, allium, Allium tenuissimum L.] / 350

401. Yejiu [野韭, allium, Allium tenuissimum L.] / 351

- **Root Edible**

  New Supplements

  402. Ganlu'er [甘露儿, Chinese artichoke Stachys sieboldii Miq., Stachys sieboldii Miq.] / 352

  403. Digua'er Miao [地瓜儿苗, lycopus lucidus, Lycopus lucidus Turcz.] / 352

- **Root and Leaf Edible**

  Original Ones

  404. Zesuan [泽蒜, allium macrostemon, Allium macrostemon Bunge] / 353

  New Supplements

  405. Louzicong [楼子葱, allium cepa, Allium cepa L. var. prolife rum (Moench) Regel] / 354

  406. Xiejiu [薤韭, Chinese chive, Allium hookeri] / 355

  407. Shuiluobo [水萝卜, summer radish, Brassicaceae] / 355

  408. Yemanjing [野蔓菁, wild turnip, Brassica rapa Linn.] / 356

- **Leaf and Fruit Edible**

  Original Ones

  409. Jicai [荠菜, shepherd's purse, Capsella bursa-pastoris (L.) Medic.] / 357

  410. Zisu [紫苏, perilla frutescens, Perilla frutescens (L.) Britt.] / 358

  411. Renzi [荏子, perilla frutescens, Perilla frutescens (L.) Britt.] / 359

  New Supplements

  412. Huicai [灰菜, chenopodium album, Chenopodium album L.] / 360

  413. Dingxiang Qie'er [丁香茄儿, calonyction muricatum, Calonyction muricatum (L.) G. Don] / 361

- **Root and Fruit Edible**

  Original Ones

  414. Shanyao [山药, common yam rhizome, Dioscorea polystachya Turcz.] / 362

草 部

叶可食

✻ 《本草》原有

Volume 1　The First Half
Herbaceous Plant
Leaf Edible
Original Ones

1. 刺蓟菜

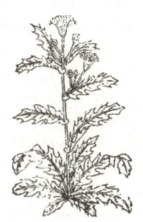

本草[1]名小蓟，俗名青刺蓟，北人呼为千针草。出冀州[2]，生平泽中，今处处有之。苗高尺余，叶似苦苣叶，茎叶俱有刺，而叶不皱，叶中心出花头，如红蓝花[3]而青紫色。性凉，无毒。一云味甘，性温。

救饥：采嫩苗叶煤熟[4]，水浸淘净，油盐调食，甚美。除风热。

治病：文具《本草·草部》[5]大小蓟条下。

【注释】

[1] 中药的统称，下同。

[2] 古代州名。在今河北冀州市一带。

[3] 红花菜的别名，见本书第8条。

[4] 处理野菜的一种方法，将野菜用水煮开，用来祛除异味或减少有毒物质。

[5] 此指宋代张存惠整理刊行的《重修政和经史证类备用本草》(简称《政和本草》)。下同。

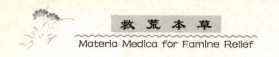

1. Cijicai [刺蓟菜, field thistle herb, Cirsium arvense (L.) Scop. var. integrifolium Wimm. et Grab.]

The materia medica[1] of Cijicai [刺蓟菜, field thistle herb, Cirsium arvense (L.) Scop. var. integrifolium Wimm. et Grab.], also named Xiaoji and Qingciji, Qianzhencao, with its origin in Jizhou[2] and growing in swamps, can be commonly seen everywhere presently. Its seedlings are one Chi high and its leaves are like those of Kuju [苦苣, endive, Cichorium endivia L.]. Both of its stems and leaves are spinose and its leaves are not rugose. Its flower head, like Honglanhua[3] [红蓝花, Tulipa, Carthamus tinctorius L.] but violaceous, stands out of the leaves. It is cold in nature and non-toxic. It is also believed to be sweet in taste and warm in nature.

For famine relief: Collect young leaves, blanch[4] and elutriate them in hot water, and then flavor them with oil and salt. It is delicious and has the function of dispelling wind-heat.

For disease treatment: See the clause of Daji [大蓟, Japanese thistle herb, Carduus crispus L.] and Xiaoji [小蓟, field thistle herb, Herba Cirsii] in *Materia Medica · Herbaceous Plant*[5].

【Notes】

[1] The general term for medicinals. Similarly hereinafter.

[2] The name of an ancient county. It is presently located in Jizhou City of Hebei Province.

[3] Another name for Honghuacai [红花菜, Chinese astragalus, Astragali Sinici Herba]. See the 8th clause of this book.

[4] A method to process edible wild herbs by boiling them in hot water to remove undesirable odor or toxicity. Similarly hereinafter.

[5] Here it refers to *Chong Xiu Zhenghe Jing Shi Zheng Lei Beiji Bencao* [《重修政和经史证类备急本草》, *Revised Zhenghe Classified Materia Medica from Historical Classics for Emergency*] compiled by Zhang Cunhui of Song Dynasty. Similarly hereinafter.

2. 大 蓟

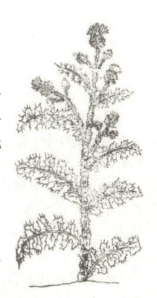

旧不著所出州土,云生山谷中,今郑州山野间亦有之。苗高三四尺[1]。茎五棱,叶似大花苦苣菜叶,茎叶俱多刺,其叶多皱。叶中心开淡紫花。味苦,性平,无毒。根有毒。

救饥:采嫩苗叶煠熟,水淘去苦味,油盐调食。

治病:文具《本草·草部》大小蓟条下。

【注释】

[1] 明代牙尺,一尺相当于现在35.8厘米。下同。

2. Daji [大蓟, Japanese thistle herb, Carduus crispus L.]

There is no record about its origin in ancient times except its growing place being in valley. Presently it can be found in the mountainous regions and plains of Zhengzhou. Its seedlings are 3 ~ 4 Chi[1] high and the stems are five-ridged. Its leaves are like those of Kujucai [苦苣菜, common sowthistle, Sonchus L.] and both of its stems and leaves are spinose. With rugose leaves and lilac capitula, it is bitter in taste, neutral in nature, and toxic in the root part only.

For famine relief: Collect young leaves, blanch them and remove the bitterness by elutriating them with water, and then flavor them with oil and salt.

For disease treatment: See the clause of Daji [大蓟, Japanese thistle herb, Carduus crispus L.] and Xiaoji [小蓟, field thistle herb, Herba Cirsii] in *Materia Medica · Herbaceous Plant.*

[Notes]

[1] The length measure in Ming Dynasty. One Chi equals 35.8 centimeter nowadays. Similarly hereinafter.

3. 山苋菜

本草名牛膝，一名百倍，俗名脚斯蹬，又名对节菜。生河内川谷及临朐、江淮、闽粤、关中、苏州皆有之，然皆不及怀州[1]者为真，蔡州者最长大柔润，今钧州山野中亦有之。苗高二尺已来，茎方，青紫色，其茎有节如鹤膝，又如牛膝状，以此名之。叶似苋菜叶而长。颇尖艄，叶皆对生。开花作穗。根味苦、酸，性平，无毒。叶味甘、微酸。恶[2]萤火、陆英、龟甲，畏[3]白前。

救饥：采苗叶煠熟，换水浸去酸味，淘净，油盐调食。

治病：文具《本草·草部》牛膝条下。

【注释】

[1] 古代州名。今河南焦作、沁阳、武陟、获嘉、修武、博爱等地。

[2] 中药学术语。指一种药物能减弱另一种药物的性能。下同。

[3] 中药学术语。指药物之间的相互抑制作用，一种药物的毒性或副作用能被另一种药物消减。下同。

3. Shanxiancai [山苋菜, twotoothed achyranthes root, Achyranthes bidentata Blume]

Shanxiancai [山苋菜, twotoothed achyranthes root, Achyranthes bidentata Blume], also named Niuxi, Baibei, Jiaosideng and Duijiecai, grows in the valley of Henei Prefecture and other places like Linqu, Jianghuai, Minyue, Guanzhong and Suzhou, while the most genuine region of it is Huaizhou[1]. It is high, soft and lustrous if originated from Caizhou. Presently it can be found in the mountainous regions and plains of Junzhou. It is violaceous, about two Chi high, with stems being square and knobs on its stems. Its shape is like a crane knee or a cow knee, from which it is named. Its pointed opposite leaves are like those of Xiancai [苋菜, edible amaranth, Amaranthus mangostanus L.], but much longer than the latter. Its inflorescence is spicate. Its roots are bitter and sour in taste, neutral in nature and non-toxic. Its leaves are sweet and slightly sour in taste. It is in mutual inhibition[2] with Yinghuo［萤火, firefly, Luciola］, Luying［陆英, Java elder fruit, Sambuci Fructus］, and Guijia［龟甲, tortoise shell, Carapax et Plastrum Testudinis］ and in the mutual restraint[3] with Baiqian［白前, willowleaf rhizome, Rhizoma Cynanchi Stauntonii］.

For famine relief: Collect young leaves and seedlings, blanch and soak them in fresh water, remove the sourness by elutriating them with water, and flavor them with oil and salt.

For disease treatment: See the clause of Niuxi［牛膝, twotoothed achyranthes root, Radix Achyranthis Bidentatae］in *Materia Medica · Herbaceous Plant.*

【Notes】

［1］The name of an ancient county. Presently it refers to the areas of Jiaozuo, Qinyang, Wuzhi, Huojia, Xiuwu and Boai in Henan Province.

［2］A term from the Chinese materia medica. It refers to one medicinal's weakening the action of another one when used together. Similarly hereinafter.

［3］A term from the Chinese materia medica. It refers to mutual restraint between two medicinals, namely, one medicinal's toxicity or side-effect being reduced by another medicinal. Similarly hereinafter.

4. 款冬花

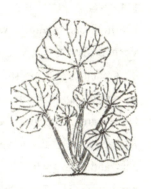

一名橐吾，一名颗东，一名虎须，一名菟奚，一名氐冬。生常山[1]山谷及上党水傍，关中、蜀北宕昌、秦州、雄州皆有，今钧州密县山谷间亦有之。茎青，微带紫色。叶似葵叶，甚大而丛生；又似石葫芦叶，颇团。开黄花，根紫色。《图经》[2]云："叶如荷而斗直，大者容一升，小者容数合[3]，俗呼为蜂斗叶，又名水斗叶。"此物不避冰雪，最先春前生，雪中出花，世谓之钻冻。又云："有叶似萆薢，开黄花，青紫萼，去土一二寸，初出如菊花萼，通直而肥实无子，陶隐居所谓出高丽[4]、百济[5]者，近此类也。"其叶味苦，花味辛、甘，性温，无毒。杏仁为之使，得紫菀良，恶皂荚、消石、玄参，畏贝母、辛夷、麻黄、黄芩、黄连、青葙。

　　救饥：采嫩叶煠熟，水浸淘去苦味，油盐调食。

　　治病：文具《本草·草部》条下。

【注释】

［1］山名，即恒山，在今河北曲阳县西北。

［2］指《本草图经》，宋代苏颂等编撰，共21卷。完成于1061年。

［3］合（gě）：容量单位，一升的十分之一。

［4］古代国名，为朝鲜半岛的国家。

［5］古代国名，为朝鲜半岛的国家。

4. Kuandonghua［款冬花, common coltsfoot flower, Tussilago farfara L.］

　　Kuandonghua［款冬花, common coltsfoot flower, Tussilago farfara L.］, also named Tuowu, Kedong, Huxu, Tuxi and Didong, grows in the valley of Changshan[1], the waterside of Shangdang County, and other places like Guanzhong, Dangchang area to the north of Shu, Qinzhou and Xiongzhou. Presently it can also be found in the valleys of Mixian County of Junzhou. Its stems are of indigo color and its leaves are big and clustered, like those of Kui［葵, malva, Malva verticillata L.］, round-shaped like those of Shihulu［石葫芦, Herb of Chinese Pothos, Pothos chinensis］. Its flowers are yellow and its roots are purple. *Tu Jing*[2] says, "Its leaves are steep like those of lotus. Its bigger leaves can hold one Sheng of water and smaller ones several Ge[3] of water, also named Fengdou leaves (Japanese butterbur) and Shuidou leaves (bailer-shaped leaves)." This plant is cold-resistant, being able to sprout before spring and blossom even in snowtime, and commonly called Zuandong (cold-drilling). *Tu Jing* also says, "Its leaves are like those of Bixie［草薢, poison yam, Rhizoma Dioscoreae Hypoglaucae］. Its flowers are yellow and calyx indigo. It sprouts calyx like the chrysanthemum when it grows 1~2 Cun above the ground, straight and strong, without seeds. Tao Yinju once stated that it is like the plant from Gaoli[4] and Baiji[5] very much." Its leaves are bitter and flowers spicy and sweet in taste. Its nature is mild and non-toxic. Regarding compatibility, Xingren［杏仁, bitter apricot seed, Semen Armeniacae Amarum] is its assistance and Ziwan [紫菀, tatarian aster root, Radix Asteris] can enhance its efficacy. It is averse to Zaojia [皂荚, soap pod, Gleditsia sinensis Lam.], Xiaoshi [消石, saltpeter, Sal Nitri] and Xuanshen [玄参, kakuda figwort root, Radix Scrophulariae], and restrained by Beimu [贝母, fritillaria, Bulbus Fritillaria], Xinyi [辛夷, Flos Magnoliae, Biond Magnolia Flower], Mahuang [麻黄, Herba Ephedrae, Ephedra], Huangqin [黄芩, Radix Scutellariae, Baical Skullcap Root], Huanglian [黄连, Rhizoma Coptidis, Golden Thread] and Qingxiang [青葙, Semen Celosiae, Feather Cockscomb Seed].

For famine relief: Collect young leaves, blanch and soak them in fresh water, remove the sourness by elutriating them with water, and flavor them with oil and salt.

For disease treatment: See the clauses in *Materia Medica · Herbaceous Plant*.

【Notes】

[1] The name of a mountain. Presently it is located in the northwest of Quyang County, Hebei Province.

[2] It refers to *Ben Cao Tu Jing* [《本草图经》, *Illustrated Classics of Materia Medica*], 21 volumes, compiled by Susong and other scholars in Song Dynasty in 1061.

[3] Pronounced "ge", a unit of capacity, equaling 1/10 of one Sheng.

[4] The name of an ancient country, located in Chaoxian Peninsula.

[5] The name of an ancient country, located in Chaoxian Peninsula.

5. 萹 蓄

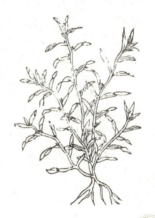

亦名萹竹,生东莱山谷,今在处有之,布地生道傍。苗似石竹,叶微阔,嫩绿如竹。赤茎如钗股[1]。节间花出甚细,淡桃红色。结小细子。根如蒿根。苗叶味苦,性平,一云味甘,无毒。

救饥:采苗叶煠熟,水浸淘净,油盐调食。

治病:文具《本草·草部》条下。

【注释】

［1］古代妇女用以固定发髻的头饰,因形状细长,常用来形容花叶的枝杈。

5. Bianxu [萹蓄, common knotgrass herb, Polygonum aviculare L.]

Bianxu [萹蓄, common knotgrass herb, Polygonum aviculare L.], also named Pianzhu, grows in the valleys of Donglai and nowadays can be seen everywhere. Its plants often grow along the roadside. Its young plants are like Shizhu [石竹, Chinese pink, Dianthus chinensis L.]. Its leaves are broad and of light malachite green. Its red stems are like Chaigu[1]. Its small pink flowers scatter among the branch knots. Its fruit is tiny and its roots are like the artemisia roots. Its plants are bitter in taste and mild in nature. It is also said to be sweet in taste and non-toxic.

For famine relief: Collect young seedlings and leaves, blanch, soak and clean them in fresh water, and flavor them with oil and salt.

For disease treatment: See the clauses in Materia Medica · Herbaceous Plant.

【Notes】

[1] A kind of hairpin in ancient times for women to fix their buns. It is long and narrow so people often use this term to refer to branches.

6. 大 蓝

生河内平泽,今处处有之,人家园圃中多种。苗高尺余。叶类白菜叶,微厚而狭窄尖艄,淡粉青色。茎叉稍间开黄花,结小荚,其子黑色。《本草》谓菘蓝可以为靛染青,以其叶似菘菜,故名菘蓝。又名马蓝,《尔雅》[1]所谓"葳,马蓝"是也。味苦,性寒,无毒。

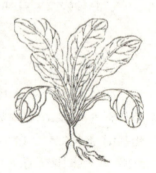

救饥:采叶煤熟,水浸去苦味,油盐调食。

治病:文具《本草·草部》蓝实条下。

【注释】

［1］文字训诂书,为儒家经典之一,约成书于秦汉时期,作者不详。

6. Dalan [大蓝, leaf and stem of true indigo, Isatis tinctoria L.]

Dalan [大蓝, leaf and stem of true indigo, Isatis tinctoria L.] grows in the flat wetlands and can be found everywhere nowadays like the nursery gardens of common people. Its plants are one Chi high and its cyan leaves are like those of Baicai [白菜, Chinese cabbage, Brassica rapa L. var. glabra Regel], only being thicker, narrower and sharper. The yellow flowers scatter among the scape and branches. It produces small legumes and black seeds. *Materia Medica* says that Songlan [菘蓝, woad, Isatis indigotica Fort], another name for Dalan, can be made into indigo indium to dye cyan color. Its leaves are like Songcai so it is called Songlan. It is also called Malan as stated in *Er Ya*[1] [《尔雅》, *Literary Expositor*] "The so-called Zhen is actually Malan." It is bitter in taste, cold in nature and non-toxic.

For famine relief: Collect and blanch leaves, remove the bitterness by soaking them in water, and flavor them with oil and salt.

For disease treatment: See the clause of Lanshi [蓝实, indigoplant fruit, Fructus Polygoni Tingtorii] in *Materia Medica · Herbaceous Plant*.

[Notes]

[1] One of the ancient Confucius classics containing commentaries on classics, names, etc. It is probably compiled during Qin and Han periods with the author unknown.

7. 石竹子

本草名瞿麦,一名巨句麦,一名大菊,一名大兰,又名杜母草、燕麦、蕎麦。生太山[1]川谷,今处处有之。苗高一尺已来。叶似独扫叶而尖小,又似小竹叶而细窄。茎亦有节。梢间开红白花而结蒴,内有小黑子。味苦、辛,性寒,无毒。蘘草、牡丹为之使,恶螵蛸。

救饥:采嫩苗叶煤熟,水浸淘净,油盐调食。

治病:文具《本草·草部》瞿麦条下。

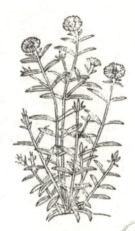

【注释】

[1] 山名,即今山东境内的泰山。

7. Shizhuzi [石竹子, Chinese pink, Dianthus chinensis L.]

Shizhuzi [石竹子, Chinese pink, Dianthus chinensis L.], also named Qumai, Jujumai, Daju, Dalan, Dumucao, Yanmai and Yuemai, grows in the valleys of Taishan[1] and can be seen everywhere presently. Its plants are about one Chi high and its leaves are like those of Dusao [独扫, kochia, Kochiae Fructus], and also like young bamboos, but sharper and narrower than the latter. There are knots on its stems and red and white flowers among the branches. Its fruit is called Shuoguo, namely capsule, with small black seeds inside. Its seeds are bitter and pungent in taste, cold in nature and non-toxic. Regarding compatibility, Rangcao [蘘草, Rhizome of Mioga Ginger, Zingiber mioga Thunb. Rosc.] and Mudan [牡丹, subshrubby peony, Paeonia suffruticosa Andr] are its assistance, and it is averse to Piaoxiao [螵蛸, mantis egg-case, Ootheca Mantidis].

For famine relief: Collect and blanch young leaves, soak and clean them with water, and flavor them with oil and salt.

For disease treatment: See the clause of Qumai [瞿麦, Herba Dianthi, Lilac Pink Herb] in *Materia Medica · Herbaceous Plant*.

【Notes】

[1] The name of a mountain, referring to Mountain Tai in Shandong Province nowadays.

8. 红花菜

本草名红蓝花,一名黄蓝。出梁、汉及西域,沧魏亦种之,今处处有之。苗高二尺许。茎叶有刺,似刺蓟叶而润泽,窊面。稍结梂彙,亦多刺。开红花,蕊出梂上,圃人采之,采已复出,至尽而罢。梂中结实,白颗如小豆大。其花暴干,以染真红,及作胭脂。花味辛,性温,无毒。叶味甘。

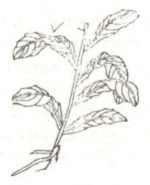

救饥：采嫩叶煠熟，油盐调食。子可笮[1]作油用。

治病：文具《本草·草部》红蓝花条下。

【注释】

[1] 方言，即压榨。

8. Honghuacai [红花菜, safflower, Carthamus tinctorius L.]

Honghuacai [红花菜, safflower, Carthamus tinctorius L.], also named Honglanhua and Huanglan, grows in the regions of Liang, Han, Xiyu and Cangwei, and it can be seen everywhere presently. Its plants are two Chi high and its leaves are thorny like those of Ciji [刺蓟, field thistle herb, Herba Cirsii], but lustrous and rough. On the top of the plants there are thorny and hedgehog-shaped capitula. Its flowers are red with pistils sticking out from the capitula. The gardener can pick pistil again and again till they do not grow any more. Its white granular fruit is like beans. Its flowers can be used to dye scarlet or as rouge when sun-dried. Its flowers are pungent in taste, mild in nature and non-toxic. Its leaves are sweet in taste.

For famine relief：Collect and blanch young leaves, and flavor them with oil and salt. Its seeds can be used to Ze[1] oil.

For disease treatment：See the clause of Honglanhua [红蓝花, Safflower, Flos Carthami] in *Materia Medica · Herbaceous Plant*.

【Notes】

[1] A local language, referring to extract.

9. 萱草花

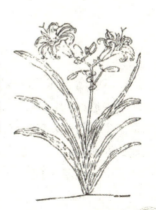

俗名川草花，本草一名鹿葱，谓生山野，花名宜男。《风土记》[1]云"怀妊妇人佩其花，生男"故也。人家园圃中多种。其叶就地丛生，两边分垂，叶似菖蒲叶而柔弱，又似粉条儿菜叶而肥大。叶间撺葶，开金黄花，味甘，无毒。根凉，亦无毒。叶味甘。

救饥：采嫩苗叶煠熟，水浸淘净，油盐调食。

治病：文具《本草·草部》条下。

【注释】

［1］西晋周处著，主要记载各个地方的风土人情，今该书已佚。

9. Xuancaohua［萱草花, day lily, Hemerocallis fulva L.］

Xuancaohua［萱草花, day lily, Hemerocallis fulva L.］, also named Chuancaohua, Lucong and Yinan, grows in the mountainous regions and the open fields. *Fengtuji*[1] says, "The pregnant woman can give birth to a boy if she wears it", and that is the reason why it is called Yinan（宜男）, meaning proper to bear a boy in Chinese. Common people often plant it in their gardens. Its clustered leaves grow along the ground, with tips drooping down. Its leaves are like those of Changpu［菖蒲, calamus, Acorus calamus L.］, but tender, and also like those of Fentiao'er Cai［粉条儿菜, scorzonera root, Scorzonerae Radix］, but larger. Among the branches and leaves there are scapes and golden yellow flowers, which are sweet in taste and non-toxic. Its roots are cool in nature and non-toxic. Its leaves are sweet in taste.

For famine relief: Collect and blanch young leaves, soak and clean them with water, and flavor them with oil and salt.

For disease treatment: See the relevant clause in *Materia Medica · Herbaceous Plant*.

［Notes］

［1］ *Fudoki*, a book compiled by Zhouchu in the Western Jin Dynasty. It is mainly about local customs and practices of different places, lost today.

10. 车轮菜

本草名车前子，一名当道，一名芣苢，一名虾蟆衣，一名牛遗，一名胜舄。《尔雅》云马舄，幽州人谓之牛舌草。生滁州及真定平泽，今处处有之。春初生苗，叶布地如匙面，累年者，长及尺余；又似玉簪叶梢大而薄。叶丛中心撺葶三四茎，作长穗，如鼠尾。花甚密，青色

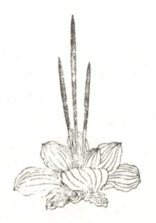

微赤。结实如葶苈子,赤黑色。生道傍。味甘、咸,性寒,无毒。一云味甘,性平。叶及根味甘,性寒。常山为之使。

救饥:采嫩苗叶煠熟,水浸去涎沫,淘净,油盐调食。

治病:文具《本草·草部》车前子条下。

10. Cheluncai [车轮菜, plantago seed, Plantago asiatica L.]

Cheluncai [车轮菜, plantago seed, Plantago asiatica L.], also named Cheqianzi, Dangdao, Fuyi, Xiamoyi, Niuyi, Shengxi, Maxi in *Er Ya* [《尔雅》, *Literary Expositor*] and Niushecao by the people from Youzhou, grows in the weedy flat wetlands of Chuzhou and Zhending, and can be seen everywhere presently. Its plants start to grow in the spring and its spoon-like leaves grow along the ground. The leaves of its perennial plants are more than one Chi long. Its leaves are like those of fragrant plantain lily, larger and thinner than the latter. Its plants send forth three or four spicate scapes among the leaves, just like the mouse tail. Its dense flowers are green, with a slight red. Its seeds are like those of Tingli [葶苈, Semen Lepidii, Semen Descurainiae], red and black. It often grows along the roadside. It is sweet and salty in taste, cold in nature and non-toxic. It is also said to be sweet in taste and mild in nature. Its leaves and roots are sweet in taste and cold in nature. Regarding compatibility, Changshan [常山, dichroa, Dichroae Radix] is its assistance.

For famine relief: Collect and blanch young leaves, soak and clean them with water, and flavor them with oil and salt.

For disease treatment: See the clause of Cheqianzi [车前子, plantago seed, Plantaginis Semen] in *Materia Medica · Herbaceous Plant*.

11. 白水荭苗

本草名荭草,一名鸿䔲。有赤白二色,《尔雅》云:"红,茏古。其大者蘬。"《郑诗》[1]云"隰有游龙"是也。所在有之,生水边下湿地。叶似蓼叶而长大,有涩毛,花开红白;又似马蓼,其茎有节而赤。味咸,性微寒,无毒。

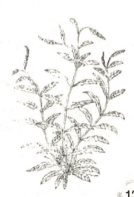

救饥：采嫩苗叶煠熟，水浸淘净，油盐调食。洗净蒸食亦可。

治病：文具《本草·草部》荭草条下。

【注释】

[1] 指《诗经·郑风》。

11. Baishuihong Miao [白水荭苗, oriental smartweed, Polygonum lapathifolium L.]

Baishuihong Miao [白水荭苗, oriental smartweed, Polygonum lapathifolium L.], also named Hongcao and Hongxie, is red and white in color. *Er Ya* [《尔雅》, *Literary Expositor*] says, "Longgu (another name for Baishuihong Miao) is red. The bigger one is called Kui (another name for Baishuihong Miao)". *Zhengshi*[1] says, "Youlong (another name for Baishuihong Miao) grows in the low wetland." It grows in the low-lying wetlands near water. Its leaves are like those of Liao [蓼, water pepper, Polygoni Hydropiperis Herba], but longer and larger than the latter, with the rough pile. Its flowers are red and white, like those of Maliao [马蓼, clematis anhweiensis, Polygonum persicaria L.]. There are knots on its red stems. It is salty in taste, slightly cold in nature and non-toxic.

For famine relief: Collect and blanch young leaves, soak and clean them with water, and flavor them with oil and salt or steam.

For disease treatment: See the clause of Hongcao [荭草, Oriental smartweed, Polygoni Orientalis Herba] in *Materia Medica · Herbaceous Plant*.

【Notes】

[1] It refers to *Shi Jing Zheng Feng* [《诗经·郑风》, *The Classics of Portry · Zheng Music*].

12. 黄 耆

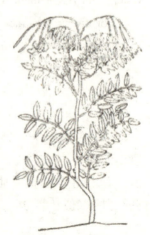

一名戴糁，一名戴椹，一名独椹，一名芰草，一名蜀脂，一名百本，一名王孙。生蜀郡山谷及白水、汉中、河东、陕西，出绵上呼为绵黄耆，今处处有之。根长二三尺。独茎，丛生枝干。其叶扶疏，作羊齿状，似槐叶微尖小；又似蒺藜叶，阔大而青白色。开黄紫花，如槐花大，结小尖角，长寸许。味甘，性微温，无毒。一云味苦，微寒。恶龟甲、白藓皮。

救饥：采嫩苗叶煤熟，换水浸淘，洗去苦味，油盐调食。药中补益，呼为羊肉。

治病：文具《本草·草部》条下。

12. Huangqi [黄耆, milkvetch root, Astragalus membranaceus (Fisch.) Bunge]

Huangqi [黄耆, milkvetch root, Astragalus membranaceus (Fisch.) Bunge], also named Daishen, Daizhen, Duzhen, Zhicao, Shuzhi, Baiben and Wangsun, grows in the valleys of Shujun and other places like Baishui, Hanzhong, Hedong and Shanxi. It is called Mianhuangqi if it grows in Mianshang County. Presently it can be seen everywhere. Its roots are 2～3 Chi long and its single stems are clustered with branches. Its scattered leaves are of the shape of sheep teeth, small and sharp like locust leaves, broad and bluish white like caltrop leaves. Its yellowish purple flowers are as big as sophora flowers and its pointed fruit is about one Cun long. It is sweet in taste, warm in nature and non-toxic. It is also said to be bitter in taste and slightly cold in nature. Regarding compatibility, it is averse to Guijia [龟甲, Tortoise Carapace and Plastron, Carapax et Plastrum Testudinis] and Baixianpi [白藓皮, dictamnus, Dictamni Cortex].

For famine relief: Collect and blanch young leaves, soak them in water and remove the bitterness, and flavor them with oil and salt. Because of its tonifying function, it is also called mutton.

For disease treatment: See the relevant clause in *Materia Medica · Herbaceous Plant*.

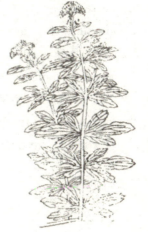

13. 威灵仙

一名能消。出商州上洛、华山并平泽，及陕西、河东、河北、河南、江湖、石州、宁化等州郡。不闻水声者良。今密县梁家冲山野中亦有之。苗高一二尺。茎方如钗股，四棱。茎多细茸白毛。叶似柳叶而阔，边有锯齿；又似旋覆花叶。其叶作层生，每层六七叶，相对排如车轮样，有六层至七层者。花浅紫色，或碧白色。作穗似蒲台子。亦有似菊花头者。结实青色，根稠密多须。味苦，性温，无毒。恶茶及面汤，以甘草、栀子代饮可也。

救饥：采叶煠熟，换水浸去苦味，再以水淘净，油盐调食。

治病：文具《本草·草部》条下。

13. Weilingxian ［威灵仙，clematis root，Eupatorium fortune Turca］

Weilingxian ［威灵仙, clematis root, Eupatorium fortune Turca］, also named Nengxiao, grows in Shangluo Mountain, Hua Mountain and the flat wetlands of Shangzhou, also in other counties like Shanxi, Hedong, Hebei, Henan, Jianghu, Shizhou and Ninghua. Its quality is better if it is planted in places without the sound of water. Presently, it can also be found in the mountainous regions and the open fields of Liangjiachong in Mixian County. Its plants are 1～2 Chi high with square stems like hairpins, covered with white piles. Its sawtooth-edged leaves are like but broader than the salix leaves, and also like the leaves of Xuanfuhua ［旋覆花, Inula Flower, Flos Inulae］. Its layered leaves grow on the stem, with 6～7 layers for each plant and 6～7 leaves for each layer, arranged in the shape of a wheel. Its fringy flowers are lilac or greenish white, like Putaizi ［蒲台子, cattail, Typha latifolia L.］, or chrysanthemum capitulum. Its fruit is green and its roots are dense and hairy. It is bitter in taste, warm in nature and non-toxic. Regarding compatibility, it is averse to tea and noodle soup. It can be taken together with Gancao ［甘草, liquorice root, Radix Glycyrrhizae］ and Zhizi ［栀子, cape jasmine fruit, Fructus Gardeniae］ to substitute tea.

For famine relief: Collect and blanch leaves, soak them in water and remove the bitterness, and flavor them with oil and salt.

For disease treatment: See the relevant clause in *Materia Medica · Herbaceous Plant*.

14. 马兜零

一名云南根,又名土青木香。生关中及信州、滁州、河东、河北、江淮、夔、浙州郡皆有,今高阜去处亦有之。春生苗如藤蔓。叶如山药叶而厚大,背白。开黄紫花,颇类枸杞花。结实如铃,作四五瓣。叶脱时,铃尚垂之,其状如马项铃,故得名。味苦,性寒。又云平,无毒。

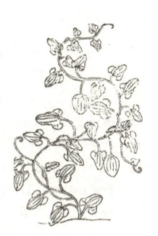

救饥:采叶煠熟,用水浸去苦味,淘净,油盐调食。

治病:文具《本草·草部》条下。

14. Madouling [马兜零, dutohmanspipe fruit, Aristolochia debilis Sieb. et Zucc.]

Madouling [马兜零, dutohmanspipe fruit, Aristolochia debilis Sieb. et Zucc.], also named Yunnangen and Tuqing Muxiang, grows in the counties like Guanzhong, Xinzhou, Chuzhou, Hedong, Hebei, Jianghuai, Kui and Zhezhou. Presently, it can also be found in the high mountains of soil. Its plants start to grow like vines in the spring. Its leaves are like and larger than Chinese yam leaves, the back of which is white. Its flowers are yellowish purple, like those of Gouqi [枸杞, barbary wolfberry fruit, Fructus Lycii]. Its fruit is like a bell, with dehiscence of 4~5 cloves, which hangs still even the leaves fall off. The shape of the fruit is like the bell tying around the horse neck and that is the reason why it is called Madouling (meaning the bell around the horse neck in Chinese). It is bitter in taste and cold in nature. It is also said to be mild in nature and non-toxic.

For famine relief: Collect and blanch leaves, soak them in water and remove the bitterness, and flavor them with oil and salt.

For disease treatment: See the relevant clause in *Materia Medica · Herbaceous Plant*.

15. 旋覆花

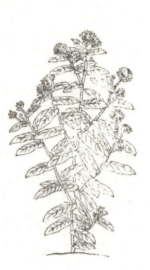

一名戴椹，一名金沸草，一名盛椹。上党田野人呼为金钱花。《尔雅》云："覆，盗庚。"出随州，生平泽川谷，今处处有之。苗多近水傍。初生大如红花叶而无刺。苗长二三尺已来。叶似柳叶稍宽大。茎细如蒿杆。开花似菊花，如铜钱大，深黄色。花味咸、甘，性温、微冷利，有小毒。叶味苦，性凉。

救饥：采叶煠熟，水浸去苦味，淘净，油盐调食。

治病：文具《本草·草部》条下。

15. Xuanfuhua [旋覆花, inula flower, Inula Britannica L.]

Xuanfuhua [旋覆花, inula flower, Inula Britannica L.] is also named Daizhen, Jinfeicao, Shengzhen and Jinqianhua by the farmers from Shangdang. *Er Ya* [《尔雅》, *Literary Expositor*] says, "Fu refers to Daogeng (another name for Xuanfuhua)." It originates from the marshes and the valleys of Suizhou and can be seen everywhere nowadays. It often grows near water. Its young plants are like Honghua [红花, safflower, Flos Carthami] without thorns, about 2~3 Chi high. Its leaves are like and broader than the salix leaves. Its stems are thin just like the artemisia ones. Its dark yellow flowers are like chrysanthemum, as big as the copper cash. Its flowers are salty and sweet in taste, warm and slightly cold in nature and slightly toxic. Its leaves are bitter in taste and cool in nature.

For famine relief: Collect and blanch leaves, soak them in water and remove the bitterness, and flavor them with oil and salt.

For disease treatment: See the relevant clause in *Materia Medica · Herbaceous Plant*.

16. 防 风

一名铜芸,一名茴草,一名百枝,一名屏风,一名蕳根,一名百蜚。生同州沙苑川泽,邯郸、琅邪、上蔡、陕西、山东,处处皆有。今中牟田野中亦有之。根土黄色,与蜀葵根相类,稍细短。茎叶俱青绿色,茎深而叶淡。叶似青蒿叶而阔大,又似米蒿叶而稀疏。茎似茴香。开细白花。结实似胡荽子而大。味甘、辛,性温,无毒。杀[1]附子毒。恶干姜、藜芦、白敛、芫花。又有石防风,亦疗头风痛。又有叉头者,令人发狂;叉尾者,发痼疾。

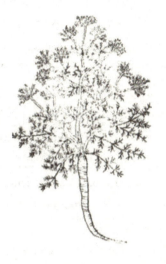

救饥:采嫩苗叶作菜茹,煤食,极爽口。

治病:文具《本草·草部》条下。

【注释】

[1] 相杀,中药配伍原则之一,即一种药物能减轻或消除另一种药物的毒性或副作用。

16. Fangfeng [防风, divaricate saposhnikovia root, Saposhnikovia divaricata (Turcz.) Schischk.]

Fangfeng [防风, divaricate saposhnikovia root, Saposhnikovia divaricata (Turcz.) Schischk.], also named Tongyun, Huicao, Baizhi, Pingfeng, Jiangen and Baifei], grows in the lakes and swamps of Tongzhou and Shayuan, and can also be seen in the places like Handan, Langya, Shangcai, Shanxi and Shandong and the fields of Zhongmu. Its khaki roots are like and shorter than those of Shukuigen [蜀葵根, hollyhock root, Althaeae Radix]. Both of its stems and leaves are turquoise in color, only the former being darker and the latter lighter. Its leaves are like and broader than those of Qinghao [青蒿, sweet wormwood herb, Herba Artemisiae Annuae], and also like and sparser than those of Mihao [米蒿, artemisia, Descurainia Sophia (L.) Webb ex Prantl]. It stems are like those of Huixiang [茴香, fennel, Fructus Foeniculi]. Its flowers are tiny and white and its fruit is like and larger than that of Husui [胡荽, coriander herb with root, Herba Coriandri Sativi cum Radice]. It is sweet and pungent in taste, warm in nature and non-toxic. Regarding compatibility, it is the antidote to[1] the toxicity of Fuzi [附子, prepared common monkshood daughter root, Radix Aconiti Lateralis Preparata] and averse to Ganjiang [干姜, dried ginger, Rhizoma Zingiberis], Lilu [藜芦, veratrum, Veratri Nigri Radix et Rhizoma], Bailian [白敛, ampelopsis, Ampelopsis Radix] and Yuanhua [芫花, genkwa, Genkwa Flos]. There are similar herbs: Shifangfeng [石防风, turpentine peucedanumk, Peucedani Terebinthacei Radix], often used to treat intermittent headache and dizziness; the kind with top furcation, making people mad if taken; the kind with bottom furcation, inducing chronic and intractable disease if taken.

For famine relief: Collect and blanch young leaves, being tasty and refreshing as food.

For disease treatment: See the relevant clause in *Materia Medica · Herbaceous Plant*.

【Notes】

[1] It refers to the mutual suppression, one of the principles of compatibility of Chinese medicines. Namely, a medicinal can reduce or dispel the toxicity or side-effect of another medicinal.

17. 郁臭苗

本草茺蔚子是也。一名益母，一名益明，一名大札，一名贞蔚，皆云蓷，益母也，亦谓蕹，臭秽。生海滨池泽，今田野处处有之。叶似荏子叶；又似艾叶而薄小，色青。茎方。节节开小白花。结子黑茶褐色，三棱，细长，味辛、甘，微温。一云微寒，无毒。

救饥：采苗叶煠熟，水浸淘净，油盐调食。

治病：文具《本草·草部》茺蔚子条下。

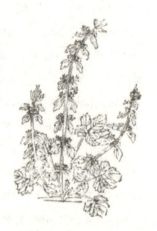

17. Yuchoumiao [郁臭苗, motherwort fruit, Lagopsis supine (Steph. ex Willd.) Ik. -Gal. ex Knorr.]

Yuchoumiao [郁臭苗, motherwort fruit, Lagopsis supine (Steph. ex Willd.) Ik. -Gal. ex Knorr.], also named Chongweizi, Yimu, Yiming, Dazha, Zhenwei and Tui (referring to Yimu or the foul smell], grows near the seasides and swamps and can be seen in the fields presently. Its leaves are like perilla leaves or argy wormwood leaves, but thinner, smaller and greener than the latter. Its stems are square with tiny white flowers. Its seeds are dark brown, triquetrum, long and thin. It is pungent and sweet in taste, and warm in nature. It is also said to be slightly cold in nature and non-toxic.

For famine relief: Collect and blanch leaves, soak them in water and make them clean, and flavor them oil and salt.

For disease treatment: See the clause of Chongweizi [茺蔚子, motherwort fruit, Fructus Leonuri] in *Materia Medica · Herbaceous Plant*.

18. 泽 漆

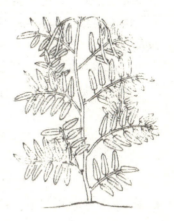

本草一名漆茎,大戟苗也。生太山川泽,及冀州、鼎州、明州,今处处有之。苗高二三尺,科叉生。茎紫赤色。叶似柳叶微细短。开黄紫花,状似杏花而瓣颇长。生时摘叶,有白汁出,亦能啮[1]人,故以为名。味苦、辛,性微寒,无毒。一云有小毒。一云性冷,微毒。小豆为之使,恶薯蓣。初尝叶味涩苦,食过回味甜。

救饥:采叶及嫩茎煠熟,水浸淘净,油盐调食。采嫩叶蒸过晒干,做茶吃亦可。

治病:文具《本草·草部》条下。

【注释】

[1] 咬、啃。这里指汁液对人的皮肤有刺激作用。

18. Zeqi [泽漆, sun spurge, Apocynum venetum L.]

Zeqi [泽漆, sun spurge, Apocynum venetum L.], also named Qijing, is actually the young plant of Daji [大戟, peking euphorbia root, Euphorbia pekinensis Rupr.]. It grows near the lakes and swamps of Taishan, and other places like Yizhou and Dingzhou and Mingzhou, and can be seen everywhere presently. Its plants are 2~3 Chi high with twigs in branches. Its stems are fuchsia and its leaves are like and shorter than salix leaves. Its yellowish purple flowers are like apricot flowers, with longer petals. The white juice flows out when its leaves are taken away from the plants, which can nibble and bite[1] people and that is the reason why it is called Zeqi. It is bitter and pungent in taste, cold in nature and non-toxic. It is also said to be cold in nature and slightly toxic. Regarding compatibility, Xiaodou [小豆, rice bean, Phaseoli Semen] is its assistance, and it is averse to Shuyu [薯蓣, common yam rhizome, Rhizoma Dioscoreae]. It tastes bitter and astringent when one tries its leaves at first, but the aftertaste is sweet.

For famine relief: Collect and blanch leaves and young stems, soak them in water and make them clean, and flavor them with oil and salt. Steam and then dry its young leaves in the sunshine, and drink like tea.

For disease treatment: See the relevant clause in *Materia Medica · Herbaceous Plant*.

【Notes】

[1] Nibble and bite. Here it refers to the skin irritation caused by the juice.

19. 酸浆草

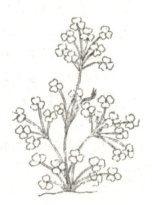

本草名酢浆草,一名醋母草,一名鸠酸草,俗为小酸茅。旧不著所出州土,今处处有之。生道傍下湿地。叶如初生小水萍,每茎端皆丛生三叶。开黄花,结黑子。南人用苗揩鍮石器[1],令白如银色光艳。味酸,性寒,无毒。

救饥:采嫩苗叶生食。

治病:文具《本草·草部》酢浆条下。

【注释】

[1]用铜做成的器皿。

19. Suanjiangcao [酸浆草, creeping wood sorrel, Oxalis corniculata L.]

Suanjiangcao [酸浆草, creeping wood sorrel, Oxalis corniculata L.] is also named Zuojiangcao, Cumucao, Jiusuancao and Xiaosuanmao, whose origin is not recorded in ancient books but can be seen everywhere presently. It grows in the low and wet places along the roadside. Its leaves are like the young pepper wort herb, with three small leaves on a petiole. Its flowers are yellow and fruit black. The southerners use its plants to polish bronze ware[1], making it shine like silver. It is sour in taste, cold in nature and non-toxic.

For famine relief: Collect young plants and leaves, and then eat them raw.

For disease treatment: See the clause of Zuojiangcao [酢浆草, creeping wood sorrel, Oxalidis Corniculatae Herba] in *Materia Medica · Herbaceous Plant.*

【Notes】

[1] The household utensils made with bronze.

20. 蛇床子

一名蛇粟,一名蛇米,一名虺床,一名思益,一名绳毒,一名枣棘,一名墙蘼,《尔雅》一名盱。生临淄川谷田野,今处处有之。苗高二三尺,青碎作丛似蒿枝。叶似黄蒿叶;又似小叶蘼芜;又似藁本叶。每枝上有花头百余,结同一窠,开白花如伞盖状。结子半黍大,黄褐色,味苦、辛、甘,无毒,性平。一云有小毒。恶牡丹、巴豆、贝母。

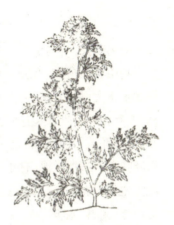

救饥:采嫩苗叶煤熟,水浸淘洗净,油盐调食。

治病:文具《本草·草部》条下。

20. Shechuangzi [蛇床子, chidium fruit, Cnidium monnieri (L.) Cuss.]

Shechuangzi [蛇床子, chidium fruit, Cnidium monnieri (L.) Cuss.], also named Shesu, Shemi, Huichuang, Siyi, Shengdu, Zaoji, Qiangmi and Xu according to *Er Ya* [《尔雅》, *Literary Expositor*], grows in the fields and valleys of Linzi and can be seen everywhere presently. Its plants are 2 ~ 3 Chi high, green and clustered like the artemisia branches. Its leaves are like those of Artemisia, Ligusticum chuanxiong Hort and Rhizoma Ligustici. There are more than 100 white flowers on each umbel, just like an umbrella. Its yellowish brown seeds are as small as half of a millet, bitter, pungent and sweet in taste, neutral in nature and non-toxic. It is also said to be slightly toxic. Regarding compatibility, it is averse to Mudan [牡丹, subshrubby peony, Paeonia suffruticosa Andr], Badou [巴豆, croton fruit, Fructus Crotonis] and Beimu [贝母, fritillaria, Bulbus Fritillaria].

For famine relief: Collect and blanch leaves and young plants, soak them in water and make them clean, and flavor them with oil and salt.

For disease treatment: See the relevant clause in *Materia Medica · Herbaceous Plant*.

21. 桔 梗

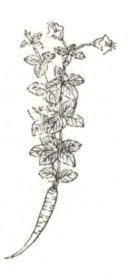

一名利如,一名房图,一名白药,一名梗草,一名荠苨。生嵩高山谷及冤句、和州、解州,今钧州密县山野亦有之。根如手指大,黄白色。春生苗,茎高尺余。叶似杏叶而长椭,四叶相对而生,嫩时亦可煮食。开花紫碧色,颇似牵牛花。秋后结子。叶名隐忍。其根有心,无心者乃荠苨也。根叶味辛、苦,性微温,有小毒。一云味苦,性平,无毒。节皮为之使,得牡砺、远志疗恚怒,得硝石、石膏疗伤寒[1]。畏白芨、龙眼、龙胆。

救饥:采叶煠熟,换水浸去苦味,淘洗净,油盐调食。

治病:文具《本草·草部》条下。

【注释】

[1] 病症名。指感受寒邪的病症。

21. Jiegeng [桔梗, platycodon root, Platycodon grandiflorus (Jacq.) A. DC.]

Jiegeng [桔梗, platycodon root, Platycodon grandiflorus (Jacq.) A. DC.], also named Liru, Fangtu, Baiyao, Gengcao and Qini, grows in the valleys of Mountain Song and other places like Yuanju, Hezhou and Xiezhou. Presently, it can be found in the mountainous regions and fields of Junzhou and Mixian of Henan Province. Its yellowish white roots are like people's fingers. Its plants are one Chi high and sprout in the spring. Its leaves, named Yinren, are like those of apricot, elliptic and quarternate arranged. Its young leaves can be eaten after being cooked. Its flowers are bluish violet like the Morning Glory. It bears fruit in autumn. Its roots have the core part while the roots of Qini [荠苨, apricot-leaved adenophora, Adenophorae Trachelioidis Radix] do not have. Its roots and leaves are pungent and bitter in taste, slightly warm in nature and slightly toxic. It is also said to be bitter in taste, neutral in nature and non-toxic. Regarding compatibility, the arthroderm is its assistance, which can treat rage if plus Muli [牡蛎, oyster shell, Concha Ostreae], Yuanzhi [远志, milkwort root, Radix Polygalae] and treat cold damage[1] if plus Xiaoshi [硝石, niter, Sal Nitri] and Shigao [石膏, gypsum, Gypsum Fibrosum]. It is restrained by Baiji [白芨, platanthera, Platantherae Tuber], Longyan [龙眼, longan aril, Arillus Longan] and Longdan [龙胆, Chinese gentian, Radix Gentianae].

For famine relief: Collect and blanch leaves, soak them in water and make them clean, and flavor them with oil and salt.

For disease treatment: See the relevant clause in *Materia Medica · Herbaceous Plant*.

【Notes】

[1] The name of a disease. Here it refers to the cold damage caused by the cold-pathogen.

22. 茴 香

一名蘹香子，北人呼为土茴香，茴、蘹声相近，故云耳。今处处有之，人家园圃多种。苗高三四尺，茎粗如笔管，傍有淡黄袴叶，拤茎而生，袴叶上发生青色细叶，似细蓬叶而长，极疏细，如丝发状，袴叶间分生叉枝。稍头开花，花头如伞盖，黄色。结子如莳萝子，微大而长，亦有线瓣，味苦、辛，性平，无毒。

救饥：采苗叶煠熟，换水淘净，油盐调食。子调和诸般食，味香美。

治病：文具《本草·草部》蘹香子条下。

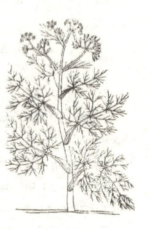

22. Huixiang［茴香, fennel, Foeniculum vulgare Mill.］

Huixiang［茴香, fennel, Foeniculum vulgare Mill.］ is also named Huaixiangzi and Tuhuixiang by northerners because of the similar Chinese sound of Hui and Huai. It can be seen everywhere presently, especially in the common people's gardens. Its plants are 3～4 Chi high and its stems are as thick as pen tubes, with yellow pant-like leaves on it. On its leaves there are green thin leaves, like bitter fleabane leaves and silky hair, longer and thinner. Among the leaves there are branches and on the top of the plants there is yellow inflorescence like an umbrella. Its fruit is like that of anethum, larger and longer, with edges along the side. It is bitter and pungent in taste, neutral in nature and non-toxic.

For famine relief: Collect and blanch leaves, soak in water and make them clean, and flavor them with oil and salt. Its fruit can be used as a seasoner for various foods, tasty and delicious.

For disease treatment: See the clause of Huaixiangzi［蘹香子, fennel, Fructus Foeniculi］in *Materia Medica · Herbaceous Plant*.

23. 夏枯草

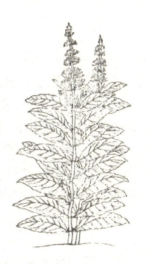

本草一名夕句,一名乃东,一名燕面。生蜀郡川谷,及河东、淮、浙、滁平泽,今祥符西田野中亦有之。苗高二三尺,其叶对节生。叶似旋覆叶,而极长大,边有细锯齿,背白,上多气脉纹路。叶端开花作穗,长二三寸许。其花紫白,似丹参花。叶味苦、微辛,性寒,无毒。土瓜为之使。俗又谓之郁臭苗,非是。

救饥:采嫩叶煤熟,换水浸淘去苦味,油盐调食。

治病:文具《本草·草部》条下。

23. Xiakucao [夏枯草, common selfheal fruit-spike, Prunella vulgaris L.]

Xiakucao [夏枯草, common selfheal fruit-spike, Prunella vulgaris L.], also named Xiju, Naidong and Yanmian, grows in the valleys of Shujun and the flat wetlands of Hedong, Huai, Zhe and Chuzhou. Presently, it can also be seen in the fields of Xiangfu County. Its plants are 2~3 Chi high, with opposite leaves like and larger than those of Xuanfuhua [旋覆花, inula flower, Flos Inulae]. There are saw teeth at the edge of its leaves, whose backsides are white and textured. There is fringy inflorescence on the top of its plant, about 2~3 Cun long. Its flowers are purplish white like those of Danshen [丹参, salvia root, Radix Salviae Miltiorrhizae]. Its leaves are bitter and slightly pungent in taste, cold in nature and non-toxic. Regarding compatibility, Tugua [土瓜, cucumber gourd, Trichosanthis Cucumeroidis Fructus] is its assistance. It is also called Yuchoumiao [郁臭苗, motherwort fruit, Fructus Leonuri] by common people, which is not right.

For famine relief: Collect and blanch young leaves, remove the bitterness by soaking them in fresh water, and flavor them with oil and salt.

For disease treatment: See the relevant clause in *Materia Medica · Herbaceous Plant*.

24. 藁 本

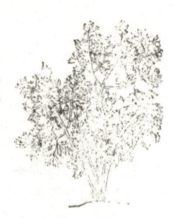

一名鬼卿，一名地新，一名微茎。生崇山山谷，及西川、河东、兖州、杭州，今卫辉辉县栲栳圈山谷间亦有之。俗名山园荽。苗高五七寸。叶似芎䕞叶细小；又似园荽叶而稀疏。茎比园荽茎颇硬直。味辛、微苦，性温、微寒，无毒。恶䕡茹，畏青葙子。

救饥：采嫩苗叶煠熟，水浸淘净，油盐调食。

治病：文具《本草·草部》条下。

24. Gaoben〔藁本，Chinese lovage，Ligusticum sinense Oliv.〕

Gaoben〔藁本，Chinese lovage，Ligusticum sinense Oliv.〕, also named Guiqing, Dixin, and Weijing, grows in the valleys of Chongshan and other places like Xichuan, Hedong, Yanzhou and Hangzhou. Presently, it can also be found in the valleys of Kaokaoquan in Weihui and Huixian. It is commonly called Shanyuansui. Its plants are 5~7 Cun high and its leaves are like and thinner than those of Xiongqiong〔芎䕞, Sichuan lovage rhizome, Rhizoma Ligustici Chuanxiong〕, and like those of Yuansui〔园荽, coriander, Coriandri Herba cum Radice〕, but sparser. Its stems are harder and straighter than those of Yuansui〔园荽, coriander, Coriandri Herba cum Radice〕. It is pungent and slightly bitter in taste, warm and slightly cold in nature and non-toxic. Regarding compatibility, it is averse to Lvru〔䕡茹, Fischer Euphorbia Root, Radix Euphorbiae Fischerianae〕 and restrained by Qingxiangzi〔青葙子, feather cockscomb seed, Semen Celosiae〕.

For famine relief: Collect and blanch young leaves, soak them in fresh water and make them clean, and flavor them with oil and salt.

For disease treatment: See the relevant clause in *Materia Medica · Herbaceous Plant*.

25. 柴 胡

一名地薰,一名山菜,一名茹草叶,一名芸蒿。生弘农川谷,及冤句、寿州、淄州、关陕、江湖间皆有。银州者为胜,今钧州密县山谷间亦有。苗甚辛香。茎青紫坚硬,微有细线楞。叶似竹叶而小。开小黄花。根淡赤色。味苦,性平,微寒,无毒。半夏为之使,恶皂荚,畏女菀、藜芦。又有苗似斜蒿,亦有似麦门冬苗而短者,开黄花,生丹州,结青子,与他处者不类。

救饥:采苗叶煠熟,换水浸淘去苦味,油盐调食。

治病:文具《本草·草部》条下。

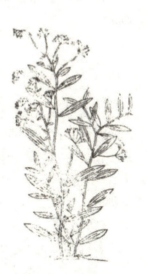

25. Chaihu [柴胡, Chinese thorowax root, Bupleurum chinense DC.]

Chaihu [柴胡, Chinese thorowax root, Bupleurum chinense DC.], also named Dixun, Shancai, Rucaoye and Yunhao, grows in the valleys of Hongnong and the lakesides of Yuanju, Shouzhou, Zizhou and Guanshan. Its quality is the best in Yinzhou. Presently, it can be seen in the valleys of Junzhou and Mixian. Its plants are spicy and its stems are indigo, hard and lined with edges. Its leaves are like the bamboo leaves but smaller. Its flowers are small and yellow, and roots light red. It is bitter in taste, neutral and slightly cold in nature and non-toxic. Regarding compatibility, Banxia [半夏, pinellia tuber, Rhizoma Pinelliae] is its assistance. Besides, it is averse to Zaojia [皂荚, soap pod, Gleditsia sinensis Lam.], mutual restraint with Nvwan [女菀, common turczaninowia herb, Turczaninowia fastigiata (Fisch.) DC.] and Lilu [藜芦, veratrum, Veratri Nigri Radix et Rhizoma]. Some kinds of its plants are like Xiehao [斜蒿, seseli, Seseli Herba]; other kinds are like Maimendong [麦门冬, ophiopogon, Ophiopogonis Radix], but shorter, originating from Danzhou, with yellow flowers and cyan fruit.

For famine relief: Collect and blanch young leaves, soak them in fresh water and make them clean, and flavor them with oil and salt.

For disease treatment: See the relevant clause in *Materia Medica · Herbaceous Plant*.

26. 漏 芦

一名野兰,俗名荚蒿。根名鹿骊根,俗呼为鬼油麻,生乔山山谷及秦州、海州、单州、曹、兖州,今钧州新郑沙岗间亦有之。苗叶就地丛生。叶似山芥菜叶而大,又多花叉,亦似白屈菜叶;又似大蓬蒿叶;及似风花菜脚叶[1]而大。叶中撺葶,上开红白花。根苗味苦、咸,性寒、大寒,无毒,连翘为之使。

救饥:采叶煠熟,水浸淘去苦味,油盐调食。

治病:文具《本草·草部》条下。

【注释】

[1]指基生叶。

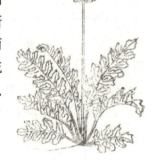

26. Loulu [漏芦, uniflower swissentaury, Rhaponticum uniflorum (L.) DC.]

Loulu [漏芦, uniflower swissentaury, Rhaponticum uniflorum (L.) DC.], also named Yelan and Jiahao, grows in the valleys of Qiaoshan and other places like Qinzhou, Haizhou, Shanzhou, Caozhou and Yanzhou. Presently it can also be seen among the sandhills in Junzhou and Xinzheng. Its roots are called Luligen or Guiyouma. Its leaves grow covering the ground like those of Shanjiecai [山芥菜, wild mustard leaf, Sinapis Folium] but larger with many leaf lobes, like those of Baiqucai [白屈菜, herb of greater celandine, Chelidonium majus L.] and Dapenghao [大蓬蒿, senecio argunensis, Senecio argunensis Turcz.], like the basal leaves[1] of Fenghuacai [风花菜, Indian rorippa herb, Rorippa globosa] but larger. There are scapes among the leaves, on top of which there are red and white flowers. Its roots and young plants are bitter and salty in taste, cold in nature and non-toxic. Regarding compatibility, Lianqiao [连翘, weeping forsythia capsule, Fructus Forsythiae] is its assistance.

For famine relief: Collect and blanch leaves, soak them in fresh water and remove the bitterness by washing, and flavor them with oil and salt.

For disease treatment: See the relevant clause in *Materia Medica · Herbaceous Plant*.

【Notes】

[1] Here it refers to the basal leaves which seem to grow out of the roots because the stems are too short.

27. 龙胆草

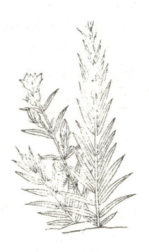

一名龙胆,一名陵游,俗呼草龙胆。生齐朐山谷,及冤句、襄州、吴兴皆有之,今钧州新郑山岗间亦有。根类牛膝,而根一本十余茎,黄白色宿根。苗高尺余,叶似柳叶而细短;又似小竹。开花如牵牛花,青碧色,似小铃形样。陶隐居[1]注云"状似龙葵,味苦如胆",因以为名。味苦,性寒、大寒,无毒。贯众、小豆为之使。恶防葵、地黄。又云:浙中又有山龙胆草,味苦涩,此同类而别种也。

救饥:采叶煠熟,换水浸淘去苦味,油盐调食。勿空腹服饵,令人溺不禁。

治病:文具《本草·草部》条下。

【注释】

[1] 陶隐居,为南朝医药学家陶弘景的别号,撰《本草经集注》。

27. Longdancao [龙胆草, Chinese Gentian, Gentiana manshurica Kitag.]

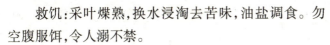
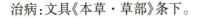

Longdancao [龙胆草, Chinese Gentian, Gentiana manshurica Kitag.], also named Longdan, Lingyou and Caolongdan, grows in the valleys of Qiqu and other places like Yuanju, Xiangzhou and Wuxing. Presently, it can also be seen among the hills of Junzhou and Xinzheng. Its perennial roots are like twotoothed achyranthes roots, on each of which there are more than ten yellowish white stems.

Its plants are one Chi high and its leaves are like the salix leaves but thinner and shorter, and also like the bamboo leaves. Its bluish violet flowers are like the Morning Glory in the shape of small bells. Tao Yinju[1] annotates that the reason for its being called Longdan is that its shape is like Longkui [龙葵, black nightshade, Solanum nigrum L.] and its taste is bitter like the bile. It is bitter in taste, cold in nature and non-toxic. Regarding compatibility, it is in mutual assistance with Guanzhong [贯众, shield-fern rhizome, Rhizoma Blechni] and Xiaodou [小豆, rice bean, Phaseoli Semen], averse to Fangkui [防葵, oreoselinum, Solanum nigrum L.] and Dihuang [地黄, unprocessed rehmannia root, Radix Rehmanniae Recens]. It is also said that there is a similar kind of herb called Shan Longdancao with bitter taste but belonging to other species.

For famine relief: Collect and blanch leaves, soak them in fresh water and remove the bitterness by washing them, and flavor them with oil and salt. It can bring about urinary incontinence if taken on an empty stomach.

For disease treatment: See the relevant clause in *Materia Medica · Herbaceous Plant*.

[Notes]

[1] The assumed name for Tao Hongjing, a medicinal scientist in the Nan Dynasty who compiled *Bencao Jingjizhu* (*Collective Commentaries on Classics of Materia Medica*).

28. 鼠 菊

本草名鼠尾草,一名蕏,一名陵翘。出黔州及所在平泽有之,今钧州新郑岗野间亦有之。苗高一二尺。叶似菊花叶,微小而肥厚;又似野艾蒿叶而脆,色淡绿。茎端作四五穗,穗似车前子穗而极疏细。开五瓣淡粉紫花,又有赤白二色花者。黔中者苗如蒿。《尔雅》谓"蕏,鼠尾",可以染皂。味苦,性微寒,无毒。

救饥:采叶煤熟,换水浸去苦味,再以水淘令净,油盐调食。

治病:文具《本草·草部》鼠尾草条下。

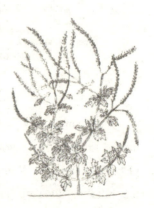

28. Shuju [鼠菊, European verbena herb, Verbena officinalis L.]

Shuju [鼠菊, European verbena herb, Verbena officinalis L.], also named Shuweicao, Qing and Lingqiao, grows in the weedy wetlands of Qianzhou. Presently, it can be seen in the hills and fields of Junzhou and Xinzheng. Its plants are 1～2 Chi high. Its green leaves are like the chrysanthemum leaves, smaller and thicker, and also like the wild mugwort leaves, more fragile. There are 4～5 fringy inflorescence on the top of its stems, like those of semen plantaginis, but smaller and sparser. Each of its flowers has 5 petals, some being pinkish purple and some being red and white. It is like artemisia if from Qianzhong and just as what *Er Ya* [《尔雅》, *Literary Expositor*] said, "Qing is the mouse tail." It can dye black color. It is bitter in taste, slightly cold in nature and non-toxic.

For famine relief: Collect and blanch leaves, soak them in fresh water, remove the bitterness by washing them, and flavor them with oil and salt.

For disease treatment: See the clause of Shuweicao [鼠尾草, European verbena herb, Herba Verbenae] *in Materia Medica · Herbaceous Plant*.

29. 前 胡

生陕西、汉、梁、江、淮、荆、襄、江宁、成州诸郡，相、孟、越、衢、婺、睦等州皆有，今密县梁家冲山野中亦有之。苗高一二尺，青白色，似斜蒿，味甚香美。叶似野菊叶而瘦细；颇似山萝卜叶亦细；又似芸蒿。开黪白花，类蛇床子花。秋间结实，根细，青紫色，一云外黑里白。味甘、辛、微苦，性微寒，无毒。半夏为之使，恶皂荚，畏藜芦。

救饥：采叶煠熟，换水浸淘净，油盐调食。

治病：文具《本草·草部》条下。

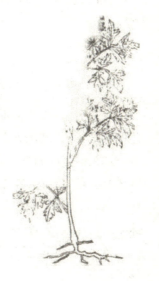

29. Qianhu [前胡, hogfennel root, Peucedanum praeruptorum Dunn]

Qianhu [前胡, hogfennel root, Peucedanum praeruptorum Dunn] grows in the counties of Shanxi, Han, Liang, Jiang, Huai, Jin, Xiang, Jiangning, Chengzhou, Xiang, Meng, Yue, Qu, Wu and Mu. Presently, it can be seen in the mountains and plains of Mixian and Liangjiachong. Its green-white plants are 1~2 Chi high, like Xiehao [斜蒿, seseli, Seseli Herba], tasting delicious. Its leaves are like the wild chrysanthemum leaves but thinner, and the chervil leaves but thinner and Chinese thorowax leaves. Its white flowers appear a little ash black like common chidium flowers. It bears fruit in autumn. Its roots are thin and of the bluish violet color. It is also said to be black in peel and white in pulp. It is sweet, pungent and slightly bitter in taste, slightly cold in nature and non-toxic. Regarding compatibility, Banxia [半夏, Pinellia Tuber, Rhizoma Pinelliae] is its assistance and it is averse to Zaojia [皂荚, soap pod, Gleditsia sinensis Lam.], restrained by Lilu [藜芦, veratrum, Veratri Nigri Radix et Rhizoma].

For famine relief: Collect and blanch leaves, soak them in fresh water and make them clean, and flavor them with oil and salt.

For disease treatment: See the relevant clause in *Materia Medica · Herbaceous Plant*.

30. 猪牙菜

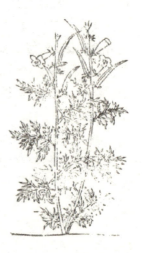

本草名角蒿,一名莪蒿,一名萝蒿,又名蘼蒿。旧云生高岗及泽田,渐洳处多有,今在处有之,生田野中。苗高一二尺。茎叶如青蒿。叶似邪蒿叶而细;又似蛇床子叶颇壮。稍间开花,红赤色,鲜明可爱。花罢结角子,似蔓菁角,长二寸许,微弯。中有子黑色,似王不留行子。味辛、苦,性温,无毒。一云性平,有小毒。

救饥:采嫩苗茎叶煠熟,水浸去苦味,淘净,油盐调食。

治病:文具《本草·草部》角蒿条下。

30. Zhuyacai [猪牙菜, Chinese incarvillea, Incarvillea sinensis Lam.]

Zhuyacai [猪牙菜, Chinese incarvillea, Incarvillea sinensis Lam.], also named Jiaohao, E'hao, Luohao and Linhao, grows in the sloping fields and the paddy fields based on ancient books. Its plants are 1～2 Chi high and its stems and leaves are like those of Qinghao [青蒿, Sweet Wormwood Herb, Herba Artemisiae Annuae]. Its leaves are like those of Xiehao [斜蒿, seseli, Seseli Herba] but thinner, and also like those of Shechuangzi [蛇床子, Chidium Fruit, Fructus Cnidii Common] but larger. On the top of its branches there are crimson flowers, bright and lovely. Its fruit is like that of Manjing [蔓菁, turnip, Brassicae Rapae Tuber et Folium], about 2 Cun long and slightly curving. Inside the fruit, there are black seeds which are like those of Wangbuliu Xing [王不留行, cow herb seed, men Vaccariae]. It is pungent and bitter in taste, warm in nature and non-toxic. It is also said to be neutral in nature and slightly toxic.

For famine relief: Collect and blanch young leaves and stems, remove the bitterness by soaking them in fresh water, wash and clean them, and flavor them with oil and salt.

For disease treatment: See the clause of Jiaohao [角蒿, Chinese incarvillea, Incarvilleae Sinensis Herba] in *Materia Medica · Herbaceous Plant*.

31. 地　榆

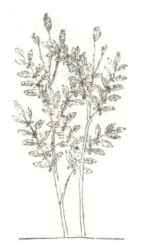

生桐柏山及冤句山谷，今处处有之，密县山野中亦有此。多宿根。其苗初生布地，后撺莛，直高三四尺。对分生叶，叶似榆叶而狭细，颇长，作锯齿状，青色。开花如椹子，紫黑色，又类豉，故名玉豉。其根外黑里红，似柳根。亦入酿酒药。烧作灰能烂石。味苦、甘、酸，性微寒。一云沉寒[1]，无毒。得发[2]良，恶麦门冬。

救饥：采嫩叶煠熟，用水浸去苦味，换水淘净，油盐调食。无茶时用叶作饮，甚解热。

治病：文具《本草·草部》条下。

【注释】

[1] 即大寒。

[2] 词义不详,待考。

31. Diyu [地榆, garden burnet root, Sanguisorba officinalis L.]

Diyu [地榆, garden burnet root, Sanguisorba officinalis L.] grows in the valleys of Tongbai Mountain and Yuanju, and can be seen everywhere presently. It also grows in the hilllands and fields of Mixian County. Its perennial plants, 3~4 Chi high if upright, grow crawling on the ground and then draw out scapes. Its opposite green leaves are like the dwarf elm leaves but thinner and longer, with saw-tooth-shaped edge. Its atropurpureus flowers are like Sangshen [桑椹, mulberry, Mori Fructus], and also like Douchi [豆豉, fermented soybean, Sojae Semen Fermentatum], which explains why it is also called Yuchi. Its roots are black outside and red inside, like the willow roots, which can be used to make the medicinal wine and break the stone into pieces if burned to ash. It is bitter, sweet and sour in taste, and slightly cold in nature. It is also said to be very cold[1] in nature and non-toxic. It produces a better effect if used together with Fa[2] and is in mutural inhibition with Maimendong [麦门冬, ophiopogon, Ophiopogon].

For famine relief: Collect and blanch young leaves and seedlings, remove the bitterness by soaking them in fresh water, wash and clean them and flavor them with oil and salt. Its leaves can be taken as tea, with the function of cooling down.

For disease treatment: See the relevant clause in *Materia Medica · Herbaceous Plant*.

【Notes】

[1] Here it means the nature of the medicinal is very cold in degree.

[2] Unclear about the meaning of this word, remaining to be verified.

32. 川 芎

一名芎藭,一名胡芎,一名香果。其苗叶名蘼芜,一名薇芜,一名茳蓠。生武功川谷、斜谷、西岭、雍州川泽及冤句。其关陕、蜀川、江东山中亦多有,以蜀川者为胜，今处处有之，人家园圃多种。苗叶似芹而叶微细窄，却有花叉；又似白芷叶亦细；又如园荽叶微壮。又有一种，叶似蛇床子叶而亦粗壮。开白花。其芎，人家种者，形块大重，实多脂润，其里色白。味辛、甘，性温，无毒。山中出者，瘦细，味苦、辛。其节大茎细状如马衔，谓之马衔芎。状如雀脑者，谓之雀脑芎，此最有力。白芷为之使，畏黄连。其蘼芜，味辛香，性温，无毒。

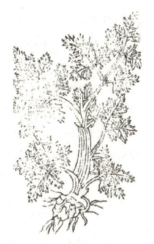

救饥：采叶煠熟，换水浸去辛味，淘净，油盐调食。亦可煮饮，甚香。

治病：文具《本草·草部》条下。

32. Chuanxiong［川芎，Sichuan lovage rhizome，Ligusticum chuanxiong S. H. Qiu et al.］

Chuanxiong［川芎，Sichuan lovage rhizome，Ligusticum chuanxiong S. H. Qiu et al.］, also named Xiongqiong, Huqiong, Xiangguo, Weiwu and Jiangli, grows in the valleys of Wugong, the swamps of Xiegu, Xiling, Yongzhou and Yuanju, and the hills of Guanshan, Shuchuan and Jiangdong. The quality is better if from the place of Shuchuan. Presently it can be seen everywhere especially in people's gardens. Its leaves are called Miwu, like those of celery but thinner and narrower with flower furcation, those of Baizhi［白芷，dahurian angelica root, Radix Angelicae Dahuricae］but thinner, and those of coriander but stronger. The leaves of another kind of it are like those of Shechuangzi［蛇床子，Chidium Fruit, Fructus Cnidii Common］but thicker and stronger. Its flowers are white. Its roots, if from common people's gardens, are big and heavy, white and lustrous like grease. It is pungent and sweet in taste, warm in nature and non-toxic. It is thin, bitter and pungent in taste if it is wild. It is called Maxianxiong if it is like Maxian with big knots and thin stems, and Quenaoxiong if it is like Quenao with stonger efficacy. Regarding compatibility, Baizhi［白芷，dahurian angelica root, Radix Angelicae Dahuricae］is its assistance and it is restrained by Huanglian［黄连，golden thread, Rhizoma Coptidis］. The part of its plants above the ground is called Miwu [蘼芜, chuanxiong leaf, Chuanxiong Folium], which is pungent in taste, warm in nature and non-toxic.

For famine relief: Collect and blanch leaves, remove the pungency by soaking them in fresh water, wash and clean them, and flavor them with oil and salt. It can also be taken like beverage after boiled in water, smelling delicious.

For disease treatment: See the relevant clause in Materia Medica · Herbaceous Plant.

33. 葛勒子秧

本草名葎草,亦名葛勒蔓,一名葛葎蔓,又名涩萝蔓,南人呼为揽藤。旧不著所出州土,今田野道傍处处有之。其苗延蔓而生,藤长丈余,茎多细涩刺。叶似草麻叶而小,亦薄,茎叶极涩,能抓挽人。茎叶间开黄白花,结子类山丝子。其叶味甘、苦,性寒,无毒。

救饥:采嫩苗叶煠熟,换水浸去苦味,淘净,油盐调食。

治病:文具《本草·草部》葎草条下。

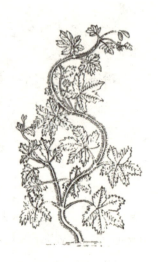

33. Gelezi Yang [葛勒子秧, Japanese hop, Humulus scandens (Lour.) Merr.]

Gelezi Yang [葛勒子秧, Japanese hop, Humulus scandens (Lour.) Merr.], also named Lvcao, Geleman, Gelvman, Seluoman and Lanteng by southerners, was not recorded about its origin in ancient times. Presently, it can be commonly seen in the fields and roadsides. Its plants creep on the ground, with cirrus more than one Zhang long and small and rough thorns on the stems. Its leaves are like those of Bima [蓖麻, Ricinuscommunis, Ricinus communis L.] but smaller and thinner. Its stems and leaves are rough enough to cling to the people who intend to draw them. Its flowers are yellowish white and its fruit is like Shansizi [山丝子, cannabis fruit, Cannabis Fructus]. Its leaves are sweet and bitter in taste, cold in nature and non-toxic.

For famine relief: Collect and blanch young plants and leaves, remove the bitterness by soaking them in fresh water, wash and clean them, and flavor them with oil and salt.

For disease treatment: See the clause of Lvcao [葎草, Japanese hop, Humuli Scandentis Herba] in *Materia Medica · Herbaceous Plant.*

34. 连 翘

一名异翘,一名兰华,一名折根,一名轵,一名三廉。《尔雅》谓之连,一名连苕。生太山山谷,及河中、江宁、泽、润、淄、兖、鼎、岳、利州、南康皆有之,今密县梁家冲山谷中亦有。科苗高三四尺,茎秆赤色。叶如榆叶大,面光,色青黄,边微细锯齿;又似金银花叶,微尖艄。开花黄色可爱。结房状似山栀子,蒴微扁而无棱瓣,蒴中有子如雀舌样,极小。其子折之,间片片相比如翘,以此得名。味苦,性平,无毒。叶亦味苦。

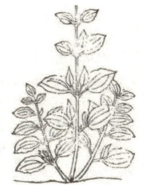

救饥:采嫩叶煠熟,换水浸去苦味,淘洗净,油盐调食。

治病:文具《本草·草部》条下。

34. Lianqiao [连翘, forsythia, Forsythia suspense (Thunb.) Vahl]

Lianqiao [连翘, forsythia, Forsythia suspense (Thunb.) Vahl], also named Yiqiao, Lanhua, Zhegen, Zhi, Sanlian, Lian and Liantiao according to *Er Ya* [《尔雅》, *Literary Expositor*], grows in the valleys of Taishan and other places like Hezhong, Jiangning, Ze, Run, Zi, Yan, Ding, Yue, Lizhou and Nankang. Presently, it can also be seen in the valleys of Liangjiangchong of Mixian County. Its plants are 3～4 Chi high with red stems. Its yellowish green leaves are like those of the elm tree, smooth and saw-tooth-edged, and also like those of Jinyinhua [金银花, lonicera, Lonicerae Flos], sharper and narrower. Its flowers are yellow and lovely. Its fruit is like Shanzhizi [山栀子, cape jasmine fruit, Gardenia jasminoides Ellis], oblate and with no ridge. Its seeds are tiny like sparrow tongues, abreast like the feature of bird's tail if bent, which justifies its name of Lianqiao. It's bitter in taste, neutral in nature and non-toxic. Its leaves are also bitter.

For famine relief: Collect and blanch young leaves, remove the bitterness by soaking them in fresh water, wash and clean them, and flavor them with oil and salt.

For disease treatment: See the relevant clause in Materia Medica · Herbaceous Plant.

35．仙灵脾

本草名淫羊藿,一名刚前,俗名黄连祖、千两金、干鸡筋、放杖草、弃杖草,俗又呼三枝九叶草。生上郡阳山山谷,及江东、陕西、泰山、汉中、湖湘、沂州等郡,并永康军皆有之,今密县山野中亦有。苗高二尺许。茎似小豆茎,极细紧。叶似杏叶颇长,近蒂皆有一缺;又似绿豆叶,亦长而光。稍间开花,白色,亦有紫色花,作碎小独头子。根紫色有须,形类黄连状。味辛,性寒,一云性温,无毒。生处不闻水声者良。薯蓣[1]、紫芝为之使。

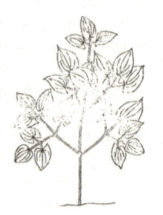

救饥:采嫩叶煠熟,水浸去邪味,淘净,油盐调食。

治病:文具《本草·草部》淫羊藿条下。

【注释】

[1] 山药别名。

35. Xianlingpi [仙灵脾, epimedium, Epimedium brevicornu Maxim.]

Xianlingpi [仙灵脾, epimedium, Epimedium brevicornu Maxim.], also named Yinyanghuo, Gangqian, Huanglianzu, Qianliangjin, Ganjijin, Fangzhangcao, Qizhangcao and Sanzhi Jiuyecao by common people, grows in the valleys of Yangshan in Shangjun and other places like Jiangdong, Shanxi, Taishan, Hanzhong, Huxiang, Yizhou and Yongkangjun. Presently, it can also be seen in the mountainous regions and fields of Mixian County. Its plants are two Chi high and its stems are thin and hard like those of Xiaodou［小豆, rice bean, Phaseoli Semen］. Its leaves are like those of apricot but longer, with a notch near the petiole, and also like those of Lvdou［绿豆, mung bean, Phaseoli Radiati Semen］, longer and smoother. On top of its branches, there are tiny white and purple flowers on the inflorescence solitarily. Its roots are purple and fibrous, like the shape of Huanglian［黄连, golden thread, Rhizoma Coptidis］. It is pungent in taste and cold in nature. It is also said to be warm in nature and non-toxic. The quality is better if it grows in the places without the sound of water. Regarding compatibility, Shuyu[1]［薯蓣, common yam rhizome, Rhizoma Dioscoreae］and Zizhi［紫芝, Chinese Ganoderma, Ganoderma Sinensis］are its assistance.

For famine relief: Collect and blanch young leaves, remove the bitterness by soaking them in fresh water, wash and clean them, and flavor them with oil and salt.

For disease treatment: See the clause of Yinyanghuo［淫羊藿, epimedium, Epimedii Herba］in *Materia Medica · Herbaceous Plant*.

【Notes】

［1］Another name for Shanyao（山药）.

36. 青 杞

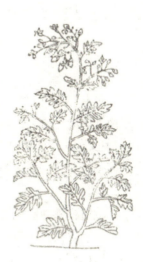

本草名蜀羊泉，一名羊泉，一名羊饴，俗名漆姑。生蜀郡山谷，及所在平泽皆有之，今祥符县西田野中亦有。苗高二尺余。叶似菊叶稍长。花开紫色。子类枸杞子，生青熟红。根如远志，无心有糁[1]，味苦，性微寒，无毒。

救饥：采嫩叶煠熟，水浸去苦味，淘洗净，油盐调食。

治病：文具《本草·草部》蜀羊泉条下。

【注释】

［1］指颗粒物。

36. Qingqi [青杞, climbing nightshade, Solanum septemlobum Bunge]

Qingqi [青杞, climbing nightshade, Solanum septemlobum Bunge], also named Shuyangquan, Yangquan, Yangyi and Qigu, grows in the valleys of Shujun and the flat wetlands within its distribution range. Presently, it can also be seen in the fields in the western part of Xiangfu County. Its plants are two Chi high and its leaves are like those of chrysanthemum but longer. Its flowers are purple and its seeds are like the Chinese wolfberry, green when growing and red when ripe. Its roots are like those of Yuanzhi [远志, Milkwort Root, Radix Polygalae], hollow and granular[1], bitter in taste, slightly cold in nature and non-toxic.

For famine relief: Collect and blanch young leaves, remove the bitterness by soaking them in fresh water, wash and clean them, and flavor them with oil and salt.

For disease treatment: See the clause of Shuyangquan [蜀羊泉, climbing nightshade, Solani Lyrati Herba] in *Materia Medica · Herbaceous Plant*.

[Notes]

[1] Here it means the central part of the root is granular.

37. 野生姜

本草名刘寄奴。生江南[1],其越州、滁州皆有之,今中牟南沙岗间亦有之。茎似艾蒿,长二三尺余。叶似菊叶而瘦细;又似野艾蒿叶亦瘦细。开花白色。结实黄白色。作细筒子蒴儿。盖蒿之类也。其子似秫而细。苗叶味苦,性温,无毒。

救饥:采嫩叶煤熟,水浸淘去苦味,油盐调食。

治病:文具《本草·草部》刘寄奴条下。

【注释】

[1] 古代地区名,泛指长江以南地区。

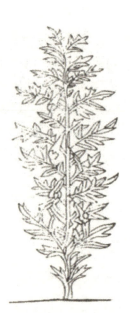

37. Yeshengjiang [野生姜, anomalous artemisia, Siphonostegia chinensis Benth.]

Yeshengjiang [野生姜, anomalous artemisia, Siphonostegia chinensis Benth.], also named Liujinu, grows in the regions of the south of the Yangtze River[1] such as Yuezhou and Chuzhou. Presently, it can also be seen in the hilllands of the south of Zhongmu. Its stems are like those of Aihao [艾蒿, mugwort, Artemisiae Argyi Folium], 2~3 Chi high. Its leaves are like those of chrysanthemum but thinner, and also like those of artemisia lavandulaefolia but thinner. Its flowers are white and its fruit is yellowish white in the shape of a tube. Probably, it belongs to the species of artemisia. Its seeds are like those of barnyard grass but smaller. Its plants and leaves are bitter in taste, warm in nature and non-toxic.

For famine relief: Collect and blanch young leaves, remove the bitterness by soaking them in fresh water, wash and clean them, and flavor them with oil and salt.

For disease treatment: See the clause of Liujinu [刘寄奴, anomalous artemisia, Artemisiae Anomalae Herba] in *Materia Medica · Herbaceous Plant.*

【Notes】

[1] The name of an ancient region, referring to the area in the south of the Yangtze River.

38. 马兰头

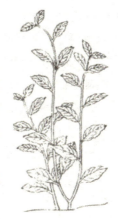

本草名马兰。旧不著所出州土。但云生泽傍,如泽兰。北人见其花,呼为紫菊,以其花似菊而紫也。苗高一二尺,茎亦紫色,叶似薄荷叶,边皆锯齿,又似地儿叶,微大。味辛,性平,无毒。又有山兰,生山侧,似刘寄奴,叶无桠,不对生,花心微黄赤。

救饥:采嫩苗叶煠熟,新汲水浸去辛味,淘洗净,油盐调食。

治病：文具《本草·草部》条下。

38. Malantou ［马兰头, kalimeris, Aster indicus L.］

Malantou ［马兰头, kalimeris, Aster indicus L.］, also named Malan and without record about its origin in ancient times, is said to grow near the water like Zelan ［泽兰, lycopus, Lycopi Herba］. Its flowers are called Ziju by northerners for its being like chrysanthemum but purple. Its plants are 1~2 Chi high and its stems are purple too. Its leaves are like those of Bohe ［薄荷, mint, Menthae Herba］ with saw-tooth-shaped edges, and also like those of sweet potatoes but larger. It is pungent in taste, neutral in nature and non-toxic. There is another kind of Shanlan, growing along the hillsides, like Liujinu ［刘寄奴, anomalous artemisia, Artemisiae Anomalae Herba］, with uncleaved and irregular leaves and yellowish red flowers.

For famine relief: Collect and blanch young leaves, remove the bitterness and pungency by soaking them in fresh water, wash and clean them, and flavor them with oil and salt.

For disease treatment: See the relevant clause in *Materia Medica · Herbaceous Plant*.

39. 豨莶

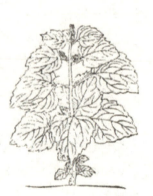

俗名粘糊菜，俗又呼火枕草。旧不著所出州郡，今处处有之。苗高三四尺，金棱银线。素根紫秸。茎叉对节而生。茎叶颇类苍耳，茎叶纹脉竖直。稍叶间开花，深黄色。又有一种苗叶似芥叶而尖狭，开花如菊，结实颇似鹤虱。科苗味苦，性寒，有小毒。

救饥：采嫩苗叶煠熟，水浸去苦味，淘洗净，油盐调食。

治病：文具《本草·草部》条下。

39. Xixian [豨莶, siegesbeckia, Sigesbeckia orientalis L.]

Xixian [豨莶, siegesbeckia, Sigesbeckia orientalis L.], also named Nianhucai and Huoxiancao, is not recorded about its origin in ancient times. Presently, it can be seen everywhere. Its plants are 3~4 Chi high, with golden-yellow ridges and silver lines. Its roots are white and its stems purple. Its branches are all opposite. Its leaves are like those of Cang'er [苍耳, xanthium herb, Xanthii Herba] with straight lines. Its dark yellow flowers are among leaves on the top of branches. There is another kind of herbs, with young leaves like those of Jiecai [芥菜, mustard leaf, Sinapis Folium] but sharper and narrower, flowers like chrysanthemum and seeds like Heshi [鹤虱, carpesium seed, Carpesii Fructus]. Its plants are bitter in taste, cold in nature and slightly toxic.

For famine relief: Collect and blanch young plants and leaves, remove the bitterness by soaking them in fresh water, wash and clean them, and flavor them with oil and salt.

For disease treatment: See the relevant clause in *Materia Medica · Herbaceous Plant*.

40. 泽泻

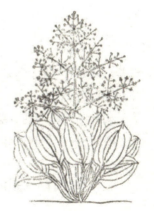

俗名水荅菜，一名水泻，一名及泻，一名芒芋，一名鹄泻。生汝南池泽，及齐州、山东、河、陕、江、淮亦有，汉中者为佳，今水边处处有之。丛生苗叶，其叶似牛舌草叶，纹脉竖直。叶丛中间撺葶，对分茎叉，茎有线楞，稍间开三瓣小白花。结实小，青细。子味甘，叶味微咸，俱无毒。

救饥：采嫩叶煠熟，水浸淘净，油盐调食。

治病：文具《本草·草部》条下。

40. Zexie [泽泻, alisma, Alisma orientale (Sam.) Juz.]

Zexie [泽泻, alisma, Alisma orientale (Sam.) Juz.], also named Shuitacai, Shuixie, Jixie, Mangyu and Huxie, grows in the marsh areas of Runan and other places like Qizhou, Shandong, He, Shan, Jiang and Huai. The quality is better if it is from Hanzhong. Presently, it can be seen near the watersides. Its clustered leaves are like those of Niushecao [牛舌草, plantago, Plantaginis Herba] with straight lines. Its scape grows out of leaves, opposite and ridged, with trivalve white flowers on top of it. Its green fruit is thin and small. Its seeds are sweet and its leaves slightly salty, both of which are non-toxic.

For famine relief: Collect and blanch young leaves, soak them in fresh water, wash and clean them, and then flavor them with oil and salt.

For disease treatment: See the relevant clause in *Materia Medica · Herbaceous Plant*.

新增
New Supplements

41．竹节菜

一名翠蝴蝶,又名翠娥眉,又名筀竹花,一名倭青草。南北皆有,今新郑县山野中亦有之。叶似竹叶,微宽短。茎淡红色,就地丛生,撺节似初生嫩苇节。稍叶间开翠碧花,状类蝴蝶,其叶味甜。

救饥:采嫩苗叶煠熟,油盐调食。

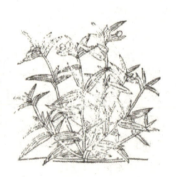

41. Zhujiecai [竹节菜, dayflower, Commelina communis L.]

Zhujiecai [竹节菜, dayflower, Commelina communis L.], also named Cuihudie, Cui'emei, Dazhuhua and Woqingcao, grows in the southern and northern parts of China. Presently, it can also be seen in the fields of Xinzhengxian. Its leaves are like those of bamboos, broader and shorter. Its red stems creep on the ground with joints sprouting out like young reed leaves. Its jade green flowers are like butterflies. Its leaves are sweet in taste.

For famine relief: Collect and blanch young leaves, and flavor them with oil and salt.

42. 独扫苗

生田野中,今处处有之。叶似竹形而柔弱细小,抪茎而生。茎叶稍间结小青子,小如粟粒。科茎老时可为扫帚。叶味甘。

救饥:采嫩苗叶煠熟,水浸淘净,油盐调食。晒干煠食,不破腹尤佳。

治病:今人多将其子亦作地肤子代用。

42. Dusaomiao [独扫苗, kochia shoot, Kochia scoparia (L.) Schrad.]

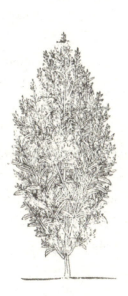

Dusaomiao [独扫苗, kochia shoot, Kochia scoparia (L.) Schrad.] grows in the field and can be seen everywhere presently. Its leaves, scattered on the stems, are like the bamboo leaves, tender and smaller. Its fruit is cyan, small as a chestnut, growing at the end of branches. Its plants can be made into brooms when old and dry. Its leaves are sweet in taste.

For famine relief: Collect and blanch young plants and leaves, soak them in fresh water, wash and clean them, and flavor them with oil and salt. It can also be taken after being dried and blanched. It is better in quality if no diarrhea happens after taken.

For disease treatment: Its fruit is also regarded as Difuzi [地肤子, kochia, Kochiae Fructus] and is used as medicinal to replace it.

43. 歪头菜

出新郑县山野中。细茎就地丛生。叶似豇豆叶而狭长,背微白,两叶并生一处。开红紫花。结角比豌豆角短小、扁瘦。叶味甜。

救饥:采叶煠熟,油盐调食。

43. Waitoucai〔歪头菜, vicia unijuga, Vicia unijuga A. Br.〕

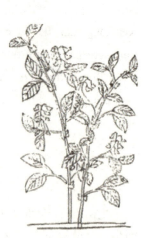

Waitoucai〔歪头菜, vicia unijuga, Vicia unijuga A. Br.〕grows in the fields of Xinzheng County. Its thin stems creep on the ground and its leaves are like those of cowpea, longer, white and bifoliolate. Its flowers are reddishly violet and its fruit is shorter, smaller and flatter than peas. Its leaves are sweet in taste.

For famine relief: Collect and blanch leaves, and flavor them with oil and salt.

44. 兔儿酸

一名兔儿浆。所在田野中皆有之。苗比水荭矮短,茎叶皆类水荭,其茎节密,其叶亦稠,比水荭叶稍薄小。味酸,性寒,无毒。

救饥:采苗叶煠熟,以新汲水浸去酸味,淘净,油盐调食。

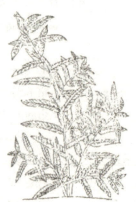

44. Tu'ersuan〔兔儿酸, amphibious polygonum, Polygonum amphibium L.〕

Tu'ersuan〔兔儿酸, amphibious polygonum, Polygonum amphibium L.〕, also named Tu'erjiang, grows in the fields of its distribution range. Its plants are shorter than Shuihong〔水荭, smartweed, Polygonum orientale L.〕, and its joint-tensed stems and thick leaves, thinner and smaller, are all like the latter. It is sour in taste, cold in nature and non-toxic.

For famine relief: Collect and blanch plants and leaves, remove the sourness by soaking them in fresh water, wash and clean them, and flavor them with oil and salt.

45. 碱 蓬

一名盐蓬。生水傍下湿地。茎似落藜,亦有线楞[1]。叶似蓬而肥壮,比蓬叶亦稀疏。茎叶间结青子,极细小。其叶味微咸,性微寒。

救饥:采苗叶煠熟,水浸去碱味,淘洗净,油盐调食。

【注释】

[1] 通"棱",指条状隆起的棱或突出的脉。

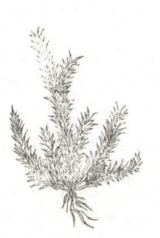

45. Jianpeng [碱蓬, suaeda, Suaeda glauca (Bunge) Bunge]

Jianpeng [碱蓬, suaeda, Suaeda glauca (Bunge) Bunge], also named Yanpeng, grows in the wetlands near water. Its stems are like those of Luoli [落藜, wild pigweed, Chenopodium album L.] with lines and ridges[1]. Its leaves are like those of curcuma rhizome but stronger and sparser. Its green fruit is tiny among the leaves. Its leaves are slightly salty and cold in nature.

For famine relief: Collect and blanch plants and leaves, remove the alkaline taste by soaking them in fresh water, wash and clean them and flavor them with oil and salt.

【Notes】

[1] Here it refers to the lines, ridges or veinlets upheaved.

46. 蒌 蒿

田野中处处有之。苗高二尺余,茎秆似艾。其叶细长,锯齿,叶㧎茎而生。味微苦,性微温。

救饥:采嫩苗叶煠熟,水浸淘净,油盐调食。

46. Lvhao [蒌蒿, common mugwort, Artemisia selengensis Turcz. ex Bess.]

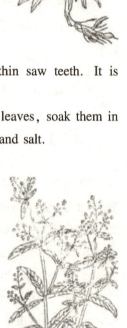

Lvhao [蒌蒿, common mugwort, Artemisia selengensis Turcz. ex Bess.] grows everywhere in the fields. Its plants are two Chi high and its stems are like those of mugwort. Its leaves, scattered on the stems, are edged with long and thin saw teeth. It is slightly bitter in taste and warm in nature.

For famine relief: Collect and blanch young plants and leaves, soak them in fresh water, wash and clean them, and flavor them with oil and salt.

47. 水萵苣

一名水菠菜。水边多生。苗高一尺许。叶似麦蓝叶而有细锯齿,两叶对生,每两叶间对叉又生两枝。稍间开青白花。结小青蓇葖,如小椒粒大。其叶味微苦,性寒。

救饥:采苗叶煠熟,水淘净,油盐调食。

47. Shuiwoju [水萵苣, water speedwell, Veronica undulate Wall. ex Jack]

Shuiwoju [水萵苣, water speedwell, Veronica undulate Wall. ex Jack], also named Shuibocai, grows near the watersides. Its plants are one Chi high and its opposite leaves are like those of Mailan [麦蓝, vaccaria, Vaccariae Semen] with saw teeth. The branches grow out of axilla of the opposite leaves. Its flowers are greenish white and its fruit is also green like Sichuan pepper. Its leaves are slightly bitter in taste and cold in nature.

For famine relief: Collect and blanch plants and leaves, wash and clean them, and flavor them with oil and salt.

48. 金盏菜

一名地冬瓜菜。生田野中。苗高二三尺。茎初微赤而有线路。叶似绵柳叶微厚,抪茎而生,茎叶稠密。开花紫色,黄心。其叶味甘、微咸。

救饥:采苗叶煠熟,水淘净,油盐调食。

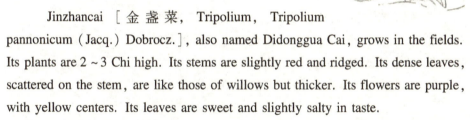

48. Jinzhancai [金盏菜, Tripolium, Tripolium pannonicum (Jacq.) Dobrocz.]

Jinzhancai [金盏菜, Tripolium, Tripolium pannonicum (Jacq.) Dobrocz.], also named Didonggua Cai, grows in the fields. Its plants are 2~3 Chi high. Its stems are slightly red and ridged. Its dense leaves, scattered on the stem, are like those of willows but thicker. Its flowers are purple, with yellow centers. Its leaves are sweet and slightly salty in taste.

For famine relief: Collect and blanch plants and leaves, wash and clean them, and flavor them with oil and salt.

49. 水辣菜

生水边下湿地中。苗高一尺余。茎圆。叶似鸡儿肠叶,头微齐短;又似马兰头叶,亦更齐短。其叶抪茎生。稍间出穗,如黄蒿穗。其叶味辣。

救饥:采嫩苗叶煠熟,换水淘去辣气,油盐调食。生亦可食。

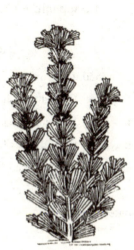

49. Shuilacai [水辣菜, Japanese artemisia, Artemisia Japonica Thunb.]

Shuilacai [水辣菜, Japanese artemisia, Artemisia Japonica Thunb.] grows in the low wetlands near the watersides. Its plants are one Chi high and its stems are round. Its leaves, scattered on the stems, are like those of Ji'erchang [鸡儿肠, aster, Asteris Radix] and Malantou [马兰头, kalimeris, Kalimeridis Herba et Radix], flatter and shorter than the latter two herbs. Its inflorescences are like the spicas of artemisia scoparia. Its leaves are pungent in taste.

For famine relief: Collect and blanch young plants and leaves, remove the pungency taste by washing them in fresh water, and then flavor them with oil and salt. It can also be taken raw.

50. 紫云菜

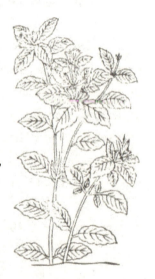

生密县付家冲山野中。苗高一二尺。茎方,紫色,对节生叉。叶似山小菜叶,颇长,拊梗对生。叶顶及叶间开淡紫花。其叶味微苦。

救饥:采嫩苗叶煠熟,水浸淘去苦味,油盐调食。

50. Ziyuncai [紫云菜, peruvian groundcherry herb, Clinopodium chinense (Benth.) Kuntze]

Ziyuncai [紫云菜, peruvian groundcherry herb, Clinopodium chinense (Benth.) Kuntze] grows in the fields of Fujiachong in Mixian County. Its plants are 1~2 Chi high and its purple stems are square with opposite branches. Its opposite leaves are like those of platycodon but longer. Its flowers are light purple at the end of branches or axilla. Its leaves are slightly bitter in taste.

For famine relief: Collect and blanch young plants and leaves, remove the bitterness taste by washing them in fresh water, and then flavor them with oil and salt.

51. 鸦 葱

生田野中。板叶尖长,搨[1]地而生,叶似初生蜀秫叶而小;又似初生大蓝叶,细窄而尖,其叶边皆曲皱。叶中攛葶,上结小菁葖,后出白英。味微辛。

救饥:采苗叶煠熟,油盐调食。

【注释】

[1] 指叶子下垂,耷拉状。

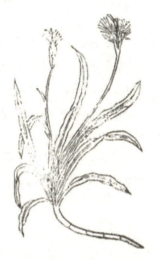

51. Yacong [鸦葱, scorzonera root, Scorzonera sinensis (Lipsch. et Krasch) Nakai]

Yacong [鸦葱, scorzonera root, Scorzonera sinensis (Lipsch. et Krasch) Nakai] grows in the fields and wilderness. Its leaves are sharp and long, hanging down[1] on the ground like those of young sorghum but smaller, and also like those of indigofera but thinner and narrower with rugose edges. Its scapes grow out of leaves and produce flower buds, which bear fruit called Baiying [白英, climbing nightshade, Solani Lyrati Herba]. It is pungent in taste.

For famine relief: Collect and blanch plants and leaves, and then flavor them with oil and salt.

【Notes】

[1] Here it refers to the drooping leaves.

52. 匙头菜

生密县山野中。作小科苗。其茎面窊背圆。叶似团匙头样,有如杏叶大,边微锯齿。开淡红花,结子黄褐色,其叶味甜。

救饥:采叶煠熟,水浸淘净,油盐调食。

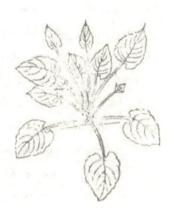

52. Shitoucai [匙头菜, violet, Viola collina Bess.]

Shitoucai [匙头菜, violet, Viola collina Bess.], very short and small, grows in the hillsides and wilderness of Mixian County. Its petioles are sunken upside and round backside. Its leaves are spoon-shaped and saw-tooth-edged, as big as apricot leaves. Its flowers are light red and its seeds are yellowish brown. Its leaves are sweet in taste.

For famine relief: Collect and blanch leaves, soak them in water, wash and clean them, and then flavor them with oil and salt.

53. 鸡冠菜

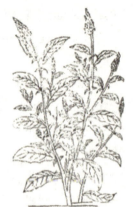

生田野中。苗高尺余。叶似青荚菜叶而窄小；又似山菜叶而窄艄。稍间出穗，似兔儿尾穗，却微细小。开粉红花。结实如苋菜子。苗叶味苦。

救饥：采苗叶煤熟，水浸淘去苦气[1]，油盐调食。

【注释】

[1] 方言，指气味。

53. Jiguancai [鸡冠菜, feather cockscomb, Celosia argentea L.]

Jiguancai [鸡冠菜, feather cockscomb, Celosia argentea L.] grows in the fields, and its plants are more than one Chi high. Its leaves are like those of Qingjiacai [青荚菜, heterophyllous patrinia, Patriniae Heterophyllae Radix] but narrower, and also like those of Shancai [山菜, Chinese thorowax root, Radix Bupleuri] but thinner. Its spicas grow out of branches, like those of Tu'erwei [兔儿尾, longifolia, Veronica longifolia L.] but smaller. Its flowers are pink and its seeds are like those of Xiancai [苋菜, amaranth, Amaranthi Caulis et Folium]. Its plants and leaves are bitter in taste.

For famine relief: Collect and blanch plants and leaves, remove the bitterness[1] by soaking them in water, and then flavor them with oil and salt.

【Notes】

［1］ Here it refers to the bitter odour.

54. 水蔓菁

一名地肤子。生中牟县南沙岗中。苗高一二尺，叶仿佛似地瓜儿叶，却甚短小，卷边窊面；又似鸡儿肠叶，颇尖艄。稍头出穗，开淡藕丝褐花。叶味甜。

救饥：采苗叶煤熟，油盐调食。

治病：今人亦将其子作地肤子用。

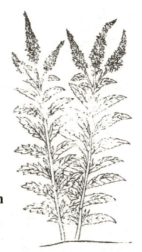

54. Shuimanjing［水蔓菁, kochia, Pseudolysimachion linariifolia Pall. ex Link subsp. dilatata （Nakai et Kitag.）Hong］

Shuimanjing［水蔓箐, kochia, Pseudolysimachion linariifolia Pall. ex Link subsp. dilatata（Nakai et Kitag.）Hong］, also named Difuzi, grows on the sandhills in the south of Zhongmu County. Its plants are 1~2 Chi high and its leaves are like those of sweet potatoes but shorter, edge-curved and concave, and also like those of Ji'erchang［鸡儿肠, aster, Asteris Radix］but sharper and narrower. Its spicas bear brown flowers, which are of pale pinkish gray color. Its leaves are sweet in taste.

For famine relief: Collect and blanch plants and leaves, and then flavor them with oil and salt.

For disease treatment: Its seeds are used as medicinal to replace Difuzi［地肤子, kochia, Kochiae Fructus］.

55. 野园荽

生祥符西北田野中。苗高一尺余。苗、叶、结实皆似家胡荽。但细小瘦窄，味甜，微辛香。

救饥：采嫩苗叶煤熟，油盐调食。

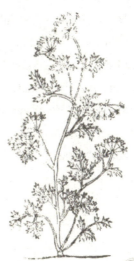

55. Yeyuansui［野园荽, wild coriander, Umbelliferae］

Yeyuansui［野园荽, wild coriander, Umbelliferae］grows in the fields of the northwest of Xiangfu County. Its plants are one Chi high. Its plants, leaves and fruit are all like those of Jiahusui［家胡荽, coriander, Coriandri Herba cum Radice］, but thinner and narrower. It is sweet and slightly pungent in taste.

For famine relief: Collect and blanch young plants and leaves, and then flavor them with oil and salt.

56. 牛尾菜

生辉县鸦子口山野间。苗高二三尺。叶似龙须菜叶，叶间分生叉枝，及出一细丝蔓；又似金刚刺叶而小，纹脉皆竖。茎叶梢间开白花。结子黑色。其叶味甘。

救饥：采嫩叶煠熟，水浸淘净，油盐调食。

56. Niuweicai［牛尾菜, riparian greenbrier root and rhizome, Smilax riparia A. DC.］

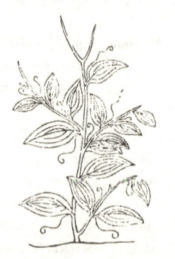

Niuweicai［牛尾菜, riparian greenbrier root and rhizome, Smilax riparia A. DC.］grows in the hillsides and wilderness of Yazikou of Huixian County. Its plants are 2～3 Chi high. Its leaves are like asparagus, with a small silky cirrus out of branches, and also like those of Jingangci［金刚刺, chinaroot, Smilacis Chinae Rhizoma］but smaller with straight lines. Its flowers are white out of the branches and leaves. Its fruit is black. Its leaves are sweet in taste.

For famine relief: Collect and blanch young leaves, soak them in water, wash and clean them, and then flavor them with oil and salt.

57. 山萮菜

生密县山野中。苗初搨地生。其叶之茎，背圆面㓕。叶似初出冬蜀葵叶稍小，五花叉，锯齿边，又似蔚臭苗叶而硬厚颇大。后撺茎叉，茎深紫色，稍叶颇小。味微辣。

救饥：采苗叶煤熟，换水浸淘净，油盐调食。

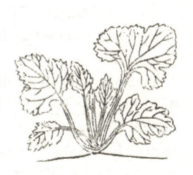

57. Shanyucai [山萮菜, Eutrema yunnanense, Eutrema yunnanense Franch.]

Shanyucai [山萮菜, Eutrema yunnanense, Eutrema yunnanense Franch.] grows in the hilllands and fields of Mixian County. Its plants creep on the ground. Its petioles are round backside and concave upside. Its leaves are like those of Dongshukui [冬蜀葵, hollyhock, Althaeae Radix] but smaller, five cracked and saw-tooth-edged, and also like those of Weichoumiao [蔚臭苗, motherwort fruit, Fructus Leonuri] but harder, thicker and larger. Its scapes are dark purple with tiny leaves at the tip of it. It is slightly pungent in taste.

For famine relief: Collect and blanch plants and leaves, soak them in fresh water, wash and clean them, and then flavor them with oil and salt.

58. 绵丝菜

生辉县山野中。苗高一二尺。叶似兔儿尾叶，但短小；又似柳叶菜叶，亦比短小。稍头攒生小菁葖，开黪白花。其叶味甜。

救饥：采嫩苗叶煤熟，水浸淘净，油盐调食。

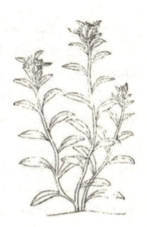

58. Miansicai [绵丝菜, silk floss, Pseudognaphalium luteoalbum (L.) Hilliard & B. L. Burtt]

Miansicai [绵丝菜, silk floss, Pseudognaphalium luteoalbum (L.) Hillard & B. L. Burtt] grows in the hilllands and fields of Huixian County. Its plants are 1~2 Chi high. Its leaves are like those of Tu'erwei [兔儿尾, longifolia, Veronica longifolia L.] but shorter, and also like those of Liuyecai [柳叶菜, willow herb, Epilobium hirsutum] but shorter. It bears small flower buds on top of branches and white flowers. Its leaves are sweet in taste.

For famine relief: Collect and blanch young plants and leaves, soak them in fresh water, wash and clean them, and then flavor them with oil and salt.

59. 米 蒿

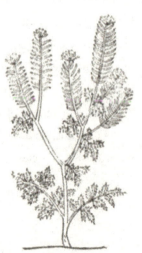

生田野中,所在处处有之。苗高尺许。叶似园荽叶微细。叶丛间分生茎叉,稍上开小青黄花。结小细角,似葶苈角儿。叶味微苦。

救饥:采嫩苗煤熟,水浸过,淘净,油盐调食。

59. Mihao [米蒿, artemisia, Descurainia Sophia (L.) Webb ex Prantl]

Mihao [米蒿, artemisia, Descurainia Sophia (L.) Webb ex Prantl] grows in the fields and places within its distribution range. Its plants are one Chi high and its leaves are like those of Yansui [芫荽, coriander, Coriandrum sativum L.] but thinner. Its inflorescence grows out of leaves, with tiny yellowish green flowers on top of it. Its fruit is small and thin, like that of Tingli [葶苈, Semen Lepidii, Semen Descurainiae]. Its leaves are slightly bitter in taste.

For famine relief: Collect and blanch young plants, soak them in fresh water, wash and clean them, and then flavor them with oil and salt.

60. 山芥菜

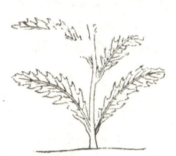

生密县山坡及岗野中。苗高一二尺。叶似家芥菜叶,瘦短微尖而多花叉。开小黄花。结小短角儿,味辣,微甜。

救饥:采苗叶拣择净,煤熟,油盐调食。

60. Shanjiecai [山芥菜, wild mustard leaf, Cruciferae]

Shanjiecai [山芥菜, wild mustard leaf, Cruciferae] grows at the hillsides and wilderness of Mixian County. Its plants are 1～2 Chi high and its leaves are like domestic ones, shorter, thinner and sharper, with more cleavages. Its flowers are tiny and yellow. Its siliques are short, slightly pungent and sweet in taste.

For famine relief: Collect and blanch plants and leaves, pick, wash and clean them, and then flavor them with oil and salt.

61. 舌头菜

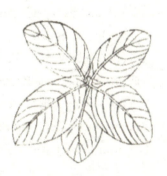

生密县山野中。苗叶揭地生。叶似山白菜叶而小,头颇团,叶面不皱,比山白菜叶亦厚,状类猪舌形,故以为名。味苦。

救饥:采叶煤熟,水浸去苦味,换水淘净,油盐调食。

61. Shetoucai [舌头菜, Kirilow Groundsel Herb, Tephroseris kirilowii]

Shetoucai [舌头菜, Kirilow Groundsel Herb, Tephroseris kirilowii] grows in the hilllands and fields of Mixian County. Its plants creep on the ground, and its leaves are like those of Shanbaicai [山白菜, aster, Asteris Radix] but smaller and thicker, with the round tip and the smooth surface. The shape of its leaves is like pork's tongue, justifying its Chinese name of Shetoucai ("shetou" meaning tongue in Chinese). It is bitter in taste.

For famine relief: Collect and blanch leaves, remove the bitterness by soaking them in fresh water, wash and clean them, and then flavor them with oil and salt.

62. 紫香蒿

生中牟县平野中。苗高一二尺。茎方紫色。叶似邪蒿叶而背白；又似野胡萝卜叶微短。茎叶稍间结小青子，比灰菜子又小。其叶味苦。

救饥：采叶煠熟，水浸去苦味，换水淘净，油盐调食。

62. Zixianghao [紫香蒿, Annuae Sweet Wormwood Herb, Artemisia]

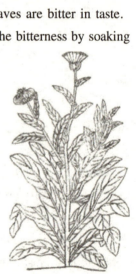

Zixianghao [紫香蒿, Annuae Sweet Wormwood Herb, Artemisia] grows in the flat fields of Zhongmu County. Its plants are 1~2 Chi high and its square stems are purple. Its leaves are like those of Xiehao [邪蒿, seseli, Seseli Herba], with the white backside, and also like those of Ye Huluobo [野胡萝卜, wild carrot, Daucus carota L.] but shorter. Its inflorescences bear green fruit, smaller than that of wild pigweeds. Its leaves are bitter in taste.

For famine relief: Collect and blanch leaves, remove the bitterness by soaking them in fresh water, wash and clean them, and then flavor them with oil and salt.

63. 金盏儿花

人家园圃中多种。苗高四五寸。叶似初生莴苣叶，比莴苣叶狭窄而厚，抪茎生叶。茎端开金黄色盏子[1]样花。其叶味酸。

救饥：采苗叶煠熟，水浸去酸味，淘净，油盐调食。

【注释】

［1］盛酒、茶的小杯子。

63. Jinzhan'er Hua［金盏儿花, Calendula, Calendula officinalis L.］

Jinzhan'er Hua［金盏儿花, Calendula, Calendula officinalis L.］ is planted in common people's nursery gardens. Its plants are 4～5 Cun high, and its leaves, scattered on the stem, are like those of Woju［莴苣, lettuce, Lactucae Sativae Caulis et Folium］but narrower and thicker. Yellow capitula grow on the top of stems, cup-shaped[1]. Its leaves are sour in taste.

For famine relief: Collect and blanch plants and leaves, remove the sourness by soaking them in fresh water, wash and clean them, and then flavor them with oil and salt.

[Notes]

［1］Here it refers to the small cup used for holding wine and tea.

64．六月菊

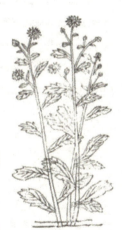

生祥符西田野中。苗高一二尺。茎似铁杆蒿茎。叶似鸡儿肠叶，但长而涩；又似马兰头叶而硬短。稍叶间开淡紫花。叶味微酸涩。

救饥：采叶煠熟，水浸去邪味，油盐调食。

64. Liuyueju［六月菊, tatarian aster root, Compositae］

Liuyueju［六月菊, tatarian aster root, Compositae］ grows in the west fields of Xiangfu. Its plants are 1～2 Chi high and its stems are like those of Tieganhao［铁杆蒿, artemisia, Artemisia gmelinii Web. ex Stechm.］. Its leaves are like those of Ji'erchang［鸡儿肠, aster, Asteris Radix］but longer and rougher, and also like those of Malantou［马兰头, kalimeris, Kalimeridis Herba et Radix］but harder and shorter. Its flowers are purple out of leaves on top of the branches. Its leaves are slightly sour and astringent.

For famine relief: Collect and blanch leaves, remove the astringency by soaking them in fresh water, and then flavor them with oil and salt.

65. 费　菜

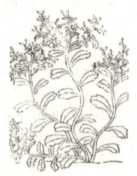

生辉县太行山车箱冲山野间。苗高尺许。叶似火焰草叶而小,头颇齐,上有锯齿。其叶抪茎而生。叶稍上开五瓣小尖淡黄花,结五瓣红小花萼儿。苗叶味酸。

救饥:采嫩苗叶煠熟,换水淘去酸味,油盐调食。

65. Feicai [费菜, phedimus aizoon, Sedum aizoon L.]

Feicai [费菜, phedimus aizoon, Sedum aizoon L.] grows in the fields of Chexiangchong of Taihang Moutain in Huixian County. Its plants are one Chi high, and its leaves are like those of Huoyancao [火焰草, Indian paintbrush, Castilleja pallida Kunth], smaller, flatter and saw-toothed. Its flowers, on the top of the branches, are light yellow with 5 acute petals and 5 pieces of red fruit. Its plants and leaves are sour in taste.

For famine relief: Collect and blanch young plants and leaves, remove the sourness by soaking them in fresh water, and then flavor them with oil and salt.

66. 千屈菜

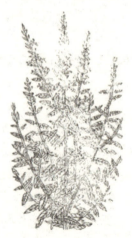

生田野中。苗高二尺许。茎方四楞。叶似山梗菜叶而不尖;又似柳叶菜叶亦短小,叶头颇齐,叶皆相对生。稍间开红紫花。叶味甜。

救饥:采嫩苗叶煠熟,水浸淘净,油盐调食。

66. Qianqucai [千屈菜, lythrum, Lythrum salicaria L.]

Qianqucai [千屈菜, lythrum, Lythrum salicaria L.] grows in the fields. Its plants are two Chi high and its stems are square. Its opposite leaves, flat-tipped, are like those of Shangengcai [山梗菜, cardinal flower, Lobelia sessilifolia Lamb.] but not so sharp, and also like those of Liuyecai [柳叶菜, swamp willow herb, Epilobii Palustris Herba] but shorter. Its flowers are reddish purple. Its leaves are sweet in taste.

For famine relief: Collect and blanch young plants and leaves, soak them in fresh water, wash and clean them, and then flavor them with oil and salt.

67. 柳叶菜

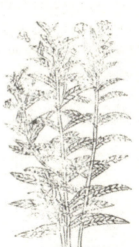

生郑州贾峪山山野中。苗高二尺余。茎淡红色。叶似柳叶而厚短，有涩毛。稍间开四瓣深红花。结细长角儿。其叶味甜。

救饥：采苗叶煠熟，油盐调食。

67. Liuyecai [柳叶菜, swamp willow herb, Epilobium hirsutum L.]

Liuyecai [柳叶菜, swamp willow herb, Epilobium hirsutum L.] grows in the hilllands and fields of Jiayu Mountain in Zhengzhou. Its plants are more than two Chi high and its stems are red. Its leaves, like those of willows, are thick and short with hairs. Its flowers are dark red among the branches and leaves, with four petals. Its fruit is thin and long. Its leaves are sweet in taste.

For famine relief: Collect and blanch plants and leaves, and then flavor them with oil and salt.

68. 婆婆指甲菜

生田野中,作地摊科。生茎细弱。叶像女人指甲;又似初生枣叶微薄。细茎,稍间结小花萼。苗叶味甘。

救饥:采嫩苗叶煠熟,油盐调食。

68. Popo Zhijiacai〔婆婆指甲菜, grasswort, Cerastium fontanum subsp. Vulgare（Hartm.）Greuter et Burdet〕

Popo Zhijiacai〔婆婆指甲菜, grasswort, Cerastium fontanum subsp. Vulgare（Hartm.）Greuter et Burdet〕grows in the fields. Its plants creep on the ground and its stems are thin and tender. Its leaves are like women's fingernails, and also like newly-born common jujube leaves but thinner. Small flower buds grow among branches. Its plants and leaves are all sweet in taste.

For famine relief: Collect and blanch young plants and leaves, and then flavor them with oil and salt.

69. 铁杆蒿

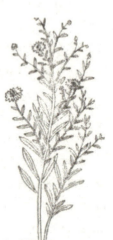

生田野中。苗茎高二三尺。叶似独扫叶,微肥短,又似扁蓄[1]叶而短小。分生茎叉,稍间开淡紫花,黄心。叶味苦。

救饥:采叶煠熟,淘去苦味,油盐调食。

【注释】

［1］即萹蓄。

69. Tieganhao〔铁杆蒿, Artemisia vestita, Aster〕

Tieganhao〔铁杆蒿, Artemisia vestita, Aster〕grows in the fields. Its plants are 2~3 Chi high and its leaves are like those of Dusao〔独扫, Broom Cypress Fruit, Belvedere Fruit〕but broader and shorter, and also like those of Bianxu[1]

[萹蓄, grass of common knot grass, Herba Polygoni Avicularis] but shorter and smaller. Its stems draw out branches which bear light purple flowers with yellow buds. Its leaves are bitter in taste.

For famine relief: Collect and blanch leaves, remove the bitterness by washing them, and then flavor them with oil and salt.

【Notes】

[1] Here it refers to the medicinal Bianxu [萹蓄, grass of common knot grass, Herba Polygoni Avicularis].

70. 山甜菜

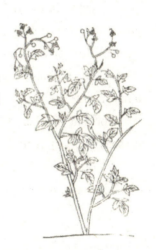

生密县韶华山山谷中。苗高二三尺。茎青白色。叶似初生绵花叶而窄,花叉颇浅。其茎叶间开五瓣淡紫花。结子如枸杞子,生则青,熟则红色。叶味苦。

救饥:采叶煠熟,换水浸,淘去苦味,油盐调食。

70. Shantiancai [山甜菜, climbing nightshade, Solanum lyratum Thunb.]

Shantiancai [山甜菜, climbing nightshade, Solanum lyratum Thunb.] grows in the valleys of Shaohuashan in Mixian County. Its plants are 2~3 Chi high and its stems are bluish white. Its leaves, lobed, are like those of cotton but narrower. Its flowers are light purple with five petals. Its fruit is like that of Chinese wolfberry, green when underripe and red when ripe. Its leaves are bitter in taste.

For famine relief: Collect and blanch leaves, remove the bitterness by soaking them in fresh water, and then flavor them with oil and salt.

71. 剪刀股

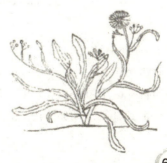

生田野中,处处有之。就地作小科苗。叶似嫩苦苣叶而细小,色颇似蓝,亦有白汁[1],茎叉稍间开淡黄花。叶味苦。

救饥:采苗叶煠熟,水浸,淘去苦味,油盐调食。
【注释】
[1]指具有白色乳汁,这是菊科菊苣族的特征。

71. Jiandaogu [剪刀股, lactuca debilis maxim, Ixeris japonica (N. L. Burman) Nakai]

Jiandaogu [剪刀股, lactuca debilis maxim, Ixeris japonica (N. L. Burman) Nakai] grows in the fields and can be seen everywhere. Its plants are short and grow along the ground. Its leaves are like those of young lettuce but thinner and smaller. It is of the color of Songlan [菘蓝, woad, Isatis tinctoria], with white juice[1]. Its inflorescences bear light yellow flowers on top of them. Its leaves are bitter in taste.

For famine relief: Collect and blanch plants and leaves, remove the bitterness by soaking them in fresh water, and then flavor them with oil and salt.

【Notes】
[1] Here it refers to the white juice, characteristic of the composite family.

72. 水苏子

生下湿地。茎淡紫色,对生茎叉,叶亦对生。其叶似地瓜叶而窄,边有花锯齿三叉,尖叶下两傍又有小叉叶。稍开花,深黄色。其叶味辛。

救饥:采苗叶煠熟,油盐调食。

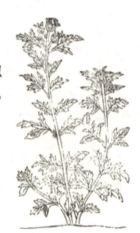

72. Shuisuzi [水苏子, bur beggarticks herb, Bidens tripartita L.]

Shuisuzi [水苏子, bur beggarticks herb, Bidens tripartita L.] grows in the low wetlands. Its stems are light purple and both of its branches and leaves are opposite. Its leaves are like those of sweet potatoes but narrower, saw-tooth-edged and trilobite. There are two small leaves under each pointed leaf. Its flowers are dark yellow on the top of branches. Its leaves are pungent in taste.

For famine relief: Collect and blanch plants and leaves, and then flavor them with oil and salt.

73. 风花菜

生田野中。苗高二尺余。叶似芥菜叶而瘦长,又多花叉。梢间开黄花如芥菜花。味辛,微苦。

救饥:采嫩苗叶煤熟,换水浸淘,去苦味,油盐调食。

73. Fenghuacai[风花菜, Indian rorippa herb, Rorippa globosa (Turca. ex Fisch. et C. A. Mey.) Hayek]

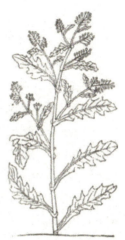

Fenghuacai[风花菜, Indian rorippa herb, Rorippa globosa (Turca. ex Fisch. et C. A. Mey.) Hayek] grows in the wilderness and fields. Its plants are two Chi high and its leaves are like those of Jiecai[芥菜, mustard leaf, Sinapis Folium] but narrower, with many lobes. Its flowers are yellow among the branches like those of Jiecai[芥菜, mustard leaf, Sinapis Folium]. It is pungent and slightly bitter in taste.

For famine relief: Collect and blanch young plants and leaves, remove the bitterness by soaking them in fresh water, and then flavor them with oil and salt.

74. 鹅儿肠

生许州水泽边。就地妥[1]茎而生。对节生叶,叶似豌豆叶而薄,又似佛指甲叶微鲱。叶间分生枝叉,开白花。结子似葶苈子。其叶味甜。

救饥:采苗叶煤熟,油盐调食。

【注释】

[1]落,垂,这里指植株匍匐的样子。

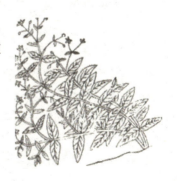

74. E'erchang [鹅儿肠, malachium, Myosoton aquaticum (L.) Moench]

E'erchang [鹅儿肠, malachium, Myosoton aquaticum (L.) Moench] grows near the marsh areas of Xuzhou. Its plants creep[1] on the ground. Its opposite leaves are like those of Laodou [䝁豆, wild soybean, Glycine ussuriensis] but thinner, and also like those of Fozhijia [佛指甲, herb of manystem stonecrop, Sedum multicaule Wall.] but sharper. It bears inflorescence out of leaves, with white flowers on it. Its seeds are like those of Tingli [葶苈, Semen Lepidii, Semen Descurainiae]. Its leaves are sweet in taste.

For famine relief: Collect and blanch plants and leaves, and then flavor them with oil and salt.

【Notes】

[1] Hang down and droop. Here it refers to the plants creeping on the ground.

75. 粉条儿菜

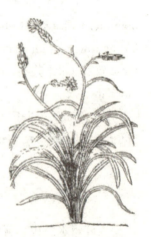

生田野中。其叶初生，就地丛生，长则四散分垂。叶似萱草叶而瘦细微短。叶间撺葶，开淡黄花。叶味甜。

救饥：采叶煠熟，淘洗净，油盐调食。

75. Fentiao'er Cai [粉条儿菜, root of Austrian serpentroot, Scorzonera albicaulis Bge.]

Fentiao'er Cai [粉条儿菜, root of Austrian serpentroot, Scorzonera albicaulis Bge.] grows in the fields, clustered on the ground when young and scattered when mature. Its leaves are like those of Xuancao [萱草, day lily, Hemerocallis Flos] but narrower and shorter. Its scapes bear light yellow flowers. Its leaves are sweet in taste.

For famine relief: Collect and blanch leaves, wash and clean them, and then

flavor them with oil and salt.

76. 辣辣菜

生荒野中，今处处有之。苗高五七寸。初生尖叶，后分枝茎，上出长叶。开细青白花。结小扁蒴，其子似米蒿子，黄色，味辣。

救饥：采嫩苗叶煠熟，水浸淘净，油盐调食。生揉[1]亦可食。

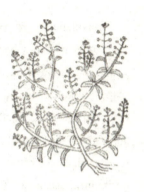

【注释】

[1] 指生食野菜的时候加盐将菜揉搓，杀出水分后食用。

76. Lalacai〔辣辣菜, garden cress, Lepidium apetalum Willd.〕

Lalacai〔辣辣菜, garden cress, Lepidium apetalum Willd.〕grows in the wilderness and is distributed everywhere presently. Its plants are 5~7 Cun high. Its newborn leaves are pointed and then the long leaves grow on its branches. Its tiny flowers are greenish white and its fruit is small and oblate. Its seeds are like those of Mihao〔米蒿, Artemisia giraldii, Artemisiadalai-lamaeKrasch〕, yellow and spicy in taste.

For famine relief: Collect and blanch young plants and leaves, soak them in water, wash and clean them, and then flavor them with oil and salt. It can also be taken after being rubbed with salt to remove the moisture[1].

【Notes】

[1] A method to process edible wild herbs when being eaten raw by rubbing the herbs with salt to remove the moisture.

77. 毛连菜

一名常十八。生田野中。苗初搨地生，后擢茎叉，高二尺许。叶似刺蓟叶而长大，稍尖，其叶边褊曲皱，上有涩毛。稍间开银褐花。味微苦。

救饥：采叶煠熟，水浸淘净，油盐调食。

77. Maoliancai［毛连菜，picris，Picris hieracioides L.］

Maoliancai［毛连菜，picris，Picris hieracioides L.］, also named Changshiba, grows in the fields. Its young plants crawl on the ground firstly and then produce scapes, about two Chi high. Its leaves is like those of Ciji［刺蓟，field thistle herb, Herba Cirsii］ but longer and larger. The top of its leaves are a little pointed, with rugose edge and rough hair. Its flowers are silver taupe on its inflorescences. It is bitter in taste.

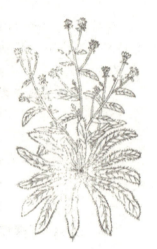

For famine relief: Collect and blanch leaves, soak them in water, wash and clean them, and then flavor them with oil and salt.

78. 小桃红

一名凤仙花，一名夹竹桃，又名海蒳，俗名染指甲草。人家园圃多种，今处处有之。苗高二尺许。叶似桃叶而窄，边有细锯齿。开红花，结实形类桃样，极小。有子似萝卜子，取之易迸散，俗名急性子。叶味苦，微涩。

救饥：采苗叶煠熟，水浸一宿做菜，油盐调食。

78. Xiaotaohong［小桃红，garden balsam flower, Impatiens balsamina L.］

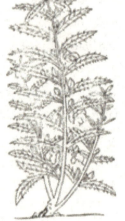

Xiaotaohong［小桃红, garden balsam flower, Impatiens balsamina L.］, also named Fengxianhua, Jiazhutao, Haina and Ranzhijia Cao (referring to grass to dye fingernails), is often planted in common people's nursery gardens. Presently it is planted everywhere. Its plants are two Chi high and its leaves are like those of peaches but narrower and saw-tooth-edged. Its flowers are red and its tiny fruit is peach-shaped. Its seeds are like those of radishes. Its pericarp is easy to crack when taking seeds out, which gives another name to it "Jixingzi", meaning short-tempered. Its leaves are bitter in taste and a bit astringent.

For famine relief: Collect and blanch plants and leaves, soak them in water for one night, and then flavor them with oil and salt.

79. 青荚儿菜

生辉县太行山山野中。苗高二尺许,对生茎叉,叶亦对生。其叶面青背白,锯齿三叉叶,脚叶花叉颇大,状似荏子叶而狭长尖䩺。茎叶稍间开五瓣小黄花,众花攒开,形如穗状。其叶味微苦。

救饥:采嫩苗叶煠熟,换水浸,淘去苦味,油盐调食。

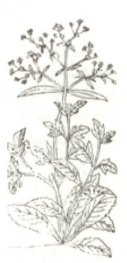

79. Qingjia'er Cai [青荚儿菜, heterophyllous patrinia, Patrinia heterophylla Bunge]

Qingjia'er Cai [青荚儿菜, heterophyllous patrinia, Patrinia heterophylla Bunge] grows in the mountain and wilderness of Taihang Mountain of Huixian County. Its plants are about two Chi high, with opposite branches and leaves. The upside of its leaves is green and backside white, saw-tooth-shaped and trifid. Its basal leaves are partite with the shape like that of Renzi [荏子, perilla, Perilla frutescens (L.) Britt.] but narrower, longer and pointed. Its yellow flowers are small and five-petaled on inflorescences, gathered and fringy. Its leaves are a little bitter in taste.

For famine relief: Collect and blanch young plants and leaves, soak them in fresh water, remove the bitterness by washing them, and then flavor them with oil and salt.

80. 八角菜

生辉县太行山山野中。苗高一尺许,苗茎甚细。其叶状类牡丹叶而大,味甜。

救饥:采嫩苗叶煠熟,水浸淘净,油盐调食。

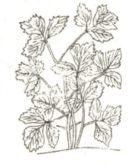

80. Bajiaocai [八角菜, umbelliferous vegetables, Umbelliferae]

Bajiaocai [八角菜, umbelliferous vegetables, Umbelliferae] grows in the wilderness of Taihang Mountain of Huixian County. Its plants are one Chi high and its stems are thin. Its leaves are like those of Mudan [牡丹, subshrubby peony, Paeonia suffruticosa Andr.] but larger, and sweet in taste.

For famine relief: Collect and blanch young plants and leaves, soak them in fresh water, wash and clean them, and then flavor them with oil and salt.

81. 耐惊菜

一名莲子草,以其花之菁葵状似小莲蓬[1]样,故名。生下湿地中。苗高一尺余。茎紫赤色,对生茎叉。叶似小桃红叶而长。稍间开细瓣白花,淡黄心。叶味苦。

救饥:采苗叶煠熟,油盐调食。

【注释】

[1] 见本书第367莲藕条。

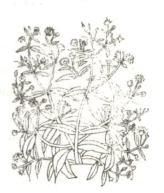

81. Naijingcai [耐惊菜, eclipta prostrata, Eclipta prostrata (L.) L.]

Naijingcai [耐惊菜, eclipta prostrata, Eclipta prostrata (L.) L.] is also named Lianzicao, for its flower buds are like Lianpeng[1] [莲蓬, lotus seedpod, Receptaculum Nelumbinis]. It grows in the low-lying wetlands. Its seedlings are about one Chi high, and its stems are purplish red with opposite branches. Its leaves are like those of Xiaotaohong [小桃红, flowering plum, Amygdalus triloba] but a little longer, bitter in taste, with thin petals and yellowish tubular flowers in the center.

For famine relief: Collect young leaves and seedlings, blanch them, and then flavor them with oil and salt.

【Notes】

[1] See the 367th clause of this book.

82. 地棠菜

生郑州南沙㘵中。苗高一二尺。叶似地棠花叶，甚大；又似初生芥菜叶，微狭而尖，味甜。

救饥：采嫩苗叶煠熟，油盐调食。

82. Ditangcai [地棠菜, figwort root, Scrophularia ningpoensis Hemsl.]

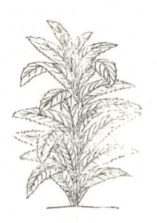

Ditangcai [地棠菜, figwort root, Scrophularia ningpoensis Hemsl.] grows in Nanshagang Prefecture of Zhengzhou. Its plants are 1~2 Chi high, and its leaves are like those of Ditanghua [地棠花, Japanese kerria flower, Kerria japonica (L.) DC.] but much bigger, or like those of young Jiecai [芥菜, leaf mustard, Brassica juncea (L.) Czern. et Coss.] but a little thinner and sharper. It is sweet in taste.

For famine relief: Collect young leaves and seedlings, blanch them, and then flavor them with oil and salt.

83. 鸡儿肠

生中牟田野中。苗高一二尺。茎黑紫色。叶似薄荷叶微小，边有稀锯齿；又似六月菊。稍叶间开细瓣淡粉紫花，黄心。叶味微辣。

救饥：采叶煠熟，换水淘去辣味，油盐调食。

83. Ji'erchang [鸡儿肠, Indian Kalimeris Herb, Kalimeris indica (L.) Sch. -Bip.]

Ji'erchang [鸡儿肠, Indian Kalimeris Herb, Kalimeris indica (L.) Sch. -Bip.] grows in the fields of Zhongmu County. Its plants are about 1~2 Chi high with black-purple stems. Its leaves are like those of Bohe [薄荷, peppermint, Herba Menthae] but a little smaller with sparse serrated margin, or like those of Liuyueju [六月菊, blanket flower, Gaillardia pulchella Foug.]. The light orchid capitula with yellow tubular flowers stand out of the leaves. Its leaves are slightly spicy in taste.

For famine relief: Collect and blanch leaves, remove the piquancy by rinsing them, and then flavor them with oil and salt.

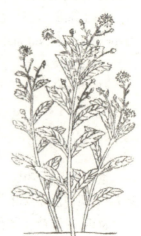

84. 雨点儿菜

生田野中。就地丛生,其茎脚紫稍青。叶如细柳叶而窄小,抪茎而生;又似石竹子叶而颇硬。稍间开小尖五瓣紫花,结角比萝卜角又大。其叶味甘。

救饥:采叶煠熟,水浸作过,淘洗令净,油盐调食。

84. Yudian'er Cai [雨点儿菜, willowleaf rhizome, Cynanchum stauntonii (Decne.) Schltr. ex Levl.]

Yudian'er Cai [雨点儿菜, willowleaf rhizome, Cynanchum stauntonii (Decne.) Schltr. ex Levl.] grows in the fields, clustered on the ground. Its stem base is purple and tip green. The leaves, which are like willow leaves but much thinner and smaller, scatter along the stems, or are like those of Shizhuzi [石竹子, Chinese pink, Dianthus

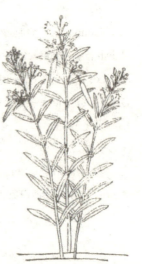

chinensis L.] but quite hard in texture. Its purple cymes with 5 little pointy petals stand out of the leaves, and the follicles are bigger than the silique of Luobo [萝卜, turnip, Raphanus sativus L.]. Its leaves are sweet in taste.

For famine relief: Collect and blanch young leaves, soak and rinse them with fresh water, and then flavor them with oil and salt.

85. 白屈菜

生田野中。苗高一二尺，初作丛生。茎叶皆青白色，茎有毛刺。稍头分叉，上开四瓣黄花。叶颇似山芥菜叶，而花叉极大；又似漏芦叶而色淡，味苦、微辣。

救饥：采叶，和净土煮熟，捞出，连土浸一宿[1]，换水淘洗净，油盐调食。

【注释】

[1] 白屈菜中可能含有不溶于水的有毒生物碱，用常规煠野菜的方法不能有效去除；采用净土吸附，可以有效去除这类有毒物质。这是中国古代采用植物吸附分离法去毒的最早记载。

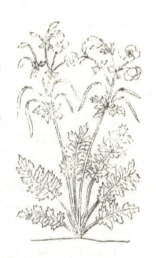

85. Baiqucai [白屈菜, celandine, Chelidonium majus L.]

Baiqucai [白屈菜, celandine, Chelidonium majus L.] grows in the fields. Its plants are about 1~2 Chi high and cluster on the ground at the early stage. Both its stems and leaves are bluish-white with burrs on the stems. The stem tips usually divaricate with quadrivalvate yellow flowers on them. Its leaves are more like those of Shanjiecai [山芥菜, wintercress, Barbarea orthoceras Ledeb.] with quite deep lobes, or like those of Loulu [漏芦, uniflower swisscentaury root, Stemmacantha uniflora (L.) Dittrich] but lighter in color. It is bitter and slightly spicy in taste.

For famine relief: Collect leaves, steam them with clean soil, soak them with the soil in water for one night[1], change the water and elutriate, and flavor them with oil and salt.

【Notes】

[1] There might be insoluble poisonous alkaloids in Baiqucai, and they can not

be effectively removed by routine blanch method. Clean soil adsorption method can be used to remove these poisonous substances effectively. It is the earliest record of botanical adsorptive separation method for detoxification in ancient China.

86. 扯根菜

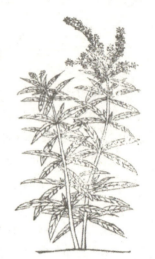

生田野中。苗高一尺许，茎色赤红。叶似小桃红叶，微窄小，色颇绿；又似小柳叶，亦短而厚窄。其叶周围攒茎而生。开碎瓣小青白花，结小花蒴，似蒺藜[1]样。叶苗味甘。

救饥：采苗叶煠熟，水浸淘净，油盐调食。

【注释】

[1] 见本书第190蒺藜条。

86. Chegencai [扯根菜, Chinese penthorum, Penthorum chinense Pursh]

Chegencai [扯根菜, Chinese penthorum, Penthorum chinense Pursh] grows in the fields. Its plants are about one Chi high with the crimson stems. Its leaves are like those of Xiaotaohong [小桃红, flowering plum, Amygdalus triloba] but quite green in color and a little narrower than the latter, or like the small willow leaves but shorter, thicker and narrower. The leaves aggregate around the stems. It has bluish white racemes with tiny petals, and the small fruit is like that of Jili[1] [蒺藜, puncturevine caltrop fruit, Tribulus terrester L.]. Its leaves and seedlings are sweet in taste.

For famine relief: Collect leaves and seedlings, blanch, soak and rinse them, and flavor them with oil and salt.

【Notes】

[1] See the 190th clause of this book.

87. 草零陵香

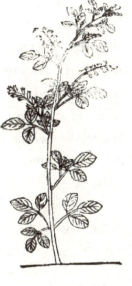

又名芫香。人家园圃中多种之。叶似苜蓿[1]叶而长大微尖。茎叶间开小淡粉紫花,作小短穗。其子小如粟粒。苗叶味苦,性平。

救饥:采苗叶煠熟,换水淘净,油盐调食。

治病:今人遇零陵香缺,多以此物代用。

【注释】

[1] 见本书第379苜蓿条。

87. Caoling Lingxiang [草零陵香, sweet clover, Melilotus officinalis (L.) Pall.]

Caoling Lingxiang [草零陵香, sweet clover, Melilotus officinalis (L.) Pall.], also named Yuanxiang, is cultivated in common people's gardens. Its leaves are like those of Muxu[1] [苜蓿, alfalfa, Medicago sativa L.] but longer, bigger and sharper than them. The short spicate racemes are light purple. Its seeds are as big as millets. The seedlings and leaves are bitter in taste and neutral in nature.

For famine relief: Collect leaves and seedlings, blanch and rinse them, and flavor them with oil and salt.

For disease treatment: Presently it is used as the substitute of Linglingxiang [零陵香, Sweet Basil herb, Ocimmum basilicum L.].

【Notes】

[1] See the 379th clause of this book.

88. 水落藜

生水边,所在处处有之。苗高尺余。茎色微红。叶似野灰菜叶而瘦小,味微苦涩,性凉。

救饥:采苗叶煠熟,换水浸淘、洗净,油盐调食。晒干煠食尤好。

88. Shuiluoli [水落藜, chenopodium serotinum, Chenopodium serotinum L.]

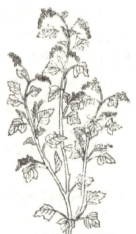

Shuiluoli [水落藜, chenopodium serotinum, Chenopodium serotinum L.] grows at the waterside and can be seen everywhere presently. Its plants are more than one Chi high with reddish stems. Its leaves are like those of Yehuicai [野灰菜, lamb's-quarters, Chenopodium album L.] but much thinner and smaller. It is slightly bitter and astringent in taste, and cool in nature.

For famine relief: Collect leaves and seedlings, blanch, soak and rinse them, and flavor them with oil and salt. It is better to blanch them after drying them in the sunshine.

89. 凉蒿菜

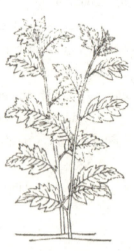

又名甘菊芽。生密县山野中。叶似菊花叶而细长尖艄，又多花叉。开黄花。其叶味甘。

救饥：采叶煠熟，换水浸淘净，油盐调食。

89. Lianghaocai [凉蒿菜, wild chrysanthemum, Dendranthema indicum (L.) Des Moul.]

Lianghaocai [凉蒿菜, wild chrysanthemum, Dendranthema indicum (L.) Des Moul.], also named Ganjuya, grows in the mountainous regions and fields of Mixian County. Its leaves are like those of Juhua [菊花, chrysanthemum, Dendranthema morifolium (Ramat.) Tzvel.] but longer and sharper. It is always partite with yellow capitula, and its leaves are sweet in taste.

For famine relief: Collect leaves, blanch, soak and elutriate them, and flavor them with oil and salt.

90. 粘鱼须

一名龙须菜。生郑州贾峪山,及新郑山野中亦有之。初先发笋,其后延蔓生茎发叶。每叶间皆分出一小叉,及出一丝蔓。叶似土茜[1]叶而大;又似金刚刺[2]叶;亦似牛尾菜叶,不涩而光泽,味甘。

救饥:采嫩笋叶煠熟,油盐调食。

【注释】

［1］见本书第 211 土茜苗条。

［2］见本书第 135 金刚刺条。

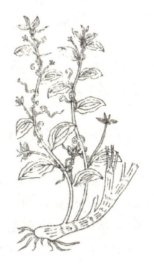

90. Nianyuxu [粘鱼须, Glabrous Greenbrier Rhizome, Smilax glabra Roxb]

Nianyuxu [粘鱼须, Glabrous Greenbrier Rhizome, Smilax glabra Roxb], also named Longxucai, grows in Jiayu Mountain of Zhengzhou. It can be found in the mountainous regions and wilderness of Xinzheng. It germinates aliform leaf sheaths at first, and then stretches out filamentous tendrils. Its leaves are like those of Tuqian[1] [土茜, India madder root, Rubia cordifolia L.] but much bigger, or like those of Jingangci[2] [金刚刺, Smilax scobinicaulis, Smilax scobinicaulis C. H. Wright] and Niuweicai [牛尾菜, Root and Rhizome of Ripqrian Greenbrier, Smilax riparia A. de Candolle]. The leaves are not rough but glossy, with sweet taste.

For famine relief: Collect young stems and leaf sheaths, blanch them, and flavor them with oil and salt.

【Notes】

［1］See the 211th clause of this book.

［2］See the 135th clause of this book.

91. 节节菜

生荒野下湿地。科苗甚小。叶似碱蓬,又更细小而稀疏。其茎多节坚硬。叶间开粉紫花。味甜。

救饥:采嫩苗拣择净,煠熟,水浸淘过,油盐调食。

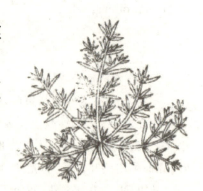

91. Jiejiecai［节节菜, Rotala indica, Rotala indica（Willd.）Koehne］

Jiejiecai［节节菜, Rotala indica, Rotala indica（Willd.）Koehne］grows in the low-lying wetland of wilderness. Its plants are very small. Its leaves are like those of Jianpeng［碱蓬, suaeda salsa, Suaeda glauca (Bunge) Bunge］but much smaller and sparser. Its stems are gnarled and hard, and its flowers are pinkish purple. It is sweet in taste.

For famine relief: Collect and trim seedlings, blanch, soak and rinse them, and then flavor them with oil and salt.

92. 野艾蒿

生田野中。苗叶类艾而细,又多花叉,叶有艾香,味苦。

救饥:采叶煠熟,水淘,去苦味,油盐调食。

92. Yeaihao［野艾蒿, artemisia lavandulaefolia, Artemisia lavandulaefolia DC.］

Yeaihao［野艾蒿, artemisia lavandulaefolia, Artemisia lavandulaefolia DC.］grows in the fields. Both the shape and the flavor of its leaves are like those of Ai［艾, mugwort, Artemisia argyi Levl. et Van.］but much thinner and more partite than the latter. It is bitter in taste.

For famine relief: Collect and blanch leaves, remove the bitterness by rinsing them, and flavor them with oil and salt.

93. 堇堇菜

一名箭头草。生田野中。苗初揭地生。叶似铍[1]箭头样,而叶蒂甚长。其后叶间撺葶,开紫花。结三瓣蒴儿,中有子,如芥子大,茶褐色。叶味甘。

救饥:采苗叶煤熟,水浸淘净,油盐调食。

治病:今人传说,根叶捣傅诸肿毒[2]。

【注释】

[1] 古代一种兵器。

[2] 指把鲜植物捣烂,敷患处,隔一定时间换药一次,使药物在较长时间内发挥作用,来治疗各种肿毒。

93. Jinjincai [堇堇菜, Tokyo violet herb, Viola philippica Cavanilles]

Jinjincai [堇堇菜, Tokyo violet herb, Viola philippica Cavanilles], also named Jiantoucao, grows in the fields. In the early growth period, its seedlings spread along the ground. Its leaves are like the heads of Pi[1] with quite long petioles. Its scapes stand out of the leaves with purple flowers during the growing period. Its fruit is tricarpellary with dark brown seeds in it. The size of the seeds is as big as that of Baijie [白芥, white mustard, Sinapis alba L.]. Its leaves are sweet in taste.

For famine relief: Collect leaves and seedlings, blanch, soak and elutriate them, and flavor them with oil and salt.

For disease treatment: Presently it is said that its roots and leaves can be used to treat pyogenic infection after pounding into pieces for external application.[2]

【Notes】

[1] A kind of knife-shaped weapon in ancient China.

[2] Pound the fresh herb into pieces; apply to the affected part to treat many kinds of pyogenic infection, change dressings at intervals to make the herbs take effect during a long period of time.

94. 婆婆纳

生田野中。苗揪地生。叶最小,如小面花[1]靥儿状,类初生菊花芽,叶又团边。微花,如云头样。味甜。

救饥:采苗叶煤熟,水浸淘净,油盐调食。

【注释】

[1] 指河南、山东、山西等地的一种面食艺术,用面粉做成各种形状的面食,蒸熟后在上面做彩绘。

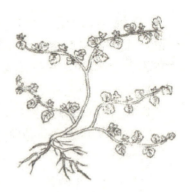

94. Popona [婆婆纳, speedwell, Veronica didyma Tenore]

Popona [婆婆纳, speedwell, Veronica didyma Tenore] grows in the fields with seedlings spreading along the ground. Its tiny ovate leaves are just like the black spot on the small Mianhua[1], or like the budding Juhua [菊花, chrysanthemums, Dendranthema morifolium (Ramat.) Tzvel.]. Its flowers are very small with the shape like cloud. It is sweet in taste.

For famine relief: Collect leaves and seedlings, blanch, soak and elutriate them, and flavor them with oil and salt.

【Notes】

[1] It refers to a kind of cooked wheaten food in Henan, Shandong, Shanxi and so on. Make wheaten food in various shapes with flour, and then apply colored drawing on them after being steamed.

95. 野茴香

生田野中。其苗初揪地生。叶似拂娘蒿[1]叶,微细小。后于叶间撺葶,分生茎叉,稍头开黄花,结细角,有小黑子。叶味苦。

救饥:采苗叶煤熟,水浸,淘去苦味,油盐调食。

【注释】

[1]见本书第112 㧕娘蒿条。

95. Yehuixiang［野茴香, wild fennel, Foeniculum vulgare Mill.］

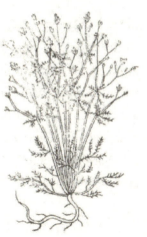

Yehuixiang［野茴香, wild fennel, Foeniculum vulgare Mill.］ grows in the fields. In the early growth period, its seedlings spread along the ground. Its leaves are like those Bunianghao[1]［㧕娘蒿, descurainia sophia, Descurainia sophia (L.) Webb ex Prantl］but a little smaller. Its scapes grow out of the leaves and branches with yellow flowers on the tips. Its fruit is thin and terete with black seeds in it. Its leaves are bitter in taste.

For famine relief: Collect young leaves and seedlings, blanch them and remove the bitterness by soaking and rinsing them, and flavor them with oil and salt.

【Notes】

[1] See the 112th clause of this book.

96. 蝎子花菜

又名虼蚤花,一名野菠菜。生田野中。苗初揭地生。叶似初生菠菜叶而瘦细,叶间撺生茎叉,高一尺余,茎有线楞。稍间开小白花。其叶味苦。

救饥:采嫩叶煤熟,水淘净,油盐调食。

96. Xiezi Huacai［蝎子花菜, limonium bicolor, Limonium bicolor (Bag.) Kuntze］

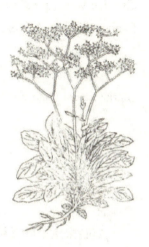

Xiezi Huacai ［蝎子花菜, limonium bicolor,

Limonium bicolor (Bag.) Kuntze], also named Gezaohua and Yebocai, grows in the fields. In the early growth period, its seedlings spread along the ground. Its leaves are like the acrospires of Bocai [菠菜, spinach, Spinacia oleracea L.] but much narrower and thinner than the latter. The ramose scapes grow out of the leaves with arris on them. It is more than one Chi high. Its flowers are small and white, and its leaves are bitter in taste.

For famine relief: Collect young leaves, blanch and rinse them, and flavor them with oil and salt.

97. 白 蒿

生荒野中。苗高二三尺。叶如细丝,似初生松针,色微青白,稍似艾香。味微辣。

救饥:采嫩苗叶煠熟,换水浸淘净,油盐调食。

97. Baihao [白蒿, virgate wormwood herb, Artemisia capillaris Thunb.]

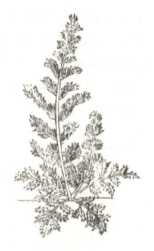

Baihao [白蒿, virgate wormwood herb, Artemisia capillaris Thunb.] grows in the wilderness. Its plants are about 2~3 Chi high. Its leaves are filament-like, and also like young pine needles with bluish white color. Its fragrance is like that of Ai [艾, mugwort, Artemisia argyi Levl. et Van.], and tastes slightly spicy.

For famine relief: Collect and blanch young leaves and seedlings, soak and elutriate them, and flavor them with oil and salt.

98. 野茼蒿

生荒野中。苗高二三尺。茎紫赤色。叶似白蒿,色微青黄;又似初生松针而葺细,味苦。

救饥:采嫩苗叶煠熟,换水浸淘净,油盐调食。

98. Yetonghao [野茼蒿, artemisia scoparia, Artemisia scoparia Waldst. et Kit.]

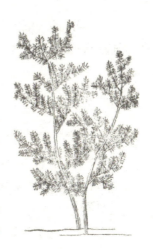

Yetonghao [野茼蒿, artemisia scoparia, Artemisia scoparia Waldst. et Kit.] grows in the wilderness. Its plants are about 2 ~ 3 Chi high with purplish red stems. Its leaves are like those of Baihao [白蒿, virgate wormwood herb, Artemisia capillaris Thunb.], bluish yellow in color, and also like young pine needles. It is bitter in taste.

For famine relief: Collect and blanch young leaves and seedlings, soak and elutriate them, and flavor them with oil and salt.

99. 野粉团儿

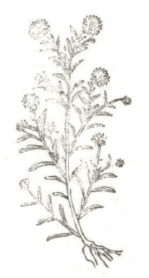

生田野中。苗高一二尺。茎似铁杆蒿茎。叶似独扫叶而小,上下稀疏。枝头分叉,开淡白花,黄心。味甜辣。

救饥:采嫩苗叶煤熟,水浸淘净,油盐调食。

99. Yefen Tuan'er [野粉团儿, kalimeris integrifolia, Kalimeris integrifolia Turcz. ex DC.]

Yefen Tuan'er [野粉团儿, kalimeris integrifolia, Kalimeris integrifolia Turcz. ex DC.] grows in the fields. Its plants are about 1 ~ 2 Chi high. Its stems are like those of Tieganhao [铁杆蒿, sacrorum, Artemisia sacrorum Ledeb.]. Its leaves are like those of Dusao [独扫, kochia scoparia, Kochia scoparia (L.) Schrad.] but much smaller than the latter, sparsely distributing on the upper and basal part of stems. It is divaricated from the top of branches. Its flowers are pale white with yellow stamens. It is sweet and spicy in taste.

For famine relief: Collect young leaves and seedlings, blanch, soak and elutriate them, and flavor them with oil and salt.

100. 蚵蛅菜

生密县山野中。科苗高二三尺许。叶似连翘叶微长；又似金银花[1]叶而尖，纹皱却少，边有小锯齿。开粉紫花，黄心。叶味甜。

救饥：采嫩苗叶煤熟，水浸，淘净，油盐调食。

【注释】

[1] 见本书239金银花条。

100. Hebocai〔蚵蛅菜, common carpesium root and leaf, Carpesium abrotanoides L.〕

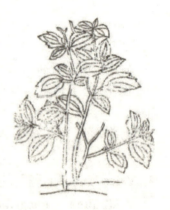

Hebocai〔蚵蛅菜, common carpesium root and leaf, Carpesium abrotanoides L.〕grows in the mountainous regions and fields of Mixian County. Its plants are about 2－3 Chi high. Its leaves are like those of Lianqiao〔连翘, weeping forsythia, Forsythia suspensa (Thunb.) Vahl〕but a little longer than the latter, or like those of Jinyinhua[1]〔金银花, honeysuckle, Lonicera japonica Thunb.〕but sharper and less rugose than the latter with irregular mucronulate-dentate margin. It blooms pinkish purple flowers with yellow stamens. Its leaves are sweet in taste.

For famine relief: Collect young leaves and seedlings, blanch, soak and elutriate them, and flavor them with oil and salt.

【Notes】

[1] See the 239th clause of this book.

101. 狗掉尾苗

生南阳府[1]马鞍山中。苗长二三尺。拖蔓而生，茎方，色青。其叶似歪头菜叶，稍大而尖艄，色深绿，纹脉微多；又似狗筋蔓[2]叶。稍间开五瓣小白花，黄心，众花攒开，其状如穗。叶味微酸。

救饥：采嫩叶煠熟，换水浸去酸味，淘净，油盐调食。

【注释】

[1] 明代府名，今河南南阳市。

[2] 见本书第138 狗筋蔓条。

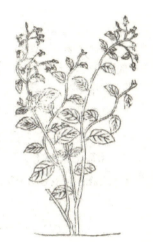

101. Goudiaowei Miao [狗掉尾苗, herba solani, Solanum lyratum Thunb.]

Goudiaowei Miao [狗掉尾苗, herba solani, Solanum lyratum Thunb.] grows in Mount Ma'an of Nanyang[1]. Its plants are about 2~3 Chi high with its vines trailing along the ground. Its scandent stems are squre in shape and green in color. Its dark green leaves are like those of Waitoucai [歪头菜, unijuga, Vicia unijuga A. Br.] but longer and sharper with more leaf veins, and also like those of Goujinman[2] [狗筋蔓, baccifera, Cucubalus baccifer L.]. Its tiny white flowers stand among branches and leaves, with five patals and yellow stamens. The spicate flowers always assemble together and the leaves taste slightly sour.

For famine relief: Collect and blanch young leaves, remove the sourness by soaking them in water, and flavor them with oil and salt.

[Notes]

[1] Prefecture in Ming Dynasty. It is presently located in Nanyang City of Henan Province.

[2] See the 138th clause of this book.

102. 石 芥

生辉县鸦子口山谷中。苗高一二尺。叶似地棠菜叶而阔短,每三叶或五叶攒生一处。开淡黄花。结黑子。苗叶味苦,微辣。

救饥:采嫩叶煤熟,换水浸去苦味,油盐调食。

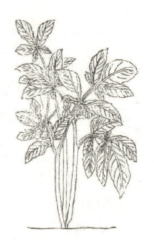

102. Shijie〔石芥, cardamine leucantha, Cardamine leucantha (Tausch) O. E. Schulz〕

Shijie〔石芥, cardamine leucantha, Cardamine leucantha (Tausch) O. E. Schulz〕grows in the valleys of Yazikou in Huixian County. Its plants are about 1~2 Chi high. Its leaves are like those of Ditangcai〔地棠菜, figwort root, Scrophularia ningpoensis Hemsl.〕but shorter and broader, with 3~5 leaves growing together (compound leaves). It bears light yellow flowers and black seeds. Its plants and leaves are bitter and slightly spicy in taste.

For famine relief: Collect and blanch young leaves, remove the bitterness by soaking them in water, and flavor them with oil and salt.

103. 獾耳菜

生中牟平野中。苗长尺余。茎多枝叉,其茎上有细线楞。叶似竹叶而短小,亦软;又似蓄叶,却颇阔大而又尖。茎叶俱有微毛。开小黪白花。结细灰青子。苗叶味甘。

救饥:采嫩苗叶煤熟,水浸淘净,油盐调食。

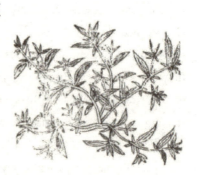

103. Huan'ercai〔獾耳菜, lithospermum arvense, Lithospermum arvense L.〕

Huan'ercai〔獾耳菜, lithospermum arvense, Lithospermum arvense L.〕

grows in the fields of Zhongmu County. Its plants are more than one Chi high. Its stems are ramose with lines and ridges on them. Its leaves are like those of a bamboo but shorter and softer, and also like those of Bianxu [萹蓄, grass of common knot Grass, Polygonum aviculare L.] but broader and sharper. Both its stems and leaves are short and strigose. It bears greyish-white flowers and greyish-green nutlets. Its plants and leaves are sweet in taste.

For famine relief: Collect and blanch seedlings and leaves, soak and rinse them, and flavor them with oil and salt.

104. 回回蒜

一名水胡椒，又名蝎虎草。生水边下湿地。苗高一尺许。叶似野艾蒿而硬，又甚花叉；又似前胡叶颇大，亦多花叉。苗茎稍头开五瓣黄花。结穗如初生桑椹子[1]而小；又似初生苍耳[2]实亦小，色青，味极辛辣。其叶味甜。

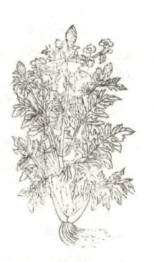

救饥：采叶煠熟，换水浸淘净，油盐调食。子可捣烂调菜用。

【注释】

［1］桑的果实。见本书第323桑椹树条。

［2］见本书第209苍耳条。

104. Huihuisuan〔回回蒜, Chinese buttercup herb, Ranunculus chinensis Bunge〕

Huihuisuan〔回回蒜, Chinese buttercup herb, Ranunculus chinensis Bunge〕, also named Shuihujiao and Xiehucao, grows in the low-lying wetlands along the waterside. Its plants are about one Chi high. Its multifid leaves are like those of wild mugworts but harder, and also like those of Qianhu〔前胡, radix peucedani, Peucedanum praeruptorum Dunn〕 but bigger. Each of its flowers, on the tip of stems and branches, is yellow with 5 petals. The green aggregate fruit is like young Sangshenzi[1] but smaller, and also like the fruit of Cang'er[2]〔苍耳,

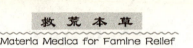

xanthium sibiricum, Xanthium sibiricum Patrin ex Widder] but smaller, and tastes very hot. Its leaves are sweet in taste.

For famine relief: Collect and blanch leaves, soak and elutriate them, and favor them with oil and salt. The pounded seeds can be used as condiment.

【Notes】

[1] It refers to the fruit of Sang [桑, mulberry, Morus alba L.]. See the 323th clause of this book.

[2] See the 209th clause of this book.

105. 地槐菜

一名小虫儿麦。生荒野中。苗高四五寸。叶似石竹子叶,极细短。开小黄白花。结小黑子。其叶味甜。

救饥:采叶煠熟,水浸淘净,油盐调食。

105. Dihuaicai [地槐菜, herba phyllanthi urinariae, Phyllanthus urinaria L.]

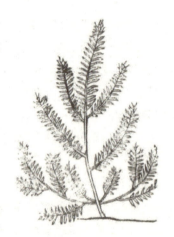

Dihuaicai [地槐菜, herba phyllanthi urinariae, Phyllanthus urinaria L.], also named Xiaochong'er Mai, grows in the wilderness. Its plants are about 4~5 Cun high. Its leaves, like those of Shizhuzi [石竹子, Chinese pink, Dianthus chinensis L.], are extremely thin and short. Its flowers are yellowish-white and its fruit is black. Its leaves are sweet in taste.

For famine relief: Collect and blanch leaves, soak and elutriate them, and flavor them with oil and salt.

106. 螺黡儿

一名地桑,又名痢见草。生荒野中。茎微红。叶似野人苋叶,微长窄而尖。开花作赤色,小细穗儿。其叶味甘。

救饥：采苗叶煠熟，水浸淘去邪味，油盐调食。

治病：今人传说治痢疾[1]，采苗用水煮服，甚效。

【注释】

[1]病症名。古代对痢疾的论述，范围较广，除包括菌痢和阿米巴痢疾外，还包括其他某些肠道疾病在内，主要症状为腹泻。

106. Luoyan'er［螺黡儿，copperleaf herb，Acalypha australis L.］

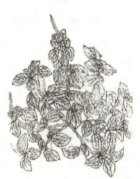

Luoyan'er［螺黡儿，copperleaf herb，Acalypha australis L.］, also named Disang or Lijiancao, grows in the wilderness. Its stems are reddish and its leaves are like those of wild Renxian［人苋，velvet flower，Amaranthus caudatus］but longer, narrower and sharper. Its inflorescences are spicate, red and thin, and its leaves are sweet in taste.

For famine relief：Collect and blanch leaves and seedlings, remove the strange taste by soaking and rinsing them in water, and flavor them with oil and salt.

For disease treatment：Presently it has good efficacy to treat dysentery[1] by decocting.

【Notes】

[1] Disease name. With the diarrhea as the main symptom, dysentery also includes many other intestinal diseases except bacillary dysentery and amoebic dysentery in ancient China.

107. 泥胡菜

生田野中。苗高一二尺，茎梗繁多。叶似水芥菜叶颇大，花叉甚深；又似风花菜叶，却比短小。叶中撺葶，分生茎叉，稍间开淡紫花，似刺蓟花。苗叶味辣。

救饥：采嫩苗叶煠熟，水浸淘净，油盐调食。

107. Nihucai［泥胡菜, hemistepta lyrata, Hemisteptia lyrata（Bunge）Fischer & C. A. Meyer］

Nihucai［泥胡菜, hemistepta lyrata, Hemisteptia lyrata（Bunge）Fischer & C. A. Meyer］grows in the fields. Its plants are about 1～2 Chi high with ramose stems. Its leaves are pinnatisect like those of Shuijiecai［水芥菜, rorippa islandica, Rorippa palustris（Linnaeus）Besser］but much bigger, and also like those of Fenghuacai［风花菜, rorippa palustris, Rorippa globosa（Turcz.）Hayek］but shorter and smaller. Its scapes draw out of leaves, branches, bearing lilac flowers which are like those of Ciji［刺蓟, field thistle herb, Herba Cirsii］. Its plants and leaves are spicy in taste.

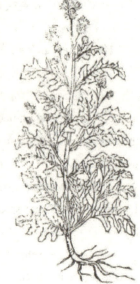

For famine relief: Collect and blanch seedlings and leaves, soak and rinse them, and flavor them with oil and salt.

108. 兔儿丝

生田野中。其苗就地拖蔓。节间生叶，如指顶大，叶边似云头样。开小黄花。苗叶味甜。

救饥：采嫩苗叶煠熟，水浸淘净，油盐调食。

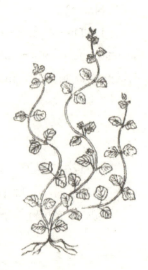

108. Tu'ersi［兔儿丝, lysimachia christinae, Lysimachia christinae Hance］

Tu'ersi［兔儿丝, lysimachia christinae, Lysimachia christinae Hance］grows in the fields with its tendrils trailing along the ground. Its leaves, scattering on the nodes, are as big as fingertips with sinuate margin. Its flowers are tiny and yellow. Its plants and leaves are sweet in taste.

For famine relief: Collect and blanch seedlings and leaves, soak and rinse them, and flavor them with oil and salt.

109. 老鹳筋

生田野中。就地拖秧而生,茎微紫色,茎叉繁稠。叶似园荽叶而头不尖;又似野胡萝卜叶而短小。叶间开五瓣小黄花。味甜。

救饥:采嫩苗叶煠熟,水浸去邪味,淘洗净,油盐调食。

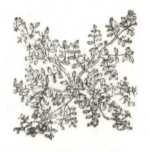

109. Laoguanjin〔老鹳筋, potentilla supina, Potentilla supina L.〕

Laoguanjin〔老鹳筋, potentilla supina, Potentilla supina L.〕grows in the fields. Its procumbent stems are pale lilac and ramose. It leaves are like those of Yuansui〔园荽, coriander herb, Coriandrum sativum L.〕with the apex less sharp, and also like those of Ye Huluobo〔野胡萝卜, wild carrot, Daucus carota L.〕but shorter and smaller. Each of its tiny flowers is yellow with 5 linear petals. It is sweet in taste.

For famine relief: Collect and blanch seedlings and leaves, remove the strange taste by soaking them in water, elutriate them, and flavor them with oil and salt.

110. 绞股蓝

生田野中,延蔓而生。叶似小蓝[1]叶,短小软薄,边有锯齿;又似痢见草[2]叶,亦软,淡绿,五叶攒生一处。开小黄花,又有开白花者。结子如豌豆大,生则青色,熟则紫黑色。叶味甜。

救饥:采叶煠熟,水浸去邪味涎沫,淘洗净,油盐调食。

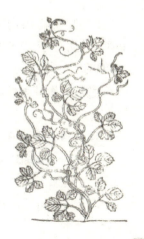

【注释】

［1］疑指蓼科蓼属蓼蓝。

［2］螺厣儿的别名。见本书第105螺厣儿条。

110. Jiaogulan［绞股蓝，Japanese cayratia herb，Cayratia japonica (Thunb.) Gagnep.］

Jiaogulan［绞股蓝，Japanese cayratia herb，Cayratia japonica (Thunb.) Gagnep.］grows in the fields with its vines creeping along the ground. Its leaves are like those of Xiaolan[1], short, soft and thin, with serrated edge, and also like those of Lijiancao[2], soft and pale green, with 5 leaves growing together (compound leaves). Its tiny flowers are yellow or white. Its fruit is as big as the pea, green when unripe and purple-black when ripe. Its leaves taste sweet.

For famine relief: Collect and blanch leaves, remove the strange taste and foam by soaking them, rinse them, and flavor them with oil and salt.

【Notes】

［1］It might refer to Liaolan［蓼蓝，indigo plant，Polygonum tinctorium Ait.］

［2］Another name for Luoyan'er［螺厣儿，copperleaf herb，Acalypha australis L.］. See the 105th clause of this book.

111. 山梗菜

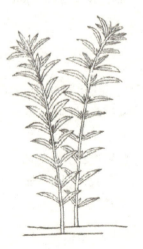

生郑州贾峪山山野中。苗高二尺许。茎淡紫色。叶似桃叶而短小，又似柳叶菜叶亦小。稍间开淡紫花。其叶味甜。

救饥：采嫩叶煠熟，淘洗净，油盐调食。

111. Shangengcai［山梗菜，lobelia sessilifolia，Lobelia sessilifolia Lamb.］

Shangengcai［山梗菜，lobelia sessilifolia，Lobelia

sessilifolia Lamb.] grows in Jiayu Mountain of Zhengzhou. Its plants are about 2 Chi high with lilac stems. Its leaves are like peach leaves but shorter and smaller, and also like salix leaves but smaller. Its flowers are lilac and its leaves are sweet in taste.

For famine relief: Collect and blanch young leaves, rinse them, and flavor them with oil and salt.

112. 拂娘蒿

生田野中。苗高二尺许。茎似黄蒿茎。其叶碎小,茸细如针,色颇黄绿,嫩则可食,老则为柴。苗叶味苦。

救饥:采嫩苗叶煠熟,换水浸淘,去蒿气,油盐调食。

112. Bunianghao [拂娘蒿, descurainia sophia, Descurainia sophia (L.) Webb ex Prantl]

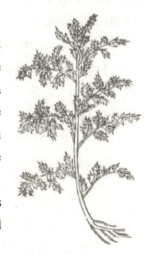

Bunianghao [拂娘蒿, descurainia sophia, Descurainia sophia (L.) Webb ex Prantl], growing in the fields, is about two Chi high. Its stems are like those of Huanghao [黄蒿, artemisia scoparia, Artemisia scoparia Waldst. et Kit.]. Its yellow-green leaves are tiny and downy, slender like needle, used for food when tender and firewood when old. Its plants and leaves are bitter in taste.

For famine relief: Collect and blanch young leaves and seedlings, remove the bitterness by soaking and elutriating them, and flavor them with oil and salt.

113. 鸡肠菜

生南阳府马鞍山荒野中。苗高二尺许。茎方,色紫。其叶对生,叶似菱[1]叶样,而无花叉;又似小灰菜[2]叶,形样微扁。开粉红花。结碗子蒴儿。叶味甜。

救饥:采苗叶煠熟,水淘净,油盐调食。

【注释】

[1] 见本书第 355 菱角条。

[2] 见本书第 412 灰菜条。

113. Jichangcai［鸡肠菜, salvia umbratica, Salvia umbratica Hance］

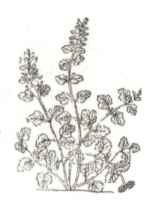

Jichangcai［鸡肠菜, salvia umbratica, Salvia umbratica Hance］grows in the wilderness of Mount Ma'an in Nanyang. Its plants are about two Chi high with quadrangular purple stems. Its opposite leaves are like those of Ling[1]［菱, water chestnut, Trapa bispinosa Roxb.］with no lobes, and also like those of Huicai[2]［灰菜, lamb's-quarters, Chenopodium album L.］but slightly oblate. Its flowers are pink and its fruit is elliptical. Its leaves taste sweet.

For famine relief: Collect plants and leaves, blanch and rinse them, and flavor them with oil and salt.

【Notes】

[1] See the 355th clause of this book.

[2] See the 412th clause of this book.

114. 水葫芦苗

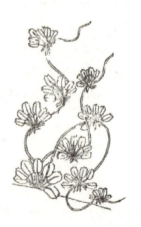

生水边。就地拖蔓而生。每节间生四叶,而叶如指顶大。其叶尖上皆作三叉,味甘。

救饥:采叶连嫩秧煠熟,水浸淘净,油盐调食。

114. Shuihulu Miao [水葫芦苗, halerpestes cymbalaris, Halerpestes sarmentosa var. multisecta (S. H. Li & Y. H. Huang) W. T. Wang]

Shuihulu Miao [水葫芦苗, halerpestes cymbalaris, Halerpestes sarmentosa var. multisecta (S. H. Li & Y. H. Huang) W. T. Wang] grows along the waterside and creeps on the ground. There are 4 leaf blades which are as big as a fingertip at each internode. Its leaves are always 3-partite and sweet in taste.

For famine relief: Collect and blanch seedlings and leaves, soak and elutriate them, and flavor them with oil and salt.

115. 胡苍耳

又名回回苍耳。生田野中。叶似皂荚[1]叶微长大;又似望江南[2]叶而小,颇硬,色微淡绿。茎有线楞。结实如苍耳[3]实,但长鞘,味微苦。

救饥:采嫩苗叶煠熟,水浸去苦味,淘净,油盐调食。

治病:今人传说,治诸般疮[4],采叶用好酒熬吃,消肿。

【注释】

[1] 见本书第309皂荚树条。
[2] 见本书第240望江南条。
[3] 见本书第209苍耳条。
[4] 病症名。皮肤感染与肌肤创伤等的总称。

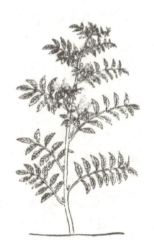

115. Hucang'er [胡苍耳, gycyrrhiza pallidilora, Glycyrrhiza pallidiflora Maxim.]

Hucang'er [胡苍耳, gycyrrhiza pallidilora, Glycyrrhiza pallidiflora Maxim.], also named Huihui Cang'er, grows in the fields. Its pale green leaves are like those of Zaojia[1][皂荚, Chinese honey locust, Gleditsia sinensis Lam.] but a little longer, and also like those of Wangjiangnan[2][望江南, coffee senna, Cassia occidentalis Linn.] but smaller and harder. Its stems are striped. Its fruit is like those of Cang'er[3][苍耳, Siberian cocklebur, Xanthium sibiricum Patrin ex Widder] but longer and sharper with the slightly bitter taste.

For famine relief: Collect and blanch seedlings and leaves, remove the bitterness by soaking them in water, elutriate them, and flavor them with oil and salt.

For disease treatment: Presently it is said to treat all kinds of sores[4]. It can subside the swelling by stewing with wine.

【Notes】

[1] See the 309th clause of this book.

[2] See the 240th clause of this book.

[3] See the 209th clause of this book.

[4] Disease name. It is a general term for pyogenic skin infections and wounds.

116. 水棘针苗

又名山油子。生田野中。苗高一二尺。茎方四楞,对分茎叉,叶亦对生。其叶似荆[1]叶而软,锯齿尖叶,茎叶紫绿。开小紫碧花。叶味辛辣、微甜,性温。

救饥:采苗叶煠熟,水淘洗净,油盐调食。

【注释】

[1] 见本书第290荆子条。

116. Shuijizhen Miao [水棘针苗, amethystea coerulea, Amethystea caerulea L.]

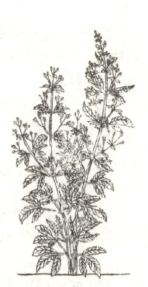

Shuijizhen Miao [水棘针苗, amethystea coerulea, Amethystea caerulea L.], also named Shanyouzi, grows in the fields. Its plants are 1~2 Chi high with quadrangular stems. Both the scapes and leaves are opposite. Its leaves are like those of Jing[1] [荆, vitex negundo, Vitex negundo L.] but softer, which are acuminate with serrate margin. Both the stems and leaves are purplish green. The tiny flowers are purplish blue. Its leaves taste pungent and spicy, slightly sweet, and warm in nature.

For famine relief: Collect plants and leaves, blanch and elutriate them, and flavor them with oil and salt.

【Notes】

[1] See the 290th clause of this book.

117. 沙 蓬

又名鸡爪菜。生田野中。苗高一尺余。初就地婆娑生,后分茎叉。其茎有细线楞。叶似独扫叶,狭窄而厚;又似石竹子叶,亦窄。茎叶稍间结小青子,小如粟粒。其叶味甘,性温。

救饥:采苗叶煠熟,水浸,淘净,油盐调食。

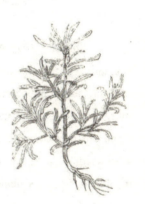

117. Shapeng [沙蓬, corispermum puberulum, Corispermum puberulum Iljin]

Shapeng [沙蓬, corispermum puberulum, Corispermum puberulum Iljin], also named Jizhuacai, grows in the fields. Its plants are more than one Chi high. In the early growth period, its plants bend and extend to the ground, and then produce shoots later. There are fine strips on the stems. Its leaves are like those of Dusao [独扫, kochia scoparia, Kochia scoparia (L.) Schrad.] but narrower and thicker, or like those of Shizhuzi [石竹子, Chinese pink, Dianthus chinensis L.] but narrower. Its green fruit, as big as chestnut, stands out of branches and leaves. Its leaves are sweet in taste and warm in nature.

For famine relief: Collect and blanch plants and leaves, soak and elutriate them, and flavor them with oil and salt.

118. 麦蓝菜

生田野中。茎叶俱深葾苣色,叶似大蓝稍叶而小,颇尖。其叶抱茎对生。每一叶间撺生一叉,茎叉稍头开小肉红花。结蒴,有子似小桃红子。苗叶味微苦。

救饥:采嫩苗叶煤熟,水浸淘净,油盐调食。

118. Mailancai [麦蓝菜, vaccaria pyramidata, Vaccaria segetalis]

Mailancai [麦蓝菜, vaccaria pyramidata, Vaccaria segetalis] grows in the fields with gray-green stems and leaves. Its leaves, opposite and amplexicaul, are like the apical leaves of Dalan [大蓝, isatis indigotica fort, Isatis indigotica Fortune] but much smaller and sharper. Its scapes stand out of axils and bear carnation tiny flowers on the top. It bears capsules, with seeds like those of Xiaotaohong [小桃红, flowering plum, Amygdalus triloba] inside. Its plants and leaves are slightly bitter in taste.

For famine relief: Collect and blanch seedlings and leaves, soak and elutriate them, and flavor them with oil and salt.

119. 女娄菜

生密县韶华山山谷中。苗高一二尺。茎叉相对分生。叶似旋覆花叶,颇短,色微深绿,抱茎对生。稍间出青蓇葖,开花微吐白蕊。结实青,子如枸杞[1]微小。其叶味苦。

救饥:采嫩苗叶煤熟,换水浸去苦味,淘净,油盐调食。

【注释】

[1] 见本书第307枸杞条。

119. Nvloucai [女娄菜, sunward melandrium herb, Silene firma Sieb. et Zucc. var. pubescens (Makino) S. Y. He]

Nvloucai [女娄菜, sunward melandrium herb, Silene firma Sieb. et Zucc. var. pubescens (Makino) S. Y. He] grows in the valleys of Shaohua Mountain in Mixian County. Its plants are 1~2 Chi high, with opposite bracts and scapes. Its dark green leaves, like those of Xuanfuhua [旋覆花, inula flower, Inula japonica Thunb.] but shorter, scatter oppositely along the stems. It bears green alabastrum and the white petals stick out of the calyx after blooming. Its fruit is green, and its seeds are like but a little smaller than Gouqi[1] [枸杞, wolfberry, Lycium chinense Mill.]. Its leaves are bitter in taste.

For famine relief: Collect and blanch seedlings and leaves, remove the bitterness by soaking them in water, elutriate them, and flavor them with oil and salt.

【Notes】

[1] See the 307th clause of this book.

120. 委陵菜

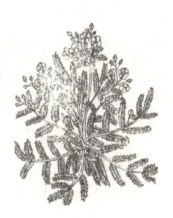

一名翻白菜。生田野中。苗初揭地生，后分茎叉，茎节稠密，上有白毛。叶仿佛类柏[1]叶，而极阔大，边如锯齿形，面青背白；又似鸡腿儿[2]叶而却窄；又类鹿蕨[3]叶亦窄。茎叶稍间开五瓣黄花。其叶味苦、微辣。

救饥：采苗叶煠熟，水浸淘净，油盐调食。

【注释】

[1] 见本书第308柏树条。

[2] 见本书第181鸡腿儿条。

[3] 见本书第133鹿蕨菜条。

120. Weilingcai [委陵菜, Chinese cinquefoil, Potentilla chinensis Ser.]

Weilingcai [委陵菜, Chinese cinquefoil, Potentilla chinensis Ser.], also named Fanbaicai, grows in the fields. In the early growth period, its seedlings spread along the ground. Its stems covered with white downs draw out branches with more nodes later. Its leaves are like those of Bai[1] [柏, cypress, Platycladus orientalis (L.) Franco] but broader with serrated edge, adaxially green and abaxially white, and also like but narrower than those of Jitui'er[2] [鸡腿儿, potentilla discolor, Potentilla discolor Bge.], or like those of Lujue[3] [鹿蕨, fern, Pteridium aquilinum (L.) Kuhn var. latiusculum (Desv.) Underw. ex Heller] but narrower. Each of its yellow flowers with 5 petals is bloomed among branches and leaves. Its plants and leaves are bitter and slightly pungent in taste.

For famine relief: Collect and blanch plants and leaves, soak and elutriate them, and flavor them with oil and salt.

【Notes】

[1] See the 308th clause of this book.

[2] See the 181th clause of this book.

[3] See the 133th clause of this book.

121. 独行菜

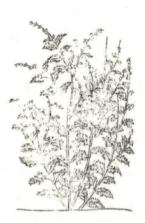

又名麦秸菜。生田野中。科苗高一尺许。叶似水棘针[1]叶,微短小;又似水苏子叶,亦短小狭窄,作瓦陇样。稍出细葶,开小黪白花。结小青蓇葖,小如绿豆粒。叶味甜,性温。

救饥:采嫩苗叶煤熟,换水淘净,油盐调食。

【注释】

[1] 见本书第116水棘针苗条。

121. Duxingcai [独行菜, garden cress, Lepidium apetalum Willd.]

Duxingcai [独行菜, garden cress, Lepidium apetalum Willd.], also named Maijiecai, grows in the fields. Its plants are about one Chi high. Its leaves are like those of Shuijizhen[1] [水棘针, amethystea coerulea, Amethystea caerulea L.] but a little shorter, and also like those of Shuisu [水苏, woundwort, Stachys japonica Miq.] but shorter and narrower, in the shape of tile ridges. The slender scapes which draw out of branches bear tiny greyish-white flowers. Its green follicles are as big as mung beans. Its leaves are sweet in taste and warm in nature.

For famine relief: Collect and blanch seedlings and leaves, elutriate them, and flavor them with oil and salt.

【Notes】

[1] See the 116th clause of this book.

122. 山 蓼

生密县山野间。苗高一二尺。叶似芍药叶而长，细窄；又似野菊花叶而硬厚；又似水胡椒[1]叶亦硬。开碎瓣白花。其叶味微辣。

救饥：采嫩叶煠熟，换水浸去辣气，作成黄色，淘洗净，油盐调食。

【注释】

[1] 回回蒜的别名，见本书第104回回蒜条。

122. Shanliao [山蓼, cematis flammula, Clematis hexapetala Pall.]

Shanliao [山蓼, cematis flammula, Clematis hexapetala Pall.] grows in the mountainous regions and fields of Mixian County. Its plants are about 1~2 Chi high. Its leaves are like those of Shaoyao [芍药, Chinese herbaceous peony, Paeonia lactiflora Pall.] but longer and narrower, and also like those of Yejuhua

[野菊花, wild chrysanthemum flower, Dendranthema indicum (L.) Des Moul.] and Shuihujiao[1] but harder and thicker. It bears white flowers with very small petals. Its leaves are slightly spicy in taste.

For famine relief: Collect and blanch young leaves, remove the spicy taste by soaking them in water, elutriate them when they turn yellow, and flavor them with oil and salt.

【Notes】

[1] Another name for Huihuisuan [回回蒜, Chinese buttercup herb, Ranunculus chinensis Bunge]. See the 104th clause of this book.

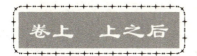

草 部

叶可食

新增

Volume 1　The Second Half
Herbaceous Plant
Leaf Edible
New Supplements

123. 花 蒿

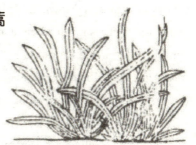

生荒野中。苗叶就地丛生。叶长三四寸,四散分垂。叶似独扫叶而长硬,其头颇齐,微有毛涩,味微辛。

救饥:采叶煠熟,水浸淘净,油盐调食。

123. Huahao [花蒿, scorzonera austriaca wild, Scorzonera austriaca Willd.]

Huahao [花蒿, scorzonera austriaca wild, Scorzonera austriaca Willd.] grows in the wilderness and clusters on the ground. Its leaves, 3~4 Cun long, scattered and sprawling, are like those of Dusao [独扫, kochia scoparia, Kochia scoparia (L.) Schrad.] but longer and harder with obtuse apex, strigillose, slightly spicy in taste.

For famine relief: Collect and blanch leaves, soak and elutriate them, and

flavor them with oil and salt.

124. 葛公菜

生密县韶华山山谷间。苗高二三尺。茎方,棱面四楞,对分茎叉。叶亦对生,叶似苏子[1]叶而小;又似荏子叶而大。梢间开粉红花。结子如小米粒而茶褐色。其叶味甜,微苦。

救饥:采叶煠熟,水浸去苦味,换水淘净,油盐调食。

【注释】

[1]见本书第342苏子苗条。

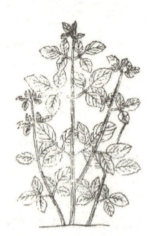

124. Gegongcai [葛公菜, danshen root, Salvia miltiorrhiza Bunge]

Gegongcai [葛公菜, danshen root, Salvia miltiorrhiza Bunge] grows in the valleys of Shaohua Mountain in Mixian County. Its plants are about 2~3 Chi high. Its stems are quadrangular, sulcate, much branched and opposite. Its opposite odd-pinnatels are like those of Suzi[1] [苏子, purple perilla, Perilla frutescens (L.) Britt.] but smaller, or like those of Renzi but much bigger. Its flowers are pinks, and its elliptic nutlets are dark brown. Its leaves are sweet and slightly bitter in taste.

For famine relief: Collect and blanch leaves, remove the bitterness by soaking them in water, elutriate them, and flavor them with oil and salt.

【Notes】

[1] See the 342th clause of this book.

125. 鲫鱼鳞

生密县韶华山山野中。苗高一二尺。茎方而茶褐色,对分茎叉。叶亦对生,叶似鸡肠菜叶颇大;又似桔梗叶而微软薄,叶面却微纹皱。梢间开粉红花。结子

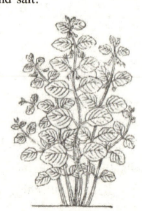

如小粟粒而茶褐色。其叶味甜。

救饥：采叶煤熟，水浸淘净，油盐调食。

125. Jiyulin［鲫鱼鳞，caryopteris terniflora，Caryopteris terniflora Maxim.］

Jiyulin［鲫鱼鳞, caryopteris terniflora, Caryopteris terniflora Maxim.］ grows in the valleys of Shaohua Mountain in Mixian County. Its plants are about 1~2 Chi high. Its stems are quadrangular and dark brown, with opposite shoots and leaves. Its leaves are like those of Jichangcai［鸡肠菜, salvia umbratica, Salvia umbratica Hance］ but much bigger, and also like those of Jiegeng［桔梗, platycodon root, Platycodon grandiflorus (Jacq.) A. DC.］ but a little softer and thinner with rugula on them. Its flowers are pinks, and its ovoid nutlets are dark brown. Its leaves are sweet in taste.

For famine relief: Collect and blanch leaves, soak and elutriate them, and flavor them with oil and salt.

126. 尖刀儿苗

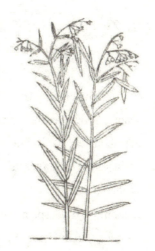

生密县梁家冲山野中。苗高二三尺。叶似细柳叶，更又细长而尖。叶皆两两抪茎对生。叶间开淡黄花。结尖角儿，长二寸许，粗如萝卜角，中有白穰及小扁黑子。其叶味甘。

救饥：采叶煤熟，水淘洗净，油盐调食。

126. Jiandao'er Miao［尖刀儿苗, paniculate swallowwort root, Cynanchum paniculatum（Bunge）Kitag.］

Jiandao'er Miao［尖刀儿苗, paniculate swallowwort root, Cynanchum paniculatum (Bunge) Kitag.］ grows in the mountainous regions and fields in Liangjiachong of Mixian County. Its plants are about 2~3 Chi high. Its leaves are like willow leaves but slenderer and sharper. Its leaves are opposite and scatter along stems. It bears yellowish green flowers among leaves. The follicles, about two Cun long, are as big as the siliques of radishes. Its black seeds are tiny and flat which are covered with white coma. Its leaves are sweet in taste.

For famine relief: Collect and blanch leaves, elutriate them, and flavor them with oil and salt.

127. 珍珠菜

生密县山野中。苗高二尺许。茎似蒿秆,微带红色。其叶状似柳叶而极细小;又似地稍瓜[1]叶。梢头出穗,状类鼠尾草[2]穗,开白花。结子小如绿豆粒,黄褐色。叶味苦涩。

救饥:采叶煠熟,换水浸去涩味,淘净,油盐调食。

【注释】

[1] 见本书第205地稍瓜条。

[2] 鼠菊的本草名。见本书第28鼠菊条。

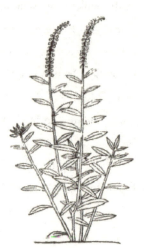

127. Zhenzhucai [珍珠菜, lysimachia clethroide duby, Lysimachia clethroides Duby]

Zhenzhucai [珍珠菜, lysimachia clethroide duby, Lysimachia clethroides Duby] grows in the mountainous regions and fields of Mixian County. Its plants are about two Chi high with dull red stems which are like those of Chrysanthemum carinatum. Its leaves are like the willow leaves but slenderer, and also like those of Dishaogua[1] [地稍瓜, cynanchum thesioides, Cynanchum thesioides (Freyn) K. Schum.]. The spica, which is like that of Shuweicao[2] [鼠尾草, European verbena herb, Herba Verbenae], stands on the top of stems with white flowers. The capsule, like mung bean, is subglobose and yellowish-brown. Its leaves are bitter and astringent in taste.

For famine relief: Collect and blanch leaves, remove the astringent flavor by soaking them in water, and flavor them with oil and salt.

[Notes]

[1] See the 205th clause of this book.

[2] The scientific name of Shuju [鼠菊, European verbena herb, Herba Verbenae]. See the 28th clause of this book.

128. 杜当归

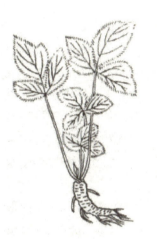

生密县山野中。苗高一尺许。茎圆而有线楞。叶似山芹菜[1]叶而硬,边有细锯齿刺;又似苍术[2]叶而大,每三叶攒生一处。开黄花。根似前胡根;又似野胡萝卜[3]根。其叶味甜。

救饥:采叶煠熟,水浸作成黄色,换水淘洗净,油盐调食。

治病:今人遇当归缺,以此药代之。

【注释】

[1] 见本书第 134 山芹菜条。

[2] 见本书第 171 苍术条。

[3] 见本书第 175 野胡萝卜条。

128. Dudanggui [杜当归, aralia cordata, Aralia continentalis Kitagawa]

Dudanggui [杜当归, aralia cordata, Aralia continentalis Kitagawa] grows in the mountainous regions and fields of Mixian County. Its plants are about one Chi high, and its stems are columniform and striped. Its leaves are like those of Shanqincai[1] [山芹菜, sanicle, Sanicula chiensis Bunge] but harder, with serrated edge, and also like but larger than those of Cangzhu[2] [苍术, atractylodes rhizome, Atractylodes Lancea (Thunb.) DC.] 3-pinnately compound. It blooms yellow flowers. Its roots are like those of Qianhu [前胡, radix peucedani, Peucedanum praeruptorum Dunn] or Ye Huluobo[3] [野胡萝卜, wild carrot, Daucus carota L.], and its leaves are sweet in taste.

For famine relief: Collect and blanch leaves, make them turn yellow by soaking them in water, elutriate them, and flavor them with oil and salt.

For disease treatment: Presently it is used as the substitute of Danggui [当归, Chinese angelica, Angelica sinensis (Oliv.) Diels].

【Notes】

[1] See the 134th clause of this book.

[2] See the 171th clause of this book.

[3] See the 175th clause of this book.

129. 风轮菜

生密县山野中。苗高二尺余。方茎四楞,色淡绿微白。叶似荏子叶而小;又似威灵仙叶微宽,边有锯齿叉,两叶对生,而叶节间又生子叶极小,四叶相攒对生。开淡粉红花。其叶味苦。

救饥:采叶煤熟,水浸去邪味,淘洗净,油盐调食。

129. Fengluncai [风轮菜, Clinopodium chinense, Clinopodium chinense (Benth.) O. Ktze.]

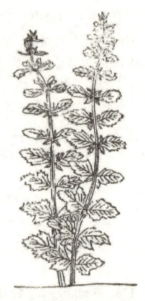

Fengluncai [风轮菜, Clinopodium chinense, Clinopodium chinense (Benth.) O. Ktze.] grows in the mountainous regions and fields of Mixian County. Its plants are more than two Chi high, and its quadrangular stems are whitish and light green. Its leaves are like but smaller than those of Renzi, and also like those of Weilingxian [威灵仙, Clematis Root, Radix Clematidis Chinese] but a little broader with crenate margin. Two opposite bracts grow out from the axil of two opposite leaves, thus the four leaves oppositely grow together. Its flowers are pale purplish pink, and its leaves are bitter in taste.

For famine relief: Collect and blanch leaves, remove the abnormal taste by soaking them in water, elutriate them, and flavor them with oil and salt.

130. 拖白练苗

生田野中。苗搨地生。叶似垂盆草叶而又小。叶间开小白花。结细黄子。

其叶味甜。

救饥：采苗叶煠熟，油盐调食。

130. Tuobailian Miao [拖白练苗, sedum polytrichoides, Sedum polytrichoides Hemsl.]

Tuobailian Miao [拖白练苗, sedum polytrichoides, Sedum polytrichoides Hemsl.] grows in the fields and creeps on the ground. Its leaves are like but smaller than those of Chuipencao [垂盆草, stringy stonecrop herb, Sedum sarmentosum Bunge]. It bears tiny white flowers and small yellow fruit. Its leaves are sweet in taste.

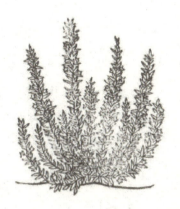

For famine relief: Collect and blanch plants and leaves, and flavor them with oil and salt.

131．透骨草

一名天芝麻。生中牟荒野中。苗高三四尺。茎方，窊面四楞，其茎脚紫，对节分生茎叉。叶似蒿叶而多花叉，叶皆对生。茎节间攒开粉红花。结子似胡麻子。叶味苦。

救饥：采嫩苗叶煠熟，水浸去苦味，淘净，油盐调食。

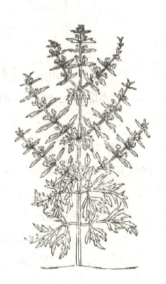

131. Tougucao [透骨草, motherwort herb, Leonurus artemisia (Laur.) S. Y. Hu]

Tougucao [透骨草, motherwort herb, Leonurus artemisia (Laur.) S. Y. Hu], also named Tianzhima, grows in the wilderness of Zhongmu. Its plants are about 3 ~ 4 Chi high. Its stems are quadrangular and shallowly sulcate, and its stem bases are purple. Both the branchlets and the leaves are opposite. Its palmatipartite leaves are like those of Lvhao [䕡蒿, seleng wormood, Artemisia selengensis Turcz. ex Bess.]. Its redish flowers assemble at internodes. Its nutlets are like semen lini and its leaves are bitter in taste.

For famine relief: Collect and blanch seedlings and leaves, remove the bitterness by soaking them in water, elutriate them, and flavor them with oil and salt.

132. 酸桶笋

生密县韶华山山涧边。初发笋叶,其后分生茎叉。科苗高四五尺。茎秆似水荭茎而红赤色。其叶似白槿[1]叶而涩;又似山格剌菜[2]叶亦涩,纹脉亦粗,味甘,微酸。

救饥:采嫩笋叶煤熟,水浸去邪味,淘净,油盐调食。

【注释】

[1] 见本书第261白槿树条。

[2] 见本书第278山格剌树条。

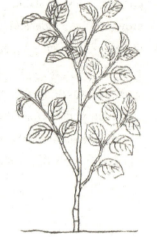

132. Suantongsun [酸桶笋, giant knotweed rhizome, Reynoutria japonica Houtt.]

Suantongsun [酸桶笋, giant knotweed rhizome, Reynoutria japonica Houtt.] grows near the streams of Shaohua Mountain in Mixian County. It germinates aliform leaf sheaths at first, and then stretches out filamentous tendrils. Its plants are about 4~5 Chi high, and its stalks are red with the shape like that of Shuihong [水荭, smartweed, Polygonum orientale L.]. Its leaves are like those of Baijin[1] [白槿, Chinese ash, Fraxinus chinensis Roxb.] or Shangela Cai[2] [山格剌菜, celastrus gemmatus, Celastrus gemmatus Loes.] but more scabrous, and its veins are thicker. It is sweet and slightly sour in taste.

For famine relief: Collect and blanch seedlings and leaves, remove the abnormal taste by soaking them in water, elutriate them, and flavor them with oil and salt.

【Notes】

[1] See the 261th clause of this book.

[2] See the 278th clause of this book.

133. 鹿蕨菜

生辉县山野中。苗高一尺许。其叶之茎背圆而面窊。叶似紫香蒿脚叶而肥阔颇硬；又似胡萝卜叶亦肥硬，味甜。

救饥：采苗叶煠熟，水浸淘净，油盐调食。

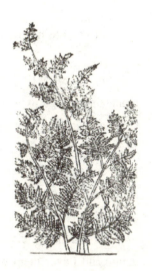

133. Lujuecai［鹿蕨菜，fern，Pteridium aquilinum（L.）Kuhn var. latiusculum（Desv.）Underw. ex Heller］

Lujuecai［鹿蕨菜，fern，Pteridium aquilinum（L.）Kuhn var. latiusculum（Desv.）Underw. ex Heller］grows in the mountainous regions and fields of Huixian County. Its plants are about one Chi high with rachises grooved adaxially and arched abaxially. The pinnas, like the basal leaves of Zixianghao［紫香蒿，annuae Sweet Wormwood Herb, Herba Artemisiae］or the leaves of Huluobo［胡萝卜，carrot，Daucus carota L. var. sativa Hoffm.］but more thicker, broader and harder, are sweet in taste.

For famine relief: Collect and blanch plants and leaves, soak and elutriate them, and flavor them with oil and salt.

134. 山芹菜

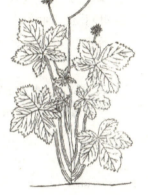

生辉县山野间。苗高一尺余。叶似野蜀葵[1]叶稍大而有五叉；又似地牡丹叶亦大。叶中撑生茎叉，稍结刺球，如鼠粘子[2]刺球而小。开花黪白色。叶味甘。

救饥：采苗叶煠熟，水浸淘净，油盐调食。

【注释】

[1] 见本书第144野蜀葵条。

[2] 指牛蒡的果实。见本书第222牛蒡子条。

134. Shanqincai〔山芹菜, sanicle, Sanicula chinensis Bunge〕

Shanqincai〔山芹菜, sanicle, Sanicula chinensis Bunge〕grows in the mountainous regions and fields of Huixian County. Its plants are more than one Chi high. Its leaves are five-forked but larger than those of Yeshukui[1]〔野蜀葵, Japanese Cryptotaenia, Cryptotaenia japonica Hassk.〕or Dimudan. Its scapes grow out of leaves, with globose fruit on top of them. The fruit, covered with uncinate bristles, is like but smaller than Shunianzi[2]. Its flowers are greyish white and its leaves are sweet in taste.

For famine relief: Collect and blanch plants and leaves, soak and elutriate them, and flavor them with oil and salt.

〔Notes〕

[1] See the 144th clause of this book.

[2] It refers to the fruit of Niubangzi〔牛蒡子, burdock, Arctium lappa L.〕. See the 222th clause of this book.

135. 金刚刺

又名老君须。生辉县鸦子口山野间。科条高三四尺。条似刺蘼花条,其上多刺。叶似牛尾菜叶;又似龙须菜叶,比此二叶俱大。叶间生细丝蔓。其叶味甘。

救饥:采叶煠熟,水浸淘净,油盐调食。

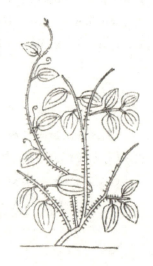

135. Jingangci〔金刚刺, smilax scobinicaulis, Smilax scobinicaulis C. H. Wright〕

Jingangci〔金刚刺, smilax scobinicaulis, Smilax scobinicaulis C. H. Wright〕, also named Laojunxu, grows in the mountainous regions and fields of Yazikou in Huixian County. Its plants are about 3~4 Chi high, and its branches, which are like those of Cimihua [刺蘪花, multiflora rose, Rosa multiflora Thunb.], are prickly. Its leaves are like but bigger than those of Niuweicai [牛尾菜, riparian greenbrier root and rhizome, Smilax riparia] or Longxucai [龙须菜, asparagus, Asparagus schoberioides Kunth]. The filamentous tendrils draw out of leaves, which are sweet in taste.

For famine relief: Collect and blanch leaves, soak and elutriate them, and flavor them with oil and salt.

136. 柳叶青

生中牟荒野中。科苗高二尺余。茎似蒿茎。叶似柳叶而短,抪茎而生。开小白花,银褐心。其叶味微辛。

救饥:采嫩叶煠熟,水浸淘净,油盐调食。

136. Liuyeqing [柳叶青, anaphalis margaritacea, Anaphalis margaritacea (L.) Benth. et Hook. f.]

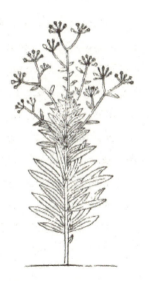

Liuyeqing [柳叶青, anaphalis margaritacea, Anaphalis margaritacea (L.) Benth. et Hook. f.] grows in the wilderness of Zhongmu. Its plants are more than two Chi high with the stems like mugworts. Its leaves are like salix leaves, but shorter, scattering on the stems. Capitulum is white with taupe tubular flowers in the center. Its leaves are slightly pungent in taste.

For famine relief: Collect and blanch young leaves, soak and elutriate them, and flavor them with oil and salt.

137. 大蓬蒿

生密县山野中。茎似黄蒿茎，色微带紫。叶似山芥菜叶而长大，极多花叉；又似风花菜叶，花叉亦多；又似漏芦叶，却微短。开碎瓣黄花。苗叶味苦。

救饥：采叶煠熟，水浸淘去苦味，油盐调食。

137. Dapenghao［大蓬蒿, senecio argunensis, Senecio argunensis Turcz.］

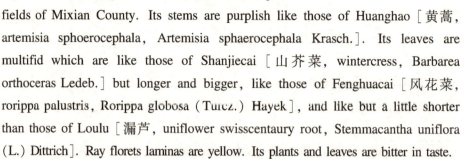

Dapenghao［大蓬蒿, senecio argunensis, Senecio argunensis Turcz.］ grows in the mountainous regions and fields of Mixian County. Its stems are purplish like those of Huanghao［黄蒿, artemisia sphoerocephala, Artemisia sphaerocephala Krasch.］. Its leaves are multifid which are like those of Shanjiecai［山芥菜, wintercress, Barbarea orthoceras Ledeb.］ but longer and bigger, like those of Fenghuacai［风花菜, rorippa palustris, Rorippa globosa (Turcz.) Hayek］, and like but a little shorter than those of Loulu［漏芦, uniflower swisscentaury root, Stemmacantha uniflora (L.) Dittrich］. Ray florets laminas are yellow. Its plants and leaves are bitter in taste.

For famine relief: Collect and blanch leaves, remove the bitterness by soaking and elutriating them, and flavor them with oil and salt.

138. 狗筋蔓

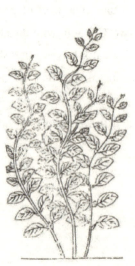

生中牟县沙岗间。小科就地拖蔓生。叶似狗掉尾[1]叶而短小；又似月芽菜[2]叶，微尖䩞而软，亦多纹脉，两叶对生。叶梢间开白花。其叶味苦。

救饥：采叶煠熟，水浸淘去苦味，油盐调食。

【注释】

［1］见本书第101狗掉尾苗条。

［2］见本书第258月芽树条。

138. Goujinman [狗筋蔓, baccifera, Cucubalus baccifer L.]

Goujinman [狗筋蔓, baccifera, Cucubalus baccifer L.] grows on the sandhills of Zhongmu and its shoots bend and trail along the ground. Its opposite leaves are like but shorter and smaller than those of Goudiaowei[1] [狗掉尾, herba solani, Solanum lyratum Thunb.], and also like those of Yueyacai[2] [月芽菜, euonymus maackii, Euonymus maackii Rupr.] but sharper, softer and papery with more veins. Its flowers are white, and its leaves are bitter in taste.

For famine relief: Collect and blanch leaves, remove the bitterness by soaking and elutriating them, and flavor them with oil and salt.

【Notes】

[1] See the 101th clause of this book.

[1] See the 258th clause of this book.

139. 兔儿伞

生荥阳[1]塔儿山荒野中。其苗高二三尺许。每科初生一茎,茎端生叶一层,有七八叶,每叶分作四叉,排生如伞盖状,故以为名。后于叶间撺生茎叉,上开淡红白花。根似牛膝而疏短,味苦,微辛。

救饥:采嫩叶煠熟,换水浸,淘去苦味,油盐调食。

【注释】

[1] 明代地名,今指河南省荥阳市。

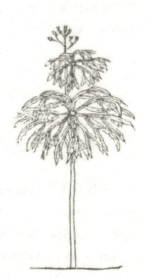

139. Tu'ersan [兔儿伞, aconiteleaf syndeilesis herb, Syneilesis aconitifolia (Bge.) Maxim.]

Tu'ersan [兔儿伞, aconiteleaf syndeilesis herb, Syneilesis aconitifolia (Bge.) Maxim.] grows in the wilderness of Ta'er Mountain in Xingyang[1]. Its plants are about 2~3 Chi high, each with only one long petiole in the early growth period. Each of its palmatifid leaves with 7~8 lobes stands on the top of petioles, and each leaf has 4 lobules. Its leaves are arranged in terminal like the canopy and so it is named. Later the scapes draw out of leaves with pale white or pale red flowers. Its roots are like those of Niuxi [牛膝, twotoothed achyranthes root, Radix Achyranthis Bidentatae] but sparser and shorter. It is bitter and slightly spicy in taste.

For famine relief: Collect and blanch young leaves, remove the bitterness by soaking and elutriating them, and flavor them with oil and salt.

【Notes】

[1] The geographic name in Ming Dynasty. Presently it refers to Xingyang City of Henan Province.

140. 地花菜

又名墓头灰。生密县山野中。苗高尺余。叶似野菊花叶而窄细；又似鼠尾草叶亦瘦细。梢叶间开五瓣小黄花。其叶味微苦。

救饥：采叶煤熟，水浸淘洗净，油盐调食。

140. Dihuacai [地花菜, atrina glass, Patrinia rupestris (Pall.) Juss. Subsp. scabra (Bunge) H. J. Wang]

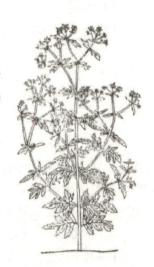

Dihuacai [地花菜, atrina glass, Patrinia rupestris (Pall.) Juss. Subsp. scabra (Bunge) H. J. Wang], also named Mutouhui, grows in the mountainous regions and fields of Mixian County. Its plants are about one Chi high. Its leaves are like those of Yejuhua [野菊花, wild chrysanthemum flower, Dendranthema indicum Des Moul.] but slenderer, and also like but thinner than those of Shuweicao [鼠尾草, European verbena herb, Herba Verbenae]. Each of its tiny flowers is yellow with five patals, and its leaves are slightly bitter in taste.

For famine relief: Collect and blanch leaves, soak and elutriate them, and

flavor them with oil and salt.

141. 杓儿菜

生密县山野中。苗高一二尺。叶类狗掉尾叶而窄,颇长,黑绿色,微有毛涩;又似耐惊菜叶而小,软薄,梢叶更小。开碎瓣淡黄白花。其叶味苦。

救饥:采叶煠熟,水浸去苦味,淘洗净,油盐调食。

141. Shao'ercai [杓儿菜, carpesium cernuum, Carpesium cernuum L.]

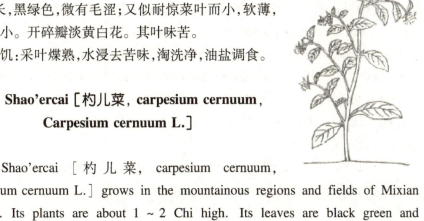

Shao'ercai [杓儿菜, carpesium cernuum, Carpesium cernuum L.] grows in the mountainous regions and fields of Mixian County. Its plants are about 1 ~ 2 Chi high. Its leaves are black green and scabridulous, which are like those of Goudiaowei [狗掉尾, herba solani, Solanum lyratum Thunb.] but narrower and longer, and like those of Naijingcai [耐惊菜, eclipta prostrata, Eclipta prostrata (L.) L.] but smaller, softer and thinner, with even smaller bracts. Both marginal florets and disk florets are tubular with yellowish white color, and its leaves are bitter in taste.

For famine relief: Collect and blanch leaves, remove the bitterness by soaking them in water, elutriate them, and flavor them with oil and salt.

142. 佛指甲

生密县山谷中。科苗高一二尺。茎微带赤黄色。其叶淡绿,背皆微带白色,叶如长匙头样,似黑豆叶而微宽;又似鹅儿肠叶甚大,皆两叶对生。开黄花。结实形如连翘,微小,中有黑子,小如粟粒。其叶味甜。

救饥:采嫩叶煠熟,换水淘洗净,油盐调食。

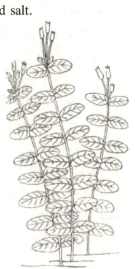

142. Fozhijia [佛指甲, hypericum ascyron, Hypericum ascyron L.]

Fozhijia [佛指甲, hypericum ascyron, Hypericum ascyron L.] grows in the valleys of Mixian County. Its plants are 1~2 Chi high and its stems are helvolus. Its opposite leaves, adaxially green and abaxially pale green with white glandular dots, are like the tips of bar spoons, like but a little broader than those of Heidou [黑豆, soybean, Glycine max (Linn.) Merr.], and like those of E'erchang [鹅儿肠, malachium, Stellariae Herba] but much larger. Its flowers are yellow and its fruit is like but a little smaller than that of Lianqiao [连翘, weeping forsythia, Forsythia suspensa (Thunb.) Vahl]. Its seeds are black with the size of millets, and its leaves are sweet in taste.

For famine relief: Collect and blanch young leaves, elutriate them, and flavor them with oil and salt.

143. 虎尾草

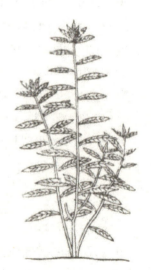

生密县山谷中。科苗高二三尺。茎圆。叶颇似柳叶而瘦短；又似兔儿尾[1]叶，亦瘦窄；又似黄精[2]叶，颇软，抪茎攒生。味甜、微涩。

救饥：采嫩苗叶煤熟，换水淘去涩味，油盐调食。

【注释】

[1] 见本书第150兔儿尾苗条。

[2] 见本书第220黄精苗条。

143. Huweicao [虎尾草, lysimachia barystachys, Lysimachia barystachys Bunge]

Huweicao [虎尾草, lysimachia barystachys, Lysimachia barystachys Bunge] grows in the valleys of Mixian County. Its plants are 2~3 Chi high with terete stems. Its leaves are like the willow leaves but thinner and shorter, like but narrower than those of Tu'erwei[1] [兔儿尾, longifolia, Veronica longifolia L.], and like those of Huangjing[2]［黄精, solomonseal rhizome, Polygonatum sibiricum Redouté］but softer, alternate or subopposite, scattering on the stems. Its plants are sweet and slightly astringent in taste.

For famine relief: Collect and blanch seedlings and leaves, remove the astringent flavor by rinsing them, and flavor them with oil and salt.

【Notes】

［1］See the 150th clause of this book.

［2］See the 220th clause of this book.

144. 野蜀葵

生荒野中，就地丛生。苗高五寸许。叶似葛勒子秧叶而厚大；又似地牡丹叶，味辣。

救饥：采嫩叶煠熟，水浸淘净，油盐调食。

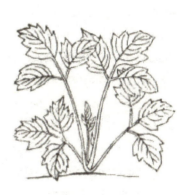

144. Yeshukui［野蜀葵, Japanese Cryptotaenia, Cryptotaenia japonica Hassk.］

Yeshukui［野蜀葵, Japanese Cryptotaenia, Cryptotaenia japonica Hassk.］grows in the fields and clusters on the ground. Its plants are about five Cun high. Its leaves are like those of Gelezi Yang［葛勒子秧, Japanese hop, Humuli Scandentis Herba］but thicker and larger, and also like those of Dimudan with slightly spicy taste.

For famine relief: Collect and blanch young leaves, soak and elutriate them, and flavor them with oil and salt.

145. 蛇葡萄

生荒野中，拖蔓而生。叶似菊[1]叶而小，花叉繁碎；又似前胡叶亦细。茎叶间开五瓣小银褐花。结子如豌豆大，生青，熟则红色。苗叶味甜。

救饥：采叶煠熟，换水浸，淘净，油盐调食。

治病：今人传说，捣根傅贴疮肿。

【注释】

[1] 见本书第238菊花条。

145. Sheputao［蛇葡萄，ampelopsis aconitifolia，Ampelopsis aconitifolia Bunge］

Sheputao［蛇葡萄, ampelopsis aconitifolia, Ampelopsis aconitifolia Bunge］ grows in the fields with tendrils trailing along the ground. Its leaves are like but smaller than those of Ju[1]［菊, chrysanthemum, Dendranthema morifolium (Ramat.) Tzvel.］with lanceolate and dense leaf blades, and also like those of Qianhu［前胡, radix peucedani, Peucedanum praeruptorum Dunn］but slenderer. Each of its flowers is tiny and silver brown with 5 petals. Its fruit, as big as the pea, is green when unripe and red when ripe. Its plants and leaves are sweet in taste.

For famine relief: Collect and blanch leaves, soak and elutriate them, and flavor them with oil and salt.

For disease treatment: Presently it is said that its roots can be used to treat sores and pyogenic infection after pounding into pieces for external application.

【Notes】

[1] See the 238th clause of this book.

146. 星宿菜

生田野中，作小科苗生。叶似石竹子叶而细小；又似米布袋[1]叶微长。稍上开五瓣小尖白花。苗叶味甜。

救饥：采苗叶煠熟，水浸淘净，油盐调食。

【注释】

[1] 见本书第216米布袋条。

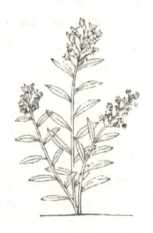

146. Xingxiucai [星宿菜, lysimachia fortunei, Lysimachia fortunei Maxim.]

Xingxiucai [星宿菜, lysimachia fortunei, Lysimachia fortunei Maxim.] grows in the fields, and its plants are short and small. Its leaves are like those of Shizhuzi [石竹子, Chinese pink, Dianthus chinensis L.] but slenderer and smaller, and also like those of Mibudai[1] [米布袋, gueldenstaedtia verna, Gueldenstaedtia verna (Georgi) Boriss. subsp. multiflora (Bunge) Tsui] but a little longer. Each of its flowers is white with 5 acute petals. Its leaves are sweet in taste.

For famine relief: Collect and blanch plants and leaves, soak and elutriate them, and flavor them with oil and salt.

【Notes】

[1] See the 216th clause of this book.

147. 水荬衣

生水泊边。叶似地稍瓜叶而窄小。每叶间皆结小青蓇葖。其叶味苦。

救饥:采苗叶煤熟,水浸淘去苦味,油盐调食。

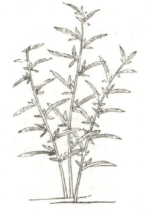

147. Shuisuoyi [水荬衣, veronica peregrina, Veronica peregrina L.]

Shuisuoyi [水荬衣, veronica peregrina, Veronica peregrina L.] grows near water. Its leaves are like those of Dishaogua [地稍瓜, cynanchum thesioides, Cynanchum thesioides (Freyn) K. Schum.] but narrower. Its axillary galls are green, and its leaves are bitter in taste.

For famine relief: Collect leaves and seedlings, blanch them and remove the bitterness by soaking and elutriating them, and flavor them with oil and salt.

148. 牛奶菜

出辉县山野中。拖藤蔓而生。叶似牛皮消叶而大；又似马兜零叶极大，叶皆对节生。梢间开青白小花。其叶味甜。

救饥：采嫩苗叶煠熟，水浸淘净，油盐调食。

148. Niunaicai［牛奶菜，marsdenia sinensis，Marsdenia sinensis Hemsl.］

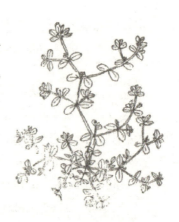

Niunaicai［牛奶菜, marsdenia sinensis, Marsdenia sinensis Hemsl.］grows in the mountainous regions and fields of Huixian County and creeps on the ground. Its opposite leaves are like but much larger than those leaves of Niupixiao［牛皮消, cynanchum caudatum, Cynanchum auriculatum Royle ex Wight］, and also like those of Madouling［马兜零, dutohmanspipe fruit, Aristolochia debilis Sieb. et Zucc.］but extremely large. Its flowers are small and green-white, and its leaves are sweet in taste.

For famine relief: Collect and blanch seedlings and leaves, soak and elutriate them, and flavor them with oil and salt.

149. 小虫儿卧单

一名铁线草。生田野中。苗揭地生。叶似苜蓿[1]叶而极小；又似鸡眼草[2]叶亦小。其茎色红。开小红花。苗味甜。

救饥：采苗叶煠熟，水浸，淘净，油盐调食。

【注释】

[1] 见本书第379 苜蓿条。

[2] 见本书第197 鸡眼草条。

149. Xiaochong'er Wodan [小虫儿卧单, euphorbia humifusa, Euphorbia humifusa Willd. ex Schlecht.]

Xiaochong'er Wodan [小虫儿卧单, euphorbia humifusa, Euphorbia humifusa Willd. ex Schlecht.], also named Tiexiancao, grows in the fields. Its stems prostrate and creep on the ground. Its leaves are like those of Muxu[1] [苜蓿, alfalfa, Medicago sativa L.] but extremely small, and also like but smaller than those of Jiyancao[2] [鸡眼草, Japan Clover Herb, Kummerowia striata (Thunb.) Schindl.]. Both its stems and flowers are red. Its plants are sweet in taste.

For famine relief: Collect and blanch plants and leaves, soak and elutriate them, and flavor them with oil and salt.

【Notes】

[1] See the 379th clause of this book.

[2] See the 197th clause of this book.

150. 兔儿尾苗

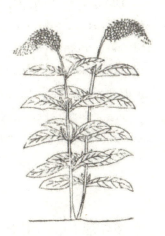

生田野中。苗高一二尺。叶似水荭叶而狭短，其尖颇齐。梢头出穗，如兔尾状。开花白色。结红菁葵，如椒目[1]大。其叶味酸。

救饥：采嫩苗叶煠熟，水浸，淘净，油盐调食。

【注释】

[1] 指花椒的果实。见本书第 252 椒树条。

150. Tu'erwei Miao [兔儿尾苗, longifolia, Veronica longifolia L.]

Tu'erwei Miao [兔儿尾苗, longifolia, Veronica longifolia L.] grows in the fields, and its plants are 1~2 Chi high. Its leaves are like those of Shuihong [水荭, smartweed, Polygonum orientale L.] but narrower and shorter with obtuse apexes. Its spiciform inflorescences are like rabbits' tails and stand on the tips of branches. Its flowers are white, and its fruit is red and as big as Jiaomu[1]. Its leaves are sour in taste.

For famine relief: Collect and blanch seedlings and leaves, soak and elutriate them, and flavor them with oil and salt.

【Notes】

[1] It refers to the fruit of Huajiao [花椒, pericarp of Tibet Pricklyash, Zanthoxylum simulans Hance]. See the 252th clause of this book.

151. 地锦苗

生田野中。小科苗高五七寸。苗叶似园荽。叶间开紫花。结小角儿。苗叶味苦。

救饥:采苗叶煠熟,水浸,淘净,油盐调食。

151. Dijinmiao [地锦苗, Herb of Common Corydalis, Corydalis edulis Maxim.]

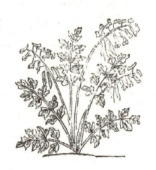

Dijinmiao [地锦苗, Herb of Common Corydalis, Corydalis edulis Maxim.] grows in the fields. Its plants, 5~7 Cun high, are short and small. Both its shoots and leaves are like those of Yuansui [园荽, coriander herb, Coriandrum sativum L.]. Its flowers are purple and its capsules are very small. Its shoots and leaves are bitter in taste.

For famine relief: Collect and blanch shoots and leaves, soak and elutriate them, and flavor them with oil and salt.

152. 野西瓜苗

俗名秃汉头。生田野中。苗高一尺许。叶似家西瓜叶而小,颇硬。叶间生蒂开五瓣银褐花,紫心黄蕊。花罢作蒴,蒴内结实,如楝子大。苗叶味微苦。

救饥:采嫩苗叶煠熟,水浸去邪味,淘过,油盐调食。

治病:今人传说,采苗捣敷疮肿,拔毒。

152. Yexigua Miao [野西瓜苗, hibiscus trionum, Hibiscus trionum Linn.]

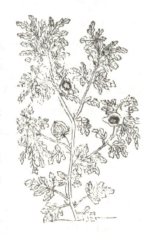

Yexigua Miao [野西瓜苗, hibiscus trionum, Hibiscus trionum Linn.], also named Tuhantou, grows in the fields. Its plants are about one Chi high. Its leaves are like those of Jiaxigua [家西瓜, watermelon, Citrullus lanatus (Thunb.) Matsum. et Nakai] but smaller and harder. The five-petal corolla is pale yellow with the purple center, and the anthers are yellow. It bears capsules after blooming and the seeds are as big as the fruit of Lian [楝, chinaberry, Melia azedarach L.]. Its plants and leaves are slightly bitter in taste.

For famine relief: Collect and blanch seedlings and leaves, remove the abnormal taste by soaking them in water, elutriate them, and flavor them with oil and salt.

For disease treatment: Presently it is said that its plants can be used to treat swollen sores and drain toxin after pounding into pieces for external application.

153. 香茶菜

生田野中。茎方，窊面四楞。叶似薄荷叶微大，抪茎对生。梢头出穗，开粉紫花，结蒴如荞麦[1]蒴而微小。叶味苦。

救饥：采叶煤熟，水浸去苦味，淘洗净，油盐调食。

【注释】

[1] 见本书第 333 荞麦苗条。

153. Xiangchacai [香茶菜, rabdosia rubescens, Rabdosia rubescens (Hemsl.) Hara]

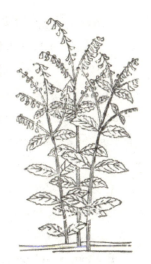

Xiangchacai [香茶菜, rabdosia rubescens, Rabdosia rubescens (Hemsl.)

Hara] grows in the fields with the stems quadrangular and sulcate. Its opposite leaves are like those of Bohe [薄荷, peppermint, Mentha canadensis L.] but a little bigger, scattered along the stem. Its panicles draw out of branches with pinkish purple flowers. Its capsules are like but a little smaller than those of Qiaomai[1] [荞麦, buckwheat, Fagopyrum esculentum Moench]. Its leaves taste bitter.

For famine relief: Collect and blanch leaves, remove the bitterness by soaking them in water, elutriate them, and flavor them with oil and salt.

【Notes】

[1] See the 333th clause of this book.

154. 蔷蘼

又名刺蘼。今处处有之。生荒野岗岭间,人家园圃中亦栽。科条青色,茎上多刺。叶似椒[1]叶而长,锯齿又细,背颇白。开红白花,亦有千叶者。味甜、淡。

救饥:采芽叶煠熟,换水浸淘净,油盐调食。

【注释】

[1] 花椒,见本书第252椒树条。

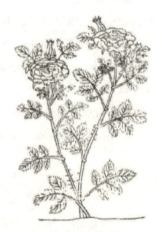

154. Qiangmi [蔷蘼, multiflora rose, Rosa multiflora Thunb.]

Qiangmi [蔷蘼, multiflora rose, Rosa multiflora Thunb.], also named Cimi, can be seen everywhere presently. It grows in the wilderness and mountain ridges, and can be seen in common people's gardens. Its branchlets are cyan and prickly. Its leaves are like but longer than those of Jiao[1] [椒, zanthoxylum simulans hance, Zanthoxylum simulans Hance] with serrulate margin, abaxially white. Its flowers are white or pink, sometimes being double petals. Its plants are sweet and bland in taste.

For famine relief: Collect and blanch shoots and leaves, soak and elutriate them, and flavor them with oil and salt.

【Notes】

［1］See the 252th clause of this book.

155. 毛女儿菜

生南阳府马鞍山中。苗高一尺许。叶似绵丝菜叶而微尖；又似兔儿尾叶而小，茎叶皆有白毛。梢间开淡黄花，如大黍粒，十数颗攒成一穗。味甘酸。

救饥：采苗叶煠熟，水浸，淘净，油盐调食。或拌米面蒸食亦可。

155. Maonv'er Cai ［毛女儿菜, gnaphalium japonicum, Gnaphalium japonicum Thunb.］

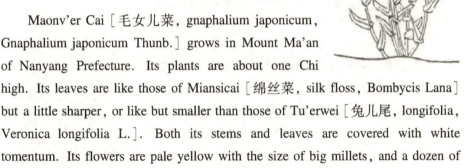

Maonv'er Cai ［毛女儿菜, gnaphalium japonicum, Gnaphalium japonicum Thunb.］ grows in Mount Ma'an of Nanyang Prefecture. Its plants are about one Chi high. Its leaves are like those of Miansicai ［绵丝菜, silk floss, Bombycis Lana］ but a little sharper, or like but smaller than those of Tu'erwei ［兔儿尾, longifolia, Veronica longifolia L.］. Both its stems and leaves are covered with white tomentum. Its flowers are pale yellow with the size of big millets, and a dozen of capitula assemble together in a dense headlike corymb. Its plants are sour in taste.

For famine relief: Collect and blanch plants and leaves, soak and elutriate them, flavor them with oil and salt, or steam them with rice and flour.

156. 牻牛儿苗

又名斗牛儿苗。生田野中。就地拖秧而生，茎蔓细弱。其茎红紫色，叶似园荽叶，瘦细而稀疏。开五瓣小紫花。结青蓇葖儿，上有一嘴，甚尖锐，如细锥子状，小儿取以为斗戏。叶味微苦。

救饥：采叶煠熟，换水浸去苦味，淘净，油盐调食。

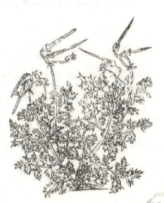

156. Mangniu'er Miao [牻牛儿苗, erodium stephanianum, Erodium stephanianum Willd.]

Mangniu'er Miao [牻牛儿苗, erodium stephanianum, Erodium stephanianum Willd.], also named Douniu'er Miao, grows in the fields. Its stems, trailing along the ground, are thin and delicate. Its shoots are reddish violet and its leaves are like those of Yuansui [园荽, coriander herb, Coriandrum sativum L.] but thinner and sparser. Each of its flowers is purple with 5 petals. Its capsules are green with apical pit shapes like awl. Children always play with it. Its leaves taste bitter.

For famine relief: Collect and blanch leaves, remove the bitterness by soaking them in water, elutriate them, and flavor them with oil and salt.

157. 铁扫帚

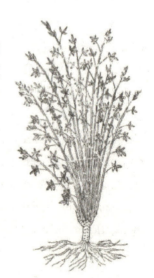

生荒野中,就地丛生。一本二三十茎,苗高三四尺。叶似苜蓿[1]叶而细长;又似细叶胡枝子[2]叶,亦短小。开小白花。其叶味苦。

救饥:采嫩苗叶煠熟,换水浸去苦味,油盐调食。

【注释】

[1] 见本书第379苜蓿条。

[2] 见本书第215胡枝子条。

157. Tiesaozhou [铁扫帚, lespedeza cuneata, Lespedeza cuneata (Dum.-Cours.) G. Don]

Tiesaozhou [铁扫帚, lespedeza cuneata, Lespedeza cuneata (Dum.-Cours.) G. Don] grows in the fields and clusters on the ground. Its plants, sprouting 20 ~ 30 shoots, are 3 ~ 4 Chi high. Its leaves are like those of Muxu[1] [苜蓿, alfalfa, Medicago sativa L.] but slenderer, and like but shorter than those of Xiye Huzhizi[2] [细叶胡枝子, lespedeza daurica, Lespedeza daurica (Laxm.) Schindl.]. Its flowers are small and white, and its leaves taste bitter.

For famine relief: Collect and blanch young leaves and seedlings, remove the bitterness by soaking them in water, and flavor them with oil and salt.

【Notes】

[1] See the 379th clause of this book.

[2] See the 215th clause of this book.

158. 山小菜

生密县山野中。科苗高二尺余，就地丛生。叶似酸浆子叶而窄小，面有细纹脉，边有锯齿，色深绿；又似桔梗叶，颇长艄，味苦。

救饥：采叶煠熟，水浸淘去苦味，油盐调食。

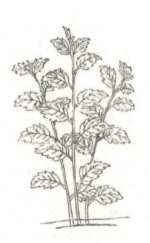

158. Shanxiaocai〔山小菜, spotted bellflower, Campanula puncatata Lam.〕

Shanxiaocai〔山小菜, spotted bellflower, Campanula puncatata Lam.〕grows in the mountainous regions and fields of Mixian County. Its plants are more than two Chi high and cluster on the ground. Its deep green leaves are like those of Suanjiang〔酸浆, winter cherry, Physalis alkekengi L.〕but narrower and smaller with veinlet and serrulate margin, and like those of Jiegeng〔桔梗, platycodon root, Platycodon grandiflorus (Jacq.) A. DC.〕but sharper and longer. It is bitter in taste.

For famine relief: Collect and blanch leaves, remove the bitterness by soaking and rinsing them in water, and flavor them with oil and salt.

159. 羊角苗

又名羊奶科，亦名合钵儿，俗名婆婆针扎儿，又名纽丝藤，一名过路黄。生田野下湿地中。拖藤蔓而生，茎色青白。叶似马兜零叶而长大；又似山药[1]叶，亦长大，面青背颇白，皆两叶相对生，茎叶折之，俱有白汁出。叶间出穗，开五瓣小白花。结角似羊角状，中有白穰。其叶味甘，微苦。

救饥：采嫩叶煠熟，换水浸去苦味邪气，淘净，油盐调食。

【注释】

［1］见本书第414山药条。

159. Yangjiaomiao ［羊角苗, cynanchum chinense, Cynanchum chinense R. Br.］

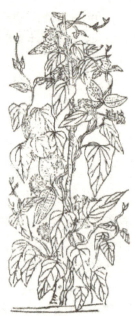

Yangjiaomiao ［羊角苗, cynanchum chinense, Cynanchum chinense R. Br.］, also named Yangnaike, Hebo'er, Popozhen zha'er, Niusiteng, Guoluhuang, grows in the low-lying wetlands and fields. Its plants trail on the ground with greenish white stems. Its opposite leaves are like those of Madouling ［马兜零, Dutohmanspipe Fruit, Fructus Aristolochiae］ or Shanyao[1] ［山药, common yam rhizome, Dioscorea opposita Thunb.］ but longer and bigger, adaxially green and abaxially whitish. It drains out white juice when the stems or leaves are broken off. The cymes draw out of leaves, and the flowers are tiny and white, with 5 petals. Its fruit is like ram's horns and the seeds are covered with white coma. Its leaves are sweet and slightly bitter in taste.

For famine relief: Collect and blanch young leaves, remove the bitterness and abnormal taste by soaking them in water, elutriate them, and flavor them with oil and salt.

【Notes】

［1］See the 414th clause of this book.

160. 耧斗菜

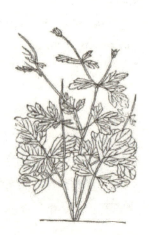

生辉县太行山山野中。小科苗就地丛生，苗高一尺许，茎梗细弱。叶似牡丹叶而小，其头颇团，味甜。

救饥：采叶煠熟，水浸，淘净，油盐调食。

160. Loudoucai [耧斗菜, aquilegia yabeana, Aquilegia yabeana Kitag.]

Loudoucai [耧斗菜, aquilegia yabeana, Aquilegia yabeana Kitag.] grows in the mountainous regions and fields of Taihang Mountain in Huixian County. Its seedlings cluster on the ground, and its plants are about one Chi high. Both its stems and petioles are thin and delicate. Its leaves are like but smaller than those of Mudan [牡丹, subshrubby peony, Paeonia suffruticosa Andr.] with obtuse apexes and sweet taste.

For famine relief: Collect and blanch leaves, soak and elutriate them, and flavor them with oil and salt.

161. 瓯 菜

生辉县山野中。就地作小科苗,生茎叉。叶似山苋菜叶而有锯齿;又似山小菜叶,其锯齿比之却小,味甜。

救饥:采嫩苗叶煤熟,水浸,淘净,油盐调食。

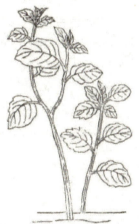

161. Oucai [瓯菜, black nightshade, Solanum nigrum L.]

Oucai [瓯菜, black nightshade, Solanum nigrum L.] grows in the mountainous regions and fields of Huixian County. Its seedlings bend to the ground and draw out shoots. Its leaves are like those of Shanxiancai [山苋菜, twotoothed achyranthes root, Achyranthes bidentata Blume] with dentate margin, and also like those of Shanxiaocai [山小菜, spotted bellflower, Campanula puncatata Lam.] with larger serration, and they taste sweet.

For famine relief: Collect and blanch seedlings and leaves, soak and elutriate them, and flavor them with oil and salt.

162. 变豆菜

生辉县太行山山野中。其苗叶初作地摊科生。叶似地牡丹叶极大,五花叉,锯齿尖。其后叶中分生茎叉,梢叶颇小,上开白花。其叶味甘。

救饥:采叶煠熟,作成黄色,换水淘净,油盐调食。

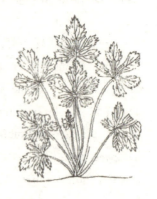

162. Biandoucai [变豆菜, sanicle, Sanicula chinensis Bunge]

Biandoucai [变豆菜, sanicle, Sanicula chinensis Bunge] grows in the mountainous regions and fields of Taihang Mountain in Huixian County, and its seedlings bend to the ground. Its leaves are, like those of Dimudan but extremely larger, five forked with serrate margin. Its scapes draw out from the center of leaves with very small leaves on its tips, and bear white flowers. Its leaves are sweet in taste.

For famine relief: Collect and blanch leaves, make them turn yellow, elutriate them, and flavor them with oil and salt.

163. 和尚菜

田野处处有之。初生揭地布叶。叶似野天茄儿[1]叶而大,背微红紫色。后撺苗高二三尺,叶似䒷[2]叶,短小而尖;又似红落藜[3]叶而色不红。结子如灰菜子[4]。叶味辛、酸,微咸。

救饥:采嫩叶煠熟,换水浸去邪味,淘净,油盐调食。或晒干煠食亦可。或云不可多食久食,令人面肿。

【注释】

[1] 见本书第217天茄儿苗条。

[2] 见本书第374䒷菜条。

[3] 见本书第345舜芒谷条。

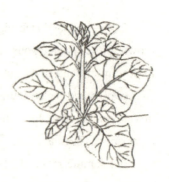

[4] 见本书第412灰菜条。

163. Heshangcai [和尚菜, adenocaulon himalaicum, Adenocaulon himalaicum Edgew.]

Heshangcai [和尚菜, adenocaulon himalaicum, Adenocaulon himalaicum Edgew.] can be seen everywhere in the fields. At the initial growth period, its leaves creep and spread on the ground. It is like that of Ye Tianqie'er[1] [野天茄儿, nightshade, Solanum nigrum L.] but bigger and abaxially reddish violet. Later its plants grow fast up to 2~3 Chi high. Its leaves are like those of Junda[2] [莙荙, spinach beet, Beta vulgaris L. var. cicla L.] but smaller and sharper, and like those of Hongluoli[3] [红落藜, chenopodium giganteum, Chenopodium giganteum D. Don] without red color. Its seeds are like those of Huicai[4] [灰菜, lamb's-quarters, Chenopodium album L.] and its leaves are pungent, sour and slightly salty in taste.

For famine relief: Collect and blanch young leaves, remove the abnormal taste by soaking them in water, elutriate them, and flavor them with oil and salt. Or blanch them after drying in the sunshine. Do not take them for a large amount or for a long time because it may lead to the swollen face.

【Notes】

[1] See the 217th clause of this book.

[2] See the 374th clause of this book.

[3] See the 345th clause of this book.

[4] See the 412th clause of this book.

根可食

《本草》原有

Root Edible

Original Ones

164. 萎蕤

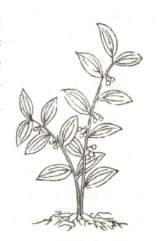

本草一名女萎,一名荧,一名地节,一名玉竹,一名马薰。生太山山谷,及舒州[1]、滁州、均州[2],今南阳府马鞍山亦有。苗高一二尺。茎斑。叶似竹叶,阔短而肥厚,叶尖处有黄点;又似百合[3]叶,却颇窄小。叶下结青子,如椒[4]粒大。其根似黄精[5]而小异,节上有须,味甘,性平,无毒。

救饥:采根,换水煮极熟,食之。

治病:文具《本草·草部》条下。

【注释】

[1] 古代州名,今安徽安庆一带。

[2] 古代州名,今湖北丹江口市

[3] 见本书第165 百合条。

[4] 见本书第252 椒树条。

[5] 见本书第220 黄精苗条。

164. Weirui [萎蕤, fragrant solomonseal rhizome, Polygonatum odoratum (Mill.) Druce]

Weirui [萎蕤, fragrant solomonseal rhizome, Polygonatum odoratum (Mill.) Druce], also named Nvwei, Ying, Dijie, Yuzhu and Maxun, grows in the valleys of Tai Mountain and other places like Shuzhou[1], Chuzhou and Junzhou[2]. Presently, it can also be seen in Ma'an Mountain of Nanyang Prefecture. Its plants are 1 ~ 2 Chi high with notate stems. Its leaves are like bamboo leaves but broader, shorter and more succulent with yellow spots on leaf apexes, and like those of Baihe[3]〔百合, lily bulb, Lilium brownii var. viridulum Baker〕but narrower and smaller. Its blue-black fruit is as big as that of Huajiao[4]〔花椒, pericarp of Tibet Pricklyash, Zanthoxylum simulans Hance〕. Its rhizomes are, like those of Huangjing[5]〔黄精, solomonseal rhizome, Polygonatum sibiricum Redouté〕but slightly different for the roots arising from stem nodes, sweet in taste, neutral in nature and non-toxic.

For famine relief: Collect rhizomes, and take them after their being fully cooked.

For disease treatment: See the clauses in *Materia Medica · Herbaceous Plant*.

【Notes】

［1］The name of an ancient county. It is presently located in Anqing of Anhui Province.

［2］The name of an ancient county. It is presently located in Danjiangkou of Hubei Province.

［3］See the 165th clause of this book.

［4］See the 252th clause of this book.

［5］See the 220th clause of this book.

165. 百　合

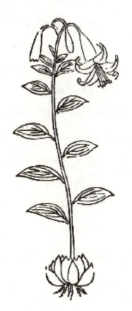

一名重箱，一名摩罗，一名中逢花，一名强瞿。生荆州山谷，今处处有之。苗高数尺，干粗如箭，四面有叶如鸡距；又似大柳叶而宽，青色稀疏。叶近茎微紫，茎端碧白。开淡黄白花，如石榴[1]蒂而大，四垂向下覆长蕊，花心有檀色，每一枝颠，须五六花。子色紫圆如梧桐子，生于枝叶间，每叶一子，不在花中，此又异也。根色白，形如松子壳，四向攒生，中间出苗；又如葫蒜，重叠生二三十瓣，味甘，性平，无毒。一云有小毒。又有一种开红花，名山丹，不堪用。

救饥：采根煮熟，食之甚益人气。又云蒸过，与蜜食之。或为粉，尤佳。

治病：文具《本草·草部》条下。

【注释】

[1] 见本书第 360 石榴条。

165. Baihe [百合, lily bulb, Lilium brownii Lilium brownii F. E. Brown var. viridulum Baker]

Baihe [百合, lily bulb, Lilium brownii var. viridulum Baker], also named Chongxiang, Moluo, Zhongfenghua and Qiangqu, grows in the valleys of Jingzhou and can be seen everywhere presently. Its plants are about several Chi high, and its stems are about the size of arrows. Its leaves, growing scatteredly on all sides like cockspurs or like big willow leaves but broader, are green and sparse. Its leaf blades which are proximal to petioles are purplish and its stem apexes are greenish white. Its yellowish white flowers are like but bigger than the calyx lobes of Shiliu[1] [石榴, pomegranate, Punica granatum L.]. Its tepals spread downward and cover its long filaments, and the anther is light red. There are 5~6 flowers on each inflorescence. Each leaf axil sends forth only one seed (bulbil), which is purple and orbicular like the phoenix tree seed. It is very strange that its seeds and do not grow in its flowers. Its white bulbs which are like pinecones grow together from all sides with seedlings drawing out from the center. And its bulbs, like Husuan [葫蒜, garlic, Allium sativum L.], overlapping with 20~30 flakes, are sweet in taste and neutral in nature and non-toxic. It is also said to be slightly toxic. Another species named Shandan bear red flowers and can not be used.

For famine relief: Collect bulbs and cook them thoroughly, and they can tonify qi. They can be used with honey after being steamed, or it is better to grind them into powder.

For disease treatment: See the clauses in *Materia Medica · Herbaceous Plant*.

【Notes】

[1] See the 360th clause of this book.

166. 天门冬

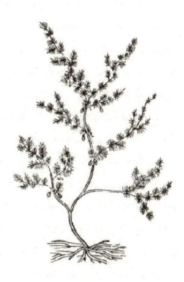

俗名万岁藤,又名娑罗树,《本草》一名颠勒,或名地门冬,或名筵门冬,或名巅棘,或名淫羊食,或名管松。生奉高山谷及建州[1]、汉州[2],今处处有之。春生藤蔓,大如钗股,长至丈余,延附草木上。叶如茴香,极尖细而疏滑,有逆刺,亦有涩而无刺者。其叶如丝杉而细散,皆名天门冬。夏生白花,亦有黄花及紫花者。秋结黑子,在其根枝傍。入伏后无花,暗结子。其根白,或黄紫色,大如手指,长二三寸,大者为胜。其生高地,根短味甜,气香者上。其生水侧下地者,叶细似蕴而微黄,根长而味多苦,气臭者下,亦可服。味苦、甘,性平、大寒,无毒。垣衣、地黄[3]及贝母为之使,畏曾青。服天门冬误食鲤鱼中毒,浮萍解之。

救饥:采根,换水浸去邪味,去心煮食。或晒干煮熟,入蜜食尤佳。

治病:文具《本草·草部》条下。

【注释】

[1] 古代州名,今福建建瓯市。
[2] 古代州名,今四川广汉、德阳、绵竹、什邡、金堂等市县地。
[3] 见本书第221 地黄苗条。

166. Tianmendong [天门冬, radix asparagi, Asparagus cochinchinensis (Lour.) Merr.]

Tianmendong [天门冬, radix asparagi, Asparagus cochinchinensis (Lour.) Merr.], also named Wansuiteng, Suoluoshu, Dianle, Dimendong, Yanmendong, Dianji, Yinyangshi and Guansong, grows in the valleys of Fenggao, Jianzhou[1] and Hanzhou[2]. Presently it can be seen everywhere. Its vines, sprouting in spring and shaping like hairpins, are more than one Zhang long, and always climb along other plants. The leaves of some species are like those of Huixiang [茴香,

fennel, Foeniculum vulgare Mill.] but extremely sharpe and thin, glabrous and spinescent. Some species is scabrous and inermous. Some species is like but smaller and sparser than that of cypress. All the species are named Tianmendong. Its flowers, blooming in summer, are white, yellow or purple. Its black fruit, bearing in autumn, grows besides the branches of its stem base. It bears fruit without blooming since the dog days begin. Its white or yellowish purple roots, 2~3 Cun long, are as big as fingers, and the bigger ones are of good quality. The species which grows in the highlands with short roots, the sweet taste and aromatic flavor are of the best quality. The species, which grows in the low-lying wetlands along the waterside with thin and small yellow leaves like those of hornworts and long roots, with bitter taste and foul smell, can also be taken. Its plants are bitter and sweet in taste, neutral in nature, extremely cold and non-toxic. Yuanyi, Dihuang[3] [地黄, unprocessed rehmannia root, Rehmannia glutinosa (Gaetn.) Libosch. ex Fisch. et Mey.] and Beimu [贝母, fritillaria, Bulbus Fritillaria] serve as the assistant herb of Tianmendong [天门冬, radix asparagi, Asparagus cochinchinensis (Lour.) Merr.], and Tianmendong is restrained by Cengqing [曾青, azurite, Azurite]. The people who are poisoned by eating Liyu [鲤鱼, carp, Cyprinus carpio L.] after taking Tianmendong can be treated by Fuping [浮萍, common ducksmeat herb, Lemna minor L.].

For famine relief: Collect roots, remove the abnormal taste by soaking them, boil them after getting rid of the stalk base and fibrous roots. Or dry and cook them thoroughly, it is better to mix with honey.

For disease treatment: See the clauses in *Materia Medica · Herbaceous Plant*.

【Notes】

[1] The name of an ancient county. It is presently located in Jian'ou City of Fujian Province.

[2] The name of an ancient county. It is presently located in the areas of Guanghan, Deyang, Mianzhu, Shifang, Jintang County.

[3] See the 221th clause of this book.

167. 章柳根

本草一名商陆,一名葛根,一名夜呼,一名白昌,一名当陆,一名章陆,《尔雅》谓之蓫薚,《广雅》谓之马尾,《易》胃之苋陆。生咸阳川谷,今处处有之。苗高三四尺。干粗似鸡冠花[1]干,微有线楞,色微紫赤。叶青如牛舌,微阔而长。根如人形者有神,亦有赤白二种,花赤根亦赤,花白根亦白。赤者不堪服食,伤人,乃至痢血[2]不已,白者堪服食。又有一种名赤昌,苗叶绝相类,不可用,须细辨之。商陆味辛、酸。一云味苦,性平,有毒。一云性冷,得大蒜良。

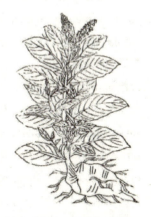

救饥:取白色根切作片子,煠熟,换水浸洗净,淡食,得大蒜良。凡制,薄切,以东流水浸二宿,捞出,与豆叶隔间入甑蒸,从午至亥。如无叶,用豆依法蒸之亦可。花白者年多,仙人采之作脯,可为下酒。

治病:文具《本草·草部》商陆条下。

【注释】

[1] 见本书第53鸡冠菜条。

[2] 病名。痢疾便中多血,称赤痢。由热毒乘血所致。

167. Zhangliugen [章柳根, pokeberry root, Phytolacca acinosa Roxb.]

Zhangliugen [章柳根, pokeberry root, Phytolacca acinosa Roxb.], also named Shanglu, Tanggen, Yehu, Baichang, Danglu, Zhanglu, Zhutang in *Er Ya* [《尔雅》, *Literary Expositor*], Mawei in *Guangya* [《广雅》, *Supplement to Literary Expositor*], and Xianlu in *I Ching* [《易经》, *The Book of Changes*], grows in the valleys of Xianyang and can be seen everywhere presently. Its plants are 3 ~ 4 Chi high and its stems are thick like those of Jiguanhua[1] [鸡冠花, feather cockscomb, *Celosia argentea* L.] with minor grooves and reddish purple color. Its green leaves are like Niushe [牛舌, plantago, *Plantago asiatica* L.] but a little broader and longer. There are 2 varieties of human-shaped roots, the white variety and the red variety, which are thought to be supernatural. The red type bears red flowers and the white type white flowers. The red type can not be taken because it leads to incontinent bloody dysentery[2] and the white type is edible. Another species, named Chichang, with the seedlings and leaves like those of the edible type, is inedible and should be carefully identified. It is pungent and sour in taste, or bitter in taste and neutral in nature with toxicity, or cold in nature and compatible with garlic.

For famine relief: Collect white roots and cut them into slices, blanch and rinse them, and take them without salt and be good to serve with garlics. To process, cut them into thin slices, soak them with eastward-flowing water for 2 nights, and steam them on soybean leaves in rice steamer from Wushi (11 a. m. to 1 p. m.) to Haishi (9 p. m. to 11 p. m.). The steam with soybean is also feasible without leaves available. Collect celestial perennial roots of white variety, and make preserved fruit as snacks that go with wine.

For disease treatment: See Shanglu Clause in *Materia Medica · Herbaceous Plant*.

【Notes】

[1] See the 53th clause of this book.

[2] A disease name. It refers to dysentery with bloody stool, which is caused by heat toxin.

168. 沙　参

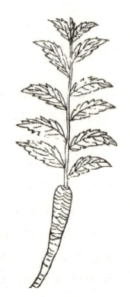

一名知母，一名苦心，一名志取，一名虎须，一名白参，一名识美，一名文希。生河内川谷及冤句、般阳[1]续山，并淄、齐、潞、随、归州[2]，而江淮、荆、湖[3]州郡皆有，今辉县太行山边亦有之。苗长一二尺，丛生崖坡间。叶似枸杞[4]叶，微长而有叉牙锯齿。开紫花。根如葵根，赤黄色，中正白实者佳。味微苦，性微寒，无毒。恶防己，反藜芦。又有杏叶沙参[5]及细叶沙参[6]，气味与此相类，但《图经》内不曾记载此二种叶苗形容，未敢并入本条，今皆另条开载。

救饥：掘根，浸洗极净，换水煮去苦味，再以水煮极熟，食之。

治病：文具《本草·草部》条下。

【注释】

［1］般阳县，出《名医别录》。西汉置，属济南郡。治所在今山东淄博市西南淄川城。

［2］古代州名，今湖北秭归、巴东、兴山三县地。

［3］古代州名，今浙江湖州市、长兴和安吉二县、德清县东部地。

［4］见本书第307枸杞条。

［5］见本书第224杏叶沙参条。

［6］见本书第180细叶沙参条。

168. Shashen［沙参, the root of straight ladybell, Adenophora stricta Miq.］

Shashen［沙参, the root of straight ladybell, Adenophora stricta Miq.］, also named Zhimu, Kuxin, Zhiqu, Huxu, Baishen, Shimei and Wenxi, grows in the mountains and river valleys of Henei, Yuanju, Xushan Mountain of Banyang[1], Zizhou, Qizhou, Luzhou, Suizhou, Guizhou[2], Jianghuaijun, Jingjun and Huzhoujun[3]. Presently it can be seen near Taihang Mountain of Huixian County. Its plants are 1~2 Chi high and cluster on the cliffs and slopes. Its leaves are like those of Gouqi[4]［枸杞, wolfberry, Lycium chinense Mill.］but a little longer with caniniform margin, and its flowers are purple. Its roots, like hollyhock roots, which are reddish yellow with white and compact center, are of good quality. It is slightly bitter in taste, slightly cold in nature and non-toxic. Shashen is averse to Fangji［防己, mealy fangji root, Stephania tetrandra］and in compatible with Lilu［藜芦, black false hellebore, Veratrum nigrum L.］. Xingye Shashen[5]［杏叶沙参, adenophora hunanensis, Adenophora hunanensis Nannf.］and Xiye Shashen[6]［细叶沙参, adenophora paniculata, Adenophora paniculata Nannf.］have the same taste and flavor as Shashen, but the shapes of its plants and leaves are not recorded in *Tu Jing Ben Cao*［《图经本草》, *Illustrated Pharmacopoeia*］. Thus both of them are recorded in the new clauses respectively without being listed here.

For famine relief: Dig roots, soak and rinse them, remove the bitterness by boiling them, and then take them after being fully cooked.

For disease treatment: See the clauses in *Materia Medica · Herbaceous Plant*.

【Notes】

[1] It belongs to Jinan Prefecture previously, and is located in Zichuan of Zibo presently.

[2] The name of an ancient county. It is presently located in Zigui, Badong, Xingshan of Hubei Province.

[3] The name of an ancient county. It is presently located in Huzhou, Changxing, Anji and east Deqing of Zhejiang Province.

[4] See the 307th clause of this book.

[5] See the 224th clause of this book.

[6] See the 180th clause of this book.

169. 麦门冬

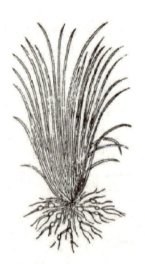

《本草》云：秦名羊韭，齐名爱韭，楚名马韭，越名羊蓍，一名禹葭，一名禹余粮。生随州、陆州及函谷堤坂肥土石间，久废处有之，今辉县山野中亦有。叶似韭叶而长，冬夏长生。根如穬麦而白色，出江宁者小润，出新安者大白。其人者苗如鹿葱，小者如韭。味甘，性平、微寒，无毒。地黄、车前为之使。恶款冬、苦瓠、苦芙。畏木耳、苦参、青襄。

救饥：采根，换水浸去邪味，淘洗净，蒸熟，去心食。

治病：文具《本草·草部》条下。

169. Maimendong [麦门冬, radix ophiopogonis, Ophiopogon japonicus (L. f.) Ker-Gawl]

Materia Medica says, "It is named Yangjiu in Qin State, Aijiu in Qi State, Majiu in Chu State, Yangshi in Yue State, and named Yujia and Yuyuliang." Maimendong [麦门冬, radix ophiopogonis, Ophiopogon japonicus (L. f.) Ker-Gawl] grows on the embankment and fertile soil of mountain slopes in Suizhou, Luzhou and Hangu. It also can be seen in deserted places and grows in the mountainous regions and fields of Huixian County presently. Its leaves are like but longer than those of Jiu〔韭, chinese chive, Allium tuberosum Rottb. ex Spreng〕, and it grows in winter and summer. Its white roots are like those of Kuangmai〔穬麦, barley, Hordeum vulgare L.〕, the species originating in Jiangning is small and glossy while the one originating in Xin'an is big and white. The big type is like Lucong〔鹿葱, lycoris squamigera, Lycoris squamigera Maxim.〕, and the small one is like Jiu〔韭, Chinese chive, Allium tuberosum Rottb. ex Spreng〕. It is sweet in taste, neutral in nature, slightly cold and non-toxic. Dihuang〔地黄, unprocessed rehmannia root, Rehmannia glutinosa Libosch. ex Fisch. et Mey.〕 and Cheqian〔车前, plantago seed, Plantago asiatica L.〕 may serve as the assistant herb of Maimendong. Maimendong is averse to Kuandong（款冬）, Kuhu（苦瓠）and Kufu（苦芙）, and it is restrained by Mu'er（木耳）, Kushen（苦参）and Qingxiang（青襄）.

For famine relief: Collect roots, remove the abnormal taste by soaking them, rinse and boil them after getting rid of the fibrous roots.

For disease treatment: See the clauses in *Materia Medica · Herbaceous Plant*.

170. 苎根

旧云闽、蜀、江、浙多有之，今许州人家田园中亦有种者。皮可绩布。苗高七八尺，一科十数茎。叶如楮[1]叶而不花叉，面青背白，上有短毛；又似苏子叶。其叶间出细穗，花如白杨[2]而长，每一朵凡十数穗，花青白色。子熟茶褐色。其根黄白色，如手指粗，宿根地中至春自生，不须藏种。荆扬间一岁二三刈，剥其皮，以竹刀刮其表，厚处自脱，得里如筋者煮之，用绩。以苎近蚕种之，则蚕不生。根味甘，性寒。

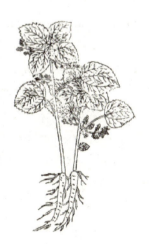

救饥：采根，刮洗去皮，煮极熟，食之甜美。

治病：文具《本草·草部》条下。

【注释】

[1] 见本书第310楮桃树条。

[2] 见本书第249白杨树条。

170. Zhugen [苎根, ramie, Boehmeria nivea (L.) Gaudich.]

It is recorded that Zhugen [苎根, ramie, Boehmeria nivea (L.) Gaudich.] grows in Fujian, Sichuan, Jiangsu and Zhejiang. Presently it is cultivated in common people's gardens in Xuzhou, and its stem bark is used for weaving. Its plants are 7~8 Chi high with a dozen canes for each. Its hispidulous leaves, adaxially green and abaxially white, are like those of Zhu[1] [楮, paper mulberry, Broussonetia papyrifera (Linn.) L'Hér. ex Vent.] with no gap, or like those of Suzi [苏子, purple perilla, Perilla frutescens (L.) Britt.]. Its panicles draw out of leaves with a dozen branches. Its flowers are greenish white and like those of Baiyang[2] [白杨, abele, Populus alba L.] but longer. Its ripe seeds are dark brown. Its roots are yellowish white with the size of fingers. Its perennial roots lay underground and sprout in spring spontaneously, so the seed preservation is unnecessary. It yields 2~3 crops one year in the areas of Jingzhou and Yangzhou. The thick part will fall off after the bark is peeled off and the surface is scraped, and you will get the vein-like ramie which can be twisted to threads after boiling. The silkworm will not grow up if it is bred surrounded by ramie. Its roots are sweet in taste and cold in nature.

For famine relief: Collect roots, remove the bark, wash and clean them, and cook them thoroughly. It tastes good.

For disease treatment: See the clauses in *Materia Medica · Herbaceous Plant*.

【Notes】

[1] See the 310th clause of this book.

[2] See the 249th clause of this book.

171. 苍 术

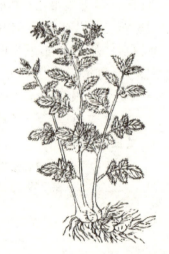

一名山蓟，一名山姜，一名山连，一名山精。生郑山[1]、汉中山谷，今近郡山谷亦有，嵩山、茅山者佳。苗淡青色，高二三尺，茎作蒿秆。叶抪茎而生，梢叶似棠[2]叶，脚叶有三五叉，皆有锯齿小刺。开花紫碧色,亦似刺蓟花,或有黄白花者。根长如指大而肥实,皮黑茶褐色。味苦、甘。一云味甘、辛,性温,无毒。防风,地榆为之使。

救饥:采根,去黑皮,薄切,浸二三宿,去苦味,煮熟食。亦作煎饵。久服轻身,延年不饥。

治病:文具《本草·草部》条下。

【注释】

［1］古代地名。今指陕西汉中。

［2］植物名,待考。

171. Cangzhu［苍术, atractylodes rhizome, Atractylodes Lancea（Thunb.）DC.］

Cangzhu［苍术, atractylodes rhizome, Atractylodes Lancea（Thunb.）DC.］, also named Shanji, Shanjiang, Shanlian and Shanjing, grows in the valleys of Zhengshan[1] and Hanzhong. Presently it can be seen in the valleys near the capital of the country and the species in Songshan Mountain and Maoshan Mountain are of good quality. Its plants are 2~3 Chi high with pale green color, and its stems are like those of Chrysanthemum carinatum. Its leaves, which are like those of Tang[2], scatter on the stems. Basal leaves are divided into 3~5 segments with serrate and spiny margin. It bears dark violet-blue flowers like those of Ciji［刺蓟, field thistle herb, Herba Cirsii］, or yellowish white flowers. Its rhizomes are as big as fingers but much thicker and stronger with dark brown bark. It is bitter and sweet in taste, or sweet and pungent in taste, warm in nature and non-toxic. Fangfeng［防风, divaricate saposhnikovia root, Saposhnikovia divaricata（Trucz.）Schischk.］ and Diyu［地榆, garden burnet root, Sanguisorba officinalis L.］ serve as the assistant herb of Cangzhu.

For famine relief: Collect roots, chip off the black bark, cut them into thin slices, remove the bitterness by soaking them for 2~3 nights, take them after they are fully boiled or serve as the bait drug. The long-term of taking it can make body light and active, prolong life without feeling hungry.

For disease treatment: See the clauses in *Materia Medica · Herbaceous Plant*.

【Notes】

［1］The geographic name in ancient China. It is presently located in Hanzhong

City of Shaanxi Province.

[2] A plant name. It remains to be verified.

172. 菖 蒲

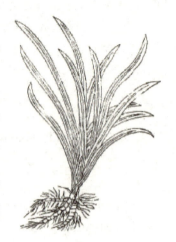

一名尧韭,一名昌阳。生上洛池泽及蜀郡严道、戎、卫[1]、衡州并嵩岳石碛上,今池泽处处有之。叶似蒲而扁,有脊,一如剑刃。其根盘屈有节,状如马鞭鞘,大根傍引三四小根,一寸九节者良,节尤密者佳,亦有十二节者,露根者不可用。又一种名兰荪,又谓溪荪,根形气色极似石上菖蒲,叶正如蒲,无脊,俗谓之菖蒲。生于水次,失水则枯。其菖蒲味辛,性温,无毒。秦皮、秦艽为之使,恶地胆、麻黄。不可犯铁,令人吐逆。

救饥:采根,肥大节稀,水浸去邪味,制造作果食之。

治病:文具《本草·草部》条下。

【注释】

[1] 古代州名,今指河南新乡、卫辉等地。

172. Changpu [菖蒲, calamus, Acorus calamus]

Changpu [菖蒲, calamus, Acorus calamus], also named Yaojiu and Changyang, grows in the swamps and the pond sides of Shangluo and Yandao in Shu Prefecture, or the rocky beach of Rongzhou, Weizhou[1], Hengzhou and Songshan Mountain. It can be seen in the swamps and the pond sides everywhere presently. Its leaves are like those of Pu [蒲, typha angustifolia, Typha orientalis Presl.], flat, middle-ribbed and ensiform. Its roots are twining and nodiferous like the stems of verbena. 3~4 rootlets draw out of the main root, the one which has nine segments in one Cun is of good quality, the one with dense segments is of the best quality, and also there is a type with twelve segments in one Cun, the roots exposed to the outside can not be used. Another species is named Lansun or Xisun, whose root color and shape are like those of Shichangpu [石菖蒲,

grassleaf sweetflag rhizome, Acorus tatarinowii], and its leaves are also like those of Shichangpu with no ribs which popularly named Changpu. It grows near the waterside and can't live without water. It is pungent in taste, warm in nature and non-toxic. Qinpi [秦皮, ash bark, Cortex Fraxinus chinensis Roxb.] and Qinjiao [秦艽, largeleaf gentian root, Gentiana macrophylla Pall.] serve as the assistant herb of Changpu, and Changpu is averse to Didan [地胆, epicauta, Meloe coarctatus Motsch.] and Mahuang [麻黄, ephedra, Ephedra sinica Stapf]. It can cause retch and vomit if contacted with iron.

For famine relief: Collect roots which are big and plump with sparse segments, remove the abnormal taste by soaking them, and make them into pastry for food.

For disease treatment: See the clauses in *Materia Medica · Herbaceous Plant*.

【Notes】

[1] The name of an ancient county. It is presently located in the places such as Xinxiang, Weihui, etc in Henan Province.

新增
New Supplements

173. 蓇子根

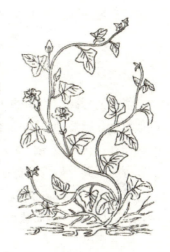

俗名打碗花,一名兔儿苗,一名狗儿秧,幽蓟[1]间谓之燕蓇根,千叶者呼为缠枝牡丹,亦名穰花。生平泽中,今处处有之。延蔓而生。叶似山药[2]叶而狭小。开花状似牵牛花,微短而圆,粉红色。其根甚多,大者如小箸粗,长一二尺,色白,味甘,性温。

救饥:采根,洗净蒸食之。或晒干杵碎,炊饭食亦好。或磨作面,作烧饼蒸食皆可。久食则头晕、破腹,间食则宜。

【注释】

[1] 明代地名。今指天津市蓟州区。

[2] 见本书第414山药条。

173. Fuzigen [葍子根, calystegia hederacea, Calystegia hederacea Wall. ex. Roxb.]

Fuzigen [葍子根, calystegia hederacea, Calystegia hederacea Wall. ex. Roxb.] is also named Dawanhua, Tu'ermiao, Gou'eryang and Yanfugen in Youji[1] area, and the double petalous variety is named Chanzhi Mudan or Ranghua. It grows in the swamps and wetlands, and can be seen everywhere presently. Its shoots are prostrate or twining, and its leaves are like but narrower and smaller than those of Shanyao[2] [山药, common yam rhizome, Dioscorea opposita Thunb.]. Its flowers are pale pink, short and ovate, and with the shape like the Morning Glory. Its white roots, ramose and slender, as big as small chopsticks, 1~2 Chi long, are sweet in taste and warm in nature.

For famine relief: Collect roots, rinse and steam them; or dry them in the sunshine, pound them into pieces, and cook them for food; or grind them into powder, make them into cakes or steam them for food. It can cause dizziness and diarrhea if taken for a long time, so it is better to use them occasionally.

【Notes】

[1] A geographic name in Ming Dynasty. It is presently located in Jizhou of Tianjin.

[2] See the 414th clause of this book.

174. 荞蒌根

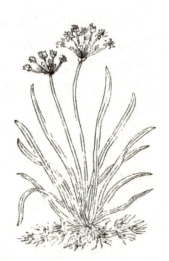

俗名面碌磭。生水边下湿地。其叶就地丛生，叶似蒲叶而肥短，叶背如剑脊样。叶丛中间撺葶，上开淡粉红花，俱皆六瓣，花头攒开如伞盖状。结子如韭花菁葖。其根如鹰爪黄连样，色似墐泥色，味甘。

救饥：采根，揩去皴毛，用水淘净，蒸熟食。或晒干，炒熟食。或磨作面蒸食皆可。

174. Maosaogen [蓤蒴根, water gladiole, Butomus umbellatus Linn.]

Maosaogen [蓤蒴根, water gladiole, Butomus umbellatus Linn.], also named Mianliuzhou, grows in the low-lying wetlands along the waterside. Its leaves, clustered on the ground, are like those of Pu [蒲, calamus, Acorus calamus] but thicker and smaller, with the ridgy midvein like a sword. Its scapes draw out of leaves and bear pale pink flowers which are six-petal and assemble like canopy. Its follicles are like the capsule of Jiu [韭, Chinese chive, Allium tuberosum Rottb. ex Spreng]. The root shape is like that of Yingzhao Huanglian [鹰爪黄连, golden thread, Coptis chinensis Franch.] with the color like the mud which is used to plug the door crack. It is sweet in taste.

For famine relief: Collect roots, remove the root hair, rinse and steam them. Or dry them in the sunshine and stir-fry or grind them into powder, and steam them for food.

175. 野胡萝卜

生荒野中。苗叶似家胡萝卜,俱细小。叶间攒生茎叉,梢头开小白花,众花攒开如伞盖状,比蛇床子花头又大。结子比蛇床子亦大。其根比家胡萝卜尤细小。味甘。

救饥:采根,洗净蒸食,生食亦可。

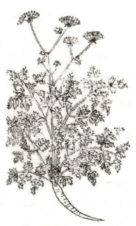

175. Ye Huluobo [野胡萝卜, wild carrot, Daucus carota L.]

Ye Huluobo [野胡萝卜, wild carrot, Daucus carota L.] grows in the wilderness, and its seedlings and leaves are like those of carrots but thinner and smaller. Its scapes stand out of leaves and bear small white flowers. Its flowers gather together like canopies. Both the umbel and the seeds are larger than those of Shechuangzi [蛇床子, common cnidium fruit, Clinopodium megalanthum (Diels) C. Y. Wu et Hsuan ex H. W. Li]. Its roots are thinner and smaller than those of carrots. It is sweet in taste.

For famine relief: Collect roots, rinse and steam them, or eat them as raw food.

176. 绵枣儿

一名石枣儿。出密县山谷中,生石间。苗高三五寸,叶似韭叶而阔,瓦陇样。叶中撺葶出穗,似鸡冠苋穗而细小,开淡粉红花,微带紫色。结小蒴儿,其子似大蓝子而小,黑色。根类独颗蒜[1];又似枣[2]形而白,味甜,性寒。

救饥:采取根,添水久煮极熟,食之。不换水煮,食后腹中鸣,有下气。

【注释】

[1] 见本书第167章柳根条。

[2] 见本书第362枣树条。

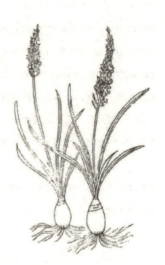

176. Mianzao'er [绵枣儿, common squill bulb, Scilla scilloides (Lindl.) Druce]

Mianzao'er [绵枣儿, common squill bulb, Scilla scilloides (Lindl.) Druce], also named Shizao'er, originates from the valleys of Mixian County and grows in the soil between stones. Its plants are 3~5 Cun high and its leaves are like those of Jiu [韭, Chinese chive, Allium tuberosum Rottb. ex Spreng] but broader with flutes. Its scapes stand out of leaves and draw out spikes which are like but smaller than those of Jiguanxian [鸡冠苋, feather cockscomb, Celosia argentea L.]. Its flowers are pale pink and purplish. It bears small capsules, and its black seeds are like those of Dalan [大蓝, isatis indigotica fort, Isatis indigotica Fortune]. Its bulbs are like Dukesuan[1] [独颗蒜, garlic, Allium sativum] or like Zao[2] [枣, jujube, Ziziphus jujuba Mill.] with white color. It is sweet in taste and cold in nature.

For famine relief: Collect bulbs, boil them for a long time, and take them after they are fully cooked. It can cause barborygmus, abdominal distention and flatus if boiled without exchanging the water.

【Notes】

[1] See the 167th clause of this book.

[2] See the 362th clause of this book.

177. 土囤儿

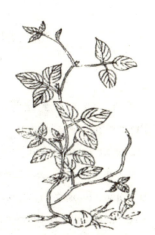

一名地栗子。出新郑山野中。细茎延蔓而生。叶似绿豆叶，微尖，每三叶攒生一处。根似土瓜儿根，微团，味甜。

救饥：采根，煮熟食之。

177. Tuluan'er [土囤儿, root of Fortune Apios, Apios fortunei Maxim.]

Tuluan'er [土囤儿, root of Fortune Apios, Apios fortunei Maxim.], also named Dilizi, grows in the mountainous regions and fields of Xinzheng. Its stems are slender and twining. Its leaves are like those of Lvdou [绿豆, mung bean, Vigna radiata (Linn.) Wilczek] but a little sharper, with three leaves growing together (compound leaves). Its root tubers are ovoid like those of Tugua'er [土瓜儿, trichosanthes cucumeroides, Trichosanthes cucumeroides (Ser.) Maxim.] and taste sweet.

For famine relief: Collect root tubers, and take them after they are fully cooked.

178. 野山药

生辉县太行山山野中。妥藤而生。其藤似葡萄[1]条稍细，藤颇紫色。其叶似家山药叶而大，微尖。根比家山药极细瘦，甚硬，皮色微赤，味微甜，性温、平，无毒。

救饥：采根，煮熟食之。

治病：今人与《本草·草部》下薯蓣同用。

【注释】

［1］见本书第350葡萄条。

178. Yeshanyao［野山药, wild yam rhizome, Dioscorea opposita Thunb.］

Yeshanyao［野山药, wild yam rhizome, Dioscorea opposita Thunb.］grows in the mountainous regions and fields of Taihang Mountain in Huixian County. Its stems are twining and purplish-red like those of Putao[1]［葡萄, grape, Vitis vinifera L.］but slenderer. Its leaves are like those of Jiashanyao［家山药, common yam rhizome, Dioscorea opposita Thunb.］but bigger and a little sharper. Its tubers are like but extremely thinner and harder than those of Jiashanyao with redish bark. It is slightly sweet in taste, warm and neutral in nature and non-toxic.

For famine relief: Collect root tubers, and take them after they are fully cooked.

For disease treatment: See the clauses in *Materia Medica · Herbaceous Plant*. It has the same usage of Shuyu［薯蓣, common yam rhizome, Dioscorea opposita Thunb.］

【Notes】

［1］See the 350th clause of this book.

179. 金瓜儿

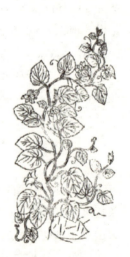

生郑州田野中。苗似初生小葫芦叶而极小，又似赤雹儿叶。茎方。茎叶俱有毛刺。每叶间出一细藤，延蔓而生。开五瓣尖碗子黄花。结子如马㼎[1]大，生青熟红。根形如鸡弹，微小，其皮土黄色，内则青白色，味微苦，性寒，与酒相反。

救饥：掘取根，换水煮，浸去苦味，再以水煮极熟，食之。

【注释】

[1] 见本书第202马㲈儿条。

179. Jingua'er［金瓜儿, thladiantha dubia, Thladiantha dubia Bunge］

Jingua'er［金瓜儿, thladiantha dubia, Thladiantha dubia Bunge］grows in the fields of Zhengzhou. Its seedlings are like those of Hulu［葫芦, bottle gourd, Lagenaria siceraria (Molina) Standl.］, and its leaves are extremely small like those of Chibao'er［赤雹儿, thladiantha dubia, Thladiantha dubia Bunge］. Both its leaves and angular stems are hirsute. Its tendrils draw out of leaves and twine around. Each of its flowers is yellow and oblong with 5 petals. Its fruit, as big as Mabao［马㲈, zehneria indica, Zehneria indica (Lour.) Keraudren］, is green when it is unripe and red when it is ripe. The root shape is like an egg but a little smaller with khaki bark and bluish-white core. It is slightly bitter in taste, cold in nature, and incompatible with rice wine.

For famine relief: Dig roots, remove the bitterness by boiling them and soaking them, and take them after they are fully cooked.

【Notes】

[1] See the 202th of this book.

180. 细叶沙参

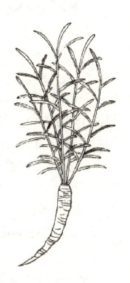

生辉县太行山山冲间。苗高一二尺,茎似蒿秆。叶似石竹子叶而细长;又似水蓑衣叶,亦细长。梢间开紫花。根似葵根而粗,如拇指大,皮色灰,中间白色,味甜,性微寒。本草有沙参,苗叶茎状,所说与此不同,未敢并入条下,今另为一条,开载于此。

救饥:掘取根,洗净,煮熟食之。

治病:与《本草·草部》沙参同用。

180. Xiye Shashen [细叶沙参, adenophora paniculata, Adenophora paniculata Nannf.]

Xiye Shashen [细叶沙参, adenophora paniculata, Adenophora paniculata Nannf.] grows in the mountainous regions and fields of Taihang Mountain in Huixian County. Its plants are 1~2 Chi high, and its stems are like those of Chrysanthemum carinatum. Its leaves are like but slenderer than those of Shizhuzi [石竹子, Chinese pink, Dianthus chinensis L.] or Shuisuoyi [水蓑衣, hygrophila salicifolia, Hygrophila salicifolia (Vahl) Nees]. It bears purple flowers. Its roots, like those of hollyhocks but thicker than the latter, as big as thumbs, with gray bark and white core, are sweet in taste and slightly cold in nature. For the seedlings, the leaves and stems of Xiye Shashen [细叶沙参, adenophora paniculata, Adenophora paniculata Nannf.] are quite different from those of Shashen [沙参, the root of straight ladybell, Adenophora stricta Miq.], so it is not included in Shashen Clause and recorded in another new clause here.

For famine relief: Dig roots, rinse and steam them, and eat them after they are fully cooked.

For disease treatment: See Shashen Clause in *Materia Medica · Herbaceous Plant*. It has the same usage of Shashen.

181. 鸡腿儿

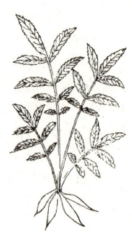

一名翻白草。出钧州山野中。苗高七八寸,细长。锯齿叶硬厚,背白,其叶似地榆叶而细长。开黄花。根如指大,长三寸许,皮赤内白,两头尖艄,味甜。

救饥:采根煮熟食,生吃亦可。

181. Jitui'er [鸡腿儿, potentilla discolor, Potentilla discolor Bge.]

Jitui'er [鸡腿儿, potentilla discolor, Potentilla discolor Bge.], also named

Fanbaicao, grows in the mountainous regions and fields of Junzhou. Its plants are 7~8 Cun high, thin and long. Its leaves are hard and thick with serrate margin, abaxially white, and like but slenderer than those of Diyu [地榆, garden burnet root, Sanguisorba officinalis L.]. Its flowers are yellow. Its fusiform roots, as big as fingers, are about three Cun long with red bark and white core. It is sweet in taste.

For famine relief: Collect roots, and eat them after they are fully cooked or when they are raw.

182. 山蔓菁

出钧州山野中。苗高一二尺。茎叶皆莴苣色。叶似桔梗叶，颇长艄而不对生；又似山小菜叶，微窄。根形类沙参，如手指粗，其皮灰色，中间白色，味甜。

救饥：采根煮熟食，生亦可食。

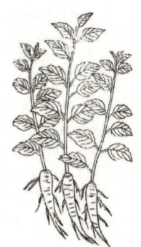

182. Shanmanjing [山蔓菁, adenophora trachelioides, Adenophora trachelioides Maxim.]

Shanmanjing [山蔓菁, adenophora trachelioides, Adenophora trachelioides Maxim.] grows in the mountainous regions and fields of Junzhou. Its plants are 1~2 Cun high, and the color of its stems and leaves is like that of Woju [莴苣, lettuce, Lactuca sativa L.]. Its leaves are like those of Jiegeng [桔梗, platycodon root, Platycodon grandiflorus (Jacq.) A. DC.] but sharper and longer without the opposite, and also like those of Shanxiaocai [山小菜, spotted bellflower, Campanula punctata Lam.] but narrower. Its roots, like those of Shashen [沙参, the root of straight ladybell, Adenophora stricta Miq.], are as big as fingers with gray bark and white core. It tastes sweet.

For famine relief: Collect roots, and eat them after they are fully cooked or when they are raw.

183. 老鸦蒜

生水边下湿地中。其叶直生,出土四垂。叶状似蒲而短,背起剑脊。其根形如蒜瓣,味甜。

救饥:采根煠熟,水浸,淘净,油盐调食。

183. Laoyasuan [老鸦蒜, lycoris, Lycoris radiata (L'Her.) Herb.]

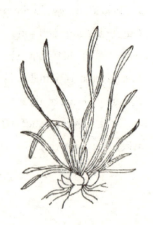

Laoyasuan [老鸦蒜, lycoris, Lycoris radiata (L'Her.) Herb.] grows in the low-lying wetlands along the waterside. Its leaves erect when sprouting and bend to the ground when growing up. Its leaves are like those of Pu [蒲, typha angustifolia, Typha orientalis Presl.] but shorter with abaxially ridgy midveins. Its bulbs are like those of garlics and taste sweet.

For famine relief: Collect and blanch bulbs, soak and rinse them, and flavor them with oil and salt.

184. 山萝卜

生山谷间,田野中亦有之。苗高五七寸,四散分生茎叶。其叶似菊叶而阔大,微有艾香,每茎五七叶排生如一大叶。稍间开紫花。根似野胡萝卜根而黪白色,味苦。

救饥:采根煠熟,水浸淘去苦味,油盐调食。

184. Shanluobo [山萝卜, scabiosa japonica, Scabiosa japonica Miq.]

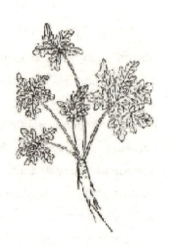

Shanluobo [山萝卜, scabiosa japonica, Scabiosa japonica Miq.] grows in the valleys, and it can be seen in the mountainous regions and wilderness. Its plants are 5~7 Cun high with scattered stems and leaves. Its leaves are like those of Ju［菊, chrysanthemum, Dendranthema morifolium（Ramat.）Tzvel.］but broader and larger with a light aroma of Ai［艾, mugwort, Artemisia argyi Levl. et Van.］. There is a big pinnatipartite leaf with 5~7 lobes on each petiole. Its purple flowers stand out of branches. Its roots are like those of Ye Huluobo［野胡萝卜, wild carrot, Daucus carota L.］with greyish-white color and bitter taste.

For famine relief: Collect and blanch roots, remove the bitterness by soaking and rinsing them, and flavor them with oil and salt.

185．地　参

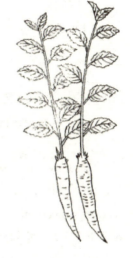

又名山蔓菁。生郑州沙岗间。苗高一二尺。叶似初生桑科[1]小叶，微短；又似桔梗叶，微长。开花似铃铎样，淡红紫色。根如拇指大，皮色苍，肉黪白色，味甜。

救饥：采根煮食。

【注释】

［1］指桑树的枝条，见本书第323桑椹树条。

185. Dishen［地参, adenophora wawreana, Adenophora wawreana Zahlbr.］

Dishen［地参, adenophora wawreana, Adenophora wawreana Zahlbr.］, also named Shanmanjing, grows on the sandhills of Zhengzhou. Its plants are 1~2 Chi high. Its leaves are like those on the twigs of Sang[1]［桑, mulberry, Morus alba L.］but a little shorter, and like those of Jiegeng［桔梗, platycodon root, Platycodon grandiflorus（Jacq.）A. DC.］but a little longer. It bears reddish-purple flowers which are like Lingduo（bell）. Its roots, as big as thumbs, with offwhite bark, and greyish-white pulp, are sweet in taste.

For famine relief: Collect and boil roots.

［Notes］

［1］See the 323th clause of this book.

186. 獐牙菜

生水边。苗初塌地生。叶似龙须菜叶而长窄,叶头颇团而不尖,其叶嫩薄;又似牛尾菜叶,亦长窄。其根如茅根[1]而嫩,皮色灰黑,味甜。

救饥:掘根,洗净煮熟,油盐调食。

【注释】

[1] 疑"茅芽根"之错漏,见本书第 233 茅芽根条。

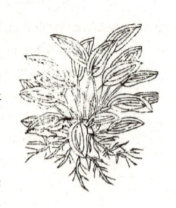

186. Zhangyacai [獐牙菜, oriental waterplantain rhizome, Alisma plantago-aquatica Linn.]

Zhangyacai [獐牙菜, oriental waterplantain rhizome, Alisma plantago-aquatica Linn.] grows along the waterside. In the early growth period, its seedlings creep on the ground. Its leaves, which are like but slenderer than those of Longxucai [龙须菜, asparagus, Asparagus schoberioides Kunth] or Niuweicai [牛尾菜, riparian greenbrier root and rhizome, Smilax riparia] with blunt apexes, are tender and thin. Its roots are tender like those of Maogen[1] [茅根, imperata, Imperata koenigii (Retz.) Beauv.] with dark gray bark, and they are sweet in taste.

For famine relief: Dig roots, rinse and boil them, and flavor them with oil and salt.

【Notes】

[1] It is suspected to be Maoyagen. See the 233th clause of this book.

187. 鸡儿头苗

生祥符西田野中。就地妥秧生。叶甚稀疏,每五叶攒生,状如一叶,其叶花叉,有小锯齿。叶间生蔓,开五瓣黄花。根叉甚多,其根形如香附子而须长,皮黑肉白,味甜。

救饥:采根,换水煮熟食。

187. Ji'ertou Miao [鸡儿头苗, potentilla reptans, Potentilla reptans L. var. sericophylla Franch.]

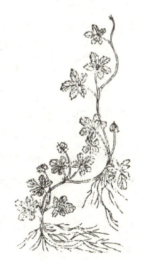

Ji'ertou Miao [鸡儿头苗, potentilla reptans, Potentilla reptans L. var. sericophylla Franch.] grows in the fields of the west of Xiangfu. Its plants trail along the ground. Its leaves are palmately divided and leaf blades pedately five-foliolate, and its lobes are parted with obtusely serrate margin. Its stolons draw out of leaves and bear five-petal yellow flowers. Its roots are much branched like those of Xiangfuzi [香附子, nutgrass galingale rhizome, Cyperus rotundus L.] with longer root hair, black root-bark and white pulp, and they are sweet in taste.

For famine relief: Collect and dig roots, and eat them after they are fully cooked.

实可食

《本草》原有

Fruit Edible

Original Ones

188. 雀 麦

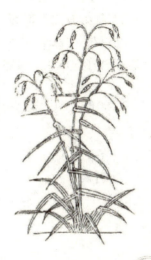

本草一名燕麦,一名蘥。生于荒野林下,今处处有之。苗似燕麦[1]而又细弱。结穗像麦穗而极细小,每穗又分作小叉穗十数个,子甚细小。味甘,性平,无毒。

救饥:采子,舂去皮,捣作面蒸食。作饼食亦可。

治病:文具《本草·草部》条下。

【注释】

[1] 见本书第 198 燕麦条。

188. Quemai [雀麦, Japanese bromegrass, Bromus japonicus Thunb. ex Murr.]

Quemai [雀麦, Japanese bromegrass, Bromus japonicus Thunb. ex Murr.], also named Yanmai and Yao, grows in the woods of wilderness, which can be seen everywhere presently. Its plants are like those of Yanmai[1] [燕麦, roegneria kamoji, Roegneria kamoji Ohwi] but slenderer. Its panicles are like but thinner and smaller than those of Mai [麦, wheat, Triticum Linn.] and bear dozens of spikelets, and its seeds are also very small. It is sweet in taste, neutral in nature and non-toxic.

For famine relief: Collect seeds, pound to peel off the seed coat, grind them into flour and steam, or make them baked wheaten cakes.

For disease treatment: See the clauses in *Materia Medica · Herbaceous Plant*.

【Notes】

[1] See the 198th clause of this book.

189. 回回米

本草名薏苡人,一名解蠡,一名屋菼,一名起实,一名赣,俗名草珠儿,又呼为西番蜀秫。生真定平泽及田野。交趾生者[1]子最大,彼土人呼为赣珠,今处处有之。苗高三四尺。叶似黍叶而稍大。开红白花,作穗子,结实青白色,形如珠而稍长,故名薏珠子。味甘,微寒,无毒。今人俗亦呼为菩提子。

救饥:采实,舂取其中人煮粥食。取叶煮饮亦香。

治病:文具《本草·草部》薏苡人条下。

【注释】

[1] 薏苡的变种,从越南引进,见本书第194川谷条。

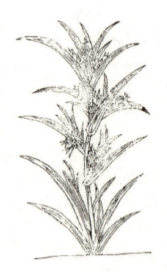

189. Huihuimi [回回米, the seed of job's tears, Coix chinensis Tod.]

Huihuimi [回回米, the seed of job's tears, Coix chinensis Tod.], also named Yiyiren, Jieli, Wutan, Qishi, Gan, Caozhu'er and Xifan Shushu, grows in the flat swamps and fields of Zhending. The species with the biggest seeds which originate in Jiaozhi[1] is called Ganzhu by local people, and presently it can be seen everywhere. Its plants are 3~4 Chi high. Its leaves are like but bigger than those of Shu [黍, millet, Panicum miliaceum L.]. The female spikelets are red while the male spikelets are yellow or white. The green-white grain is shaped like the bead but longer, so it is called Yizhuzi. It is sweet in taste, slightly cold in nature and non-toxic. Presently people always call it Putizi.

For famine relief: Collect grains, grind them and peel off the coat for cooking congee, or collect leaves, boil them for tea.

For disease treatment: See Yiyiren Clause in *Materia Medica · Herbaceous Plant*.

【Notes】

[1] One variation of Yiyi imported from Vietnam. See the 194th clause of this book.

190. 蒺藜子

本草一名旁通,一名屈人,一名止行,一名犲羽,一名升推,一名即藜,一名茨。生冯翊[1]平泽或道傍,今处处有之。布地蔓生。细叶,开小黄花,结子有三角刺人是也。性苦,辛,性温,微寒,无毒。乌头为之使。又有一种白蒺藜,出同州沙苑。开黄紫花,作荚子,结子状如腰子样,小如黍粒,补肾药多用,味甘,有小毒。

救饥:收子炒微黄,捣去刺,磨面作烧饼,或蒸食皆可。

治病:文具《本草·草部》条下。

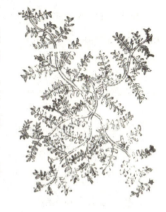

【注释】

[1] 古代郡名,今指陕西韩城市以南,渭河以北地区。

190. Jilizi [蒺藜子, puncturevine caltrop fruit, Tribulus terrester L.]

Jilizi [蒺藜子, puncturevine caltrop fruit, Tribulus terrester L.], also named Pangtong, Quren, Zhixing, Chaiyu, Shengtui, Jili and Ci, grows in the swarmps or the roadsides of Fengyi[1] and can be seen everywhere presently. Its plants are prostrate on the ground. Its leaves are slender and small, and its flowers are yellow. There are three spikes on the carpel of schizocarp. It is bitter and pungent in taste, warm and slightly cold in nature and non-toxic. Wutou [乌头, common monkshood, Aconitum carmichaelii Debx.] serves as the assistant herb of Jilizi. There is another kind of plant called Baijili [白蒺藜, flatstem milkvetch seed, Astragalus complanatus Bunge], which grows in Shayuan of Tongzhou. It bears yellowish-purple flowers and legumes with the kidney-like seeds which are as big as millets. It is sweet in taste and slightly toxic, often applied in kidney-reinforcing decoctions.

For famine relief: Collect seeds, dry-fry them to yellow, pound them to remove the spikes, grind them into flour to make wheaten cakes, or steam them for food.

For disease treatment: See the clauses in *Materia Medica · Herbaceous Plant*.

【Notes】

[1] The name of an ancient prefecture. It is presently located in the south of Hancheng and in the north of Weihe in Shaanxi Province.

191. 苘 子

本草名苘与实。处处有之。北人种以打绳索。苗高五六尺。叶似芋[1]叶而短薄,微有毛涩。开金黄花,结实壳,似蜀葵实壳而圆大,俗呼为苘馒头。子黑色如蟒豆大,味苦,性平,无毒。

救饥:采嫩苘馒头,取子生食。子坚实时收取子,浸去苦味,晒干磨面食。

治病:文具《本草·草部》苘实条下。

【注释】

[1] 见本书第365芋苗条。

191. Qingzi［苘子, abutilon, Abutilon theophrasti Medicus］

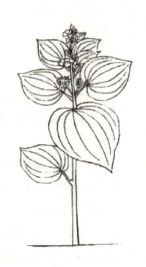

Qingzi［苘子, abutilon, Abutilon theophrasti Medicus］, also named Qingshi, can be seen everywhere. Northerners always cultivate it for making ropes. Its plants are 5~6 Chi high. Its puberulous leaves are like those of Yu[1]［芋, taro, Colocasia esculenta (L). Schott］but thinner and shorter. Its flowers are golden yellow. Its fruit, covered with hulls, commonly known as Qingmantou, is like the capsule of Shukui［蜀葵, hollyhock, Althaea rosea (Linn.) Cavan.］but larger and rounder. Its black seeds are as big as those of Laodou［䝁豆, wild soybean, Glycine soja Sieb. et Zucc.］. It is bitter in taste, neutral in nature and non-toxic.

For famine relief: Collect young fruit, eat uncooked seeds, or collect ripe seeds, remove the bitterness by soaking them, dry them up and grind them into flour.

For disease treatment: See the clause of Qingshi in *Materia Medica · Herbaceous Plant*.

【Notes】

[1] See the 365th clause of this book.

※ 新增

New Supplements

192. 稗 子

有二种,水稗生水田边,旱稗生田野中。今皆处处有之。苗叶似穄子[1],叶色深绿,脚叶颇带紫色。梢头出扁穗,结子如黍粒大,茶褐色,味微苦,性微温。

救饥:采子,捣米煮粥食,蒸食尤佳,或磨作面食皆可。

【注释】

[1] 见本书第193穄子条。

192. Baizi [稗子, barnyard millet, Echinochloa crusgalli (L.) Beauv.]

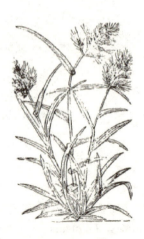

There are two kinds of Baizi [稗子, barnyard millet, Echinochloa crusgalli (L.) Beauv.]: Shuibai [水稗, panicum crus, Echinochloa phyllopogon (Stapf) Koss.] grows near the irrigated fields while Hanbai [旱稗, barnyard millet, Echinochloa hispidula (Retz.) Nees] grows in the fields. Presently it can be seen everywhere. Its upper leaves are dark green which is like that of Canzi[1] [穄子, barnyard millet, Echinochloa crusgalli (L.) Beauv. var. crusgalli], while its lower leaves are purplish. Its flat spikelets draw out of panicles, and bear dark brown caryopses which are like millets. It is slightly bitter in taste and slightly warm in nature.

For famine relief: Collect caryopses, thresh them to make congee, especially good to steam them, or grind them into flour.

【Notes】

[1] See the 193th clause of this book.

193. 穄 子

生水田中及下湿地内。苗叶似稻，但差短。梢头结穗，仿佛稗子穗。其子如黍粒大，茶褐色，味甘。

救饥：采子，捣米煮粥，或磨作面蒸食亦可。

193. Canzi [穄子, barnyard millet, Echinochloa crusgalli (L.) Beauv. var. crusgalli]

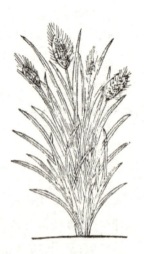

Canzi [穄子, barnyard millet, Echinochloa crusgalli (L.) Beauv. var. crusgalli] grows in the rice fields and low-lying wetlands. Its leaves are like those of Dao [稻, paddy, Oryza sativa L.] but a little shorter, and its spikes are like those of Baizi [稗子, barnyard millet, Echinochloa crusgalli (L.) Beauv.]. Its dark brown caryopses are as big as millets with sweet taste.

For famine relief: Collect caryopsis, thresh them to make congee, or grind them into flour and steam.

194. 川 谷

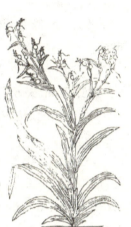

生汜水县田野中。苗高三四尺。叶似初生蜀秫叶微小。叶间丛开小黄白花,结子似草珠儿[1]微小,味甘。

救饥:采子捣为米,生用冷水淘净后,以滚水汤三五次,去水下锅,或作粥,或作炊饭食皆可。亦堪造酒。

【注释】

[1] 回回米的别名,见本书第189回回米条。

194. Chuangu [川谷, adlay, Coix lacryma-jobi L.]

Chuangu [川谷, adlay, Coix lacryma-jobi L.] grows in the fields of Sishui County with plants 3~4 Chi high. Its leaves are like those of young Shushu [蜀秫, sorghum, Sorghum bicolor (L.) Moench] but a little smaller. Its yellow-white flowers assemble among leaves, and the caryopses are like Caozhu'er[1] with sweet taste.

For famine relief: Collect and thresh caryopses, rinse them with cold water, blanch them 3~5 times with boiling water, drain them to make congee or for cooking, or make rice wine.

【Notes】

[1] Another name for Huihuimi [回回米, the seed of job's tears, Coix chinensis Tod.]. See the 189th clause of this book.

195. 莠草子

生田野中。苗叶似谷而叶微瘦。梢间结茸细毛穗。其子比谷细小,舂米类析米,熟时即收,不收即落。味微苦,性温。

救饥:采莠穗,揉取子捣米,作粥或作水饭,皆可食。

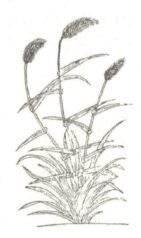

195. Youcaozi [莠草子, green bristlegrass, Setaria viridis (L.) Beauv.]

Youcaozi [莠草子, green bristlegrass, Setaria viridis (L.) Beauv.] grows in the fields, and its leaves are like those of Gu [谷, foxtail millet, Setaria italica (L.) Beauv.] but a little narrower. Its panicles are dense and its branchlets bear pubescent spikelets. Its caryopses are smaller than those of Gu [谷, foxtail millet, Setaria italica (L.) Beauv.] and as big as sagos after hulling. It should be reaped immediately when ripe or it will fall off. It is slightly bitter in taste and warm in nature.

For famine relief: Collect panicles, rub and hull them to get rice, and make congee or steam rice.

196. 野 黍

生荒野中。科苗皆类家黍而茎叶细弱。穗甚瘦小,黍粒亦极细小,味甜,性微温。

救饥:采子,舂去粗糠,或捣或磨面,蒸糕食,甚甜。

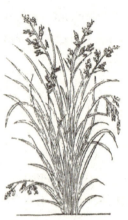

196. Yeshu［野黍, wild broom corn millet, Panicum miliaceum L.］

Yeshu［野黍, wild broom corn millet, Panicum miliaceum L.］grows in the wilderness, and its plants are like Jiashu［家黍, proso millet, Panicum miliaceum L.］, but both the stalks and the leaves are slenderer. Both the spikes and the millet grains are very thin and small. It is sweet in taste and slightly warm in nature.

For famine relief：Collect caryopses, thresh the chaff, pound or grind them into flour and make them steamed puddings. They taste very sweet.

197．鸡眼草

又名掐不齐,以其叶用指甲掐之,作劗不齐,故名。生荒野中,揭地生。叶如鸡眼大,似三叶酸浆[1]叶而圆；又似小虫儿卧单叶而大。结子小如粟粒,黑茶褐色,味微苦,气味与槐[2]相类,性温。

救饥:采子,捣取米,其米青色。先用冷水淘净,却以滚水汤三五次,去水下锅,或煮粥,或作炊饭食之,或磨面作饼食亦可。

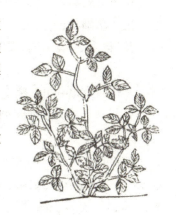

【注释】

［1］即酸浆草。见本书第19酸浆草条。

［2］见本书第320槐树芽条。

197. Jiyancao［鸡眼草, Japan clover herb, Kummerowia striata（Thunb.）Schindl.］

Jiyancao［鸡眼草, Japan clover herb, Kummerowia striata（Thunb.）Schindl.］is also named Qiabuqi for the irregular cleft nipped by finger nails. It grows in the wilderness and spreads along the ground. Its leaves, as big as chicken eyes, are obovate like those of Suanjiangcao[1]［酸浆草, creeping wood sorrel, Oxalis corniculata L.］or like but bigger than those of Xiaochong'er Wodan［小虫

儿卧单, euphorbia humifusa, Euphorbia humifusa Willd. ex Schlecht.]. Its seeds are as big as millets with black and dark brown color. It tastes slightly bitter which is like Huai[2][槐, sophora japonica, Sophora japonica Linn.] with warm nature.

For famine relief: Collect and thresh seeds, get green grains, rinse them with cold water, blanch them 3~5 times with boiling water, drain them to make congee or for cooking, or grind them into flour to make baked wheaten cakes.

【Notes】

[1] See the 19th clause of this book.

[2] See the 320th clause of this book.

198. 燕 麦

田野处处有之。其苗似麦揰,但细弱,叶亦瘦细,拼茎而生。结细长穗,其麦粒极细小。味甘。

救饥:采子,舂去皮,捣磨为面食。

198. Yanmai [燕麦, roegneria kamoji, Roegneria kamoji Ohwi]

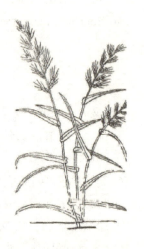

Yanmai [燕麦, roegneria kamoji, Roegneria kamoji Ohwi] grows in the fields everywhere. Its scapes, like those of wheat seedlings, draw out of stems, and its culms are thinner and more delicate with slender leaves scattering on them. Its spicas are slim and long with very small kernels. It is sweet in taste.

For famine relief: Collect seeds, pound them to peel off the seed coats, and grind them into flour.

199. 泼 盘

一名托盘。生汝南荒野中,陈蔡间多有之。苗高五七寸。茎叶有小刺。其叶仿佛似艾叶,稍团,叶背亦白,每三叶攒生一处。结子作穗,如半柿[1]大,类小盘堆石榴[2]颗状,下有蒂承,如柿蒂形,味甘酸,性温。

救饥：以泼盘颗粒红熟时采食之，彼土人取以当果。

【注释】

[1] 见本书第348 柿树条。

[2] 见本书第360 石榴条。

199. Popan〔泼盘, Japanese Raspberry Herb, Rubus parvifolius L.〕

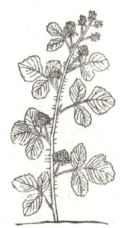

Popan〔泼盘, Japanese Raspberry Herb, Rubus parvifolius L.〕, also named Tuopan, grows in the wilderness of Runan. It can also be seen in the areas of Chen and Cai Prefecture. Its plants are 5~7 Cun high, both the stems and the leaves are covered with prickles. Its leaves are like those of Ai〔艾, mugwort, Artemisia argyi Levl. et Van.〕but slightly rounded and abaxially white. Its imparipinnate leaves are usually three-foliolate. Its spike-like aggregate fruit is as big as half Shi[1]. The fruit shapes are like many seeds of Shiliu[2] piling on the small plate with the receptacle like kaki calyx under the plate. It is sweet and sour in taste, and warm in nature.

For famine relief: Pick and eat it when its fruit is red and ripe. The local people take it as fruit.

【Notes】

[1] See the 348th clause of this book.

[2] See the 360th clause of this book.

200. 丝瓜苗

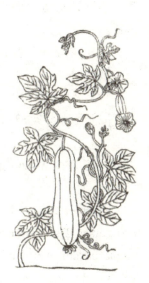

人家园篱边多种之。延蔓而生。叶似栝楼叶而花叉大，每叶间出一丝藤，缠附草木上。茎叶间开五瓣大黄花。结瓜，形如黄瓜而大，色青，嫩时可食，老则去皮，内有丝缕，可以擦洗油腻器皿，味微甜。

救饥：采嫩瓜，切碎煤熟，水浸，淘净，油盐调食。

200. Siguamiao [丝瓜苗, luffa, Luffa cylindrica (L.) Roem.]

Siguamiao [丝瓜苗, luffa, Luffa cylindrica (L.) Roem.] is cultivated in common people's gardens, twining and climbing along the fences. Its leaves are like those of Gualou (栝楼) with deeper lobes. Its tendrils draw out of each leaf and twine around other plants. It bears big yellow flowers with 5 petals for each. Shaping like Huanggua [黄瓜, cucumber, Cucumis sativus L.] but bigger than the latter, its young fruit is cyan and edible. When the fruit is overripe, the inside fibers can be used to wash greasy utensils after peeling off the pericarp.

For famine relief: Collect young fruits, cut them into small pieces and blanch them, soak and rinse them, and flavor them with oil and salt.

201. 地角儿苗

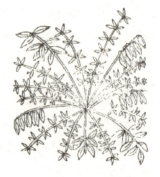

一名地牛儿苗。生田野中。揭地生,一根就分数十茎,其茎甚稠。叶似胡豆[1]叶微小,叶生茎面,每攒四叶对生作一处。茎傍另又生葶,梢头开淡紫花。结角似连翘角而小,中有子,状似䝁豆[2]颗,味甘。

救饥:采嫩角生食,硬角煮熟食豆。

【注释】

[1] 见本书第330 胡豆条。

[2] 见本书第327 䝁豆条。

201. Dijiao'er Miao [地角儿苗, oxytropis bicolor, Oxytropis bicolor Bunge]

Dijiao'er Miao [地角儿苗, oxytropis bicolor, Oxytropis bicolor Bunge], also named Diniu'ermiao, grows in the fields and spreads along the ground. A simple caudex can put forth dozens of dense branchlets (pinnately compound leaves). Its leaves are like but smaller than those of Hudou[1] [胡豆, astragalus complanatus, Astragalus complanatus Bunge]. Its leaves grow on the front of stems with 4 blades arranged at opposite sides. Its scapes draw out beside stems and bear pale pruple flowers. Its legumes are like the capsules of Lianqiao［连翘, weeping forsythia, Forsythia suspensa (Thunb.) Vahl］but smaller. Its seeds are like those of Laodou[2]［䝁豆, wild soybean, Glycine soja Sieb. et Zucc.］and taste sweet.

For famine relief: Collect legumes, eat raw tender legumes, and boil ripe legumes and eat beans.

【Notes】

［1］See the 330th clause of this book.

［2］See the 327th clause of this book.

202. 马㼎儿

生田野中。就地拖秧而生。叶似甜瓜叶极小，茎蔓亦细。开黄花。结实比鸡弹微小，味微酸。

救饥：摘取马㼎儿熟者食之。

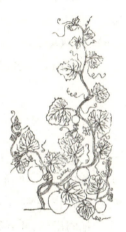

202. Mabao'er［马㼎儿, zehneria indica, Zehneria indica (Lour.) Keraudren］

Mabao'er［马㼎儿, zehneria indica, Zehneria indica (Lour.) Keraudren］grows in the fields and trails along the ground. Its leaves are like those of Tiangua［甜瓜, cucumis melon, Cucumis melo L.］but extremely small, and its tendrils are also very slender. Its flowers are yellow and its fruit is smaller than eggs with slightly sour taste.

For famine relief: Collect the ripe fruit to eat.

203. 山䔮豆

一名山豌豆。生密县山野中。苗高尺许。其茎窊面剑脊。叶似竹叶而齐短，两两对生。开淡紫花。结小角儿。其豆扁如䝁豆，味甜。

救饥：采取角儿煮食，或打取豆食皆可。

203. Shanlidou［山䔧豆, lathyrus quinquenervius, Lathyrus quinquenervius (Miq.) Litv.］

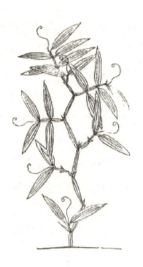

Shanlidou［山䔧豆, lathyrus quinquenervius, Lathyrus quinquenervius (Miq.) Litv.］, also named Shanwandou, grows in the mountainous regions and fields of Mixian County. Its plants are about one Chi high. Its stems and rachises are grooved adaxially like the ridge of a sword. Its leaflets are like but shorter than the bamboo leaves and oppose to each other. It bears pale purple flowers and small legumes. Its flat beans are like Laodou［荖豆, wild soybean, Glycine soja Sieb. et Zucc.］and taste sweet.

For famine relief: Collect and boil legumes, or peel the beans to eat.

204. 龙芽草

一名瓜香草。生辉县鸦子口山野间。苗高一尺余。茎多涩毛。叶形如地棠叶而宽大，叶头齐团，每五叶或七叶作一茎排生，叶茎脚上又有小芽叶，两两对生。梢间出穗，开五瓣小圆黄花。结青毛菁葖，有子大如黍粒，味甜。

救饥：收取其子，或捣或磨作面食之。

204. Longyacao［龙芽草, agrimony, Agrimonia pilosa Ldb.］

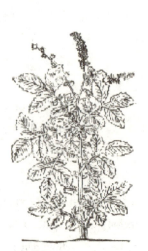

Longyacao［龙芽草, agrimony, Agrimonia pilosa Ldb.］, also named Guaxiangcao, grows in the mountainous regions and fields of Yazikou in Huixian County. Its plants are more than one Chi high and its stems are hirsute. Its leaves are like those of Ditang［地棠, figwort root, Scrophularia ningpoensis Hemsl.］but broader and bigger with round leaf apexes. Its leaf blades are interrupted imparipinnate with 5~7 leaflets arranged on rachils. Its small stipules stand beside basal rachils and oppose to each other. The spicate-raceme draws out of branches and bears round tiny yellow flowers with 5 petals for each. The fruit is wrapped in hypanthium and covered with piluses, and its seeds are as big as proso millets with sweet taste.

For famine relief: Collect seeds, and pound or grind them into flour.

205. 地稍瓜

生田野中。苗长尺许,作地摊科生。叶似独扫叶而细窄尖硬;又似沙蓬叶亦硬,周围攒茎而生。茎叶间开小白花。结角长大如莲子,两头尖艄;又似鸦嘴形,名地稍瓜,味甘。

救饥:其角嫩时,摘取煠食角。若皮硬,剥取角中嫩穰生食。

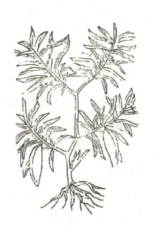

205. Dishaogua [地稍瓜, cynanchum thesioides, Cynanchum thesioides K. Schum.]

Dishaogua [地稍瓜, cynanchum thesioides, Cynanchum thesioides K. Schum.] grows in the fields. Its plants are about one Chi high and bend to the ground. Its leaves are like those of Dusao [独扫, kochia scoparia, Kochia scoparia (L.) Schrad.] but narrower and harder, and like but harder than those of Shapeng [沙蓬, corispermum puberulum, Corispermum puberulum Iljin], aggregating around stems. Its tiny white flowers stand among stems and leaves. Its follicles are fusiform as big as lotus seeds, or shape like the crow mouth, and they taste sweet.

For famine relief: Collect and blanch young follicles, shell them and eat the pulp when the pericarp turns hard.

206. 锦荔枝

又名癞葡萄。人家园篱边多种之。苗引藤蔓,延附草木生。茎长七八尺,茎有毛涩。叶似野葡萄[1]叶,而花叉多。叶间生细丝蔓。开五瓣黄碗子花。结实如鸡子大,尖艄纹皱,状似荔枝而大,生青熟黄,内有红瓤,味甜。

救饥:采荔枝黄熟者,食瓤。

【注释】

[1] 见本书第357野葡萄条。

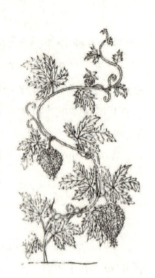

206. Jinlizhi [锦荔枝, balsam pear, Momordica charantia L.]

Jinlizhi [锦荔枝, balsam pear, Momordica charantia L.], also named Laiputao, is cultivated in common people's garden fences. Its plants are a kind of scandent liana, climbing and twining along other vegetation. Its stems are 7 ~ 8 Chi long covered with pubescence. Its leaves are like those of Yeputao[1] [野葡萄, vitis bryoniifolia, Vitis bryoniifolia Bunge] with many lobes. Its tendrils draw out of leaves and bear yellow flowers with five-obovate petals for each. The fruit, as big as the egg, fusiform and verrucose, shapes like Lizhi [荔枝, litchi, Litchi chinensis Sonn.] but bigger than the latter. It is green when it is unripe and yellow when it is ripe with red pulp inside, and tastes sweet.

For famine relief: Collect yellow ripe fruit, and eat the pulp.

【Notes】

[1] See the 357th clause of this book.

207. 鸡冠果

一名野杨梅。生密县山谷中。苗高五七寸。叶似泼盘叶而小;又似鸡儿头叶微团。开五瓣黄花。结实似红小杨梅状,味甜酸。

救饥:采取其果红熟者食之。

207. Jiguanguo〔鸡冠果, Indian mock strawberry, Duchesnea indica (Andr.) Focke〕

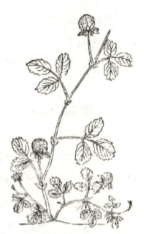

Jiguanguo〔鸡冠果, Indian mock strawberry, Duchesnea indica (Andr.) Focke〕, also named Yeyangmei, grows in the valleys of Mixian County. Its plants are 5~7 Cun high. Its leaves are like but smaller than those of Popan〔泼盘, Japanese Raspberry Herb, Rubus parvifolius L.〕, and like those of Ji'ertou Miao〔鸡儿头苗, potentilla reptans, Potentilla reptans L. var. sericophylla Franch.〕but slightly rounded. It bears five-petaled yellow flowers and the red aggregate fruit shapes like small Yangmei〔杨梅, waxberry, Myrica rubra (Lour.) S. et Zucc.〕with sweet and sour taste.

For famine relief: Collect the red ripe fruit to eat.

叶及实皆可食

✳ 《本草》原有

Leaf and Fruit Edible
Original Ones

208. 羊蹄苗

一名东方宿,一名连虫陆,一名鬼目,一名蓄,俗呼猪耳朵。生陈留川泽,今所在有之。苗初揭地生,后撺生茎叉,高二尺余。其叶狭长,颇似莴苣而色深青;又似大蓝叶微阔,茎节间紫赤色。其花青白成穗。其子三棱。根似牛蒡[1]而坚实。味苦,性寒,无毒。

救饥:采嫩苗叶煠熟,水浸淘净苦味,油盐调食。其子熟时,打子捣为米,以滚水汤三五次,淘净下锅,作水饭食,微破腹。

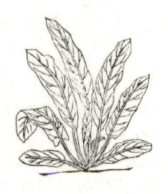

治病：文具《本草·草部》条下。

【注释】

［1］见本书第222 牛蒡子条。

208. Yangtimiao ［羊蹄苗, curly dock, Rumex crispus L.］

Yangtimiao ［羊蹄苗, curly dock, Rumex crispus L.］, also named Dongfangsu, Lianchonglu, Guimu and Xu, and generally called Zhu'erduo, grows in the streamsides and swamps and can be seen everywhere presently. In the early growth period, its seedlings spread along the ground, and then draw out the branches which are more than two Chi high. Its leaves are slender like those of Woju ［莴苣, lettuce, Lactuca sativa L.］ with dark green color, and like those of Dalan ［大蓝, isatis indigotica fort, Isatis indigotica Fortune］ but broader with purplish red internodes. Its panicles are pale green with spiciform branches. Its achenes are trigonous and its roots are like but stronger than those of Niubangzi[1] ［牛蒡子, burdock, Arctium lappa L.］. It is bitter in taste, cold in nature and non-toxic.

For famine relief：Collect young leaves and seedlings, blanch them and remove the bitterness by soaking and rinsing them, and flavor them with oil and salt. Collect and thresh the ripe fruit, blanch them 3~5 times with boiling water, rinse them and make congee. It can cause mild diarrhea sometimes.

For disease treatment：See the clauses in *Materia Medica · Herbaceous Plant.*

【Notes】

［1］ See the 222th clause of this book.

209. 苍 耳

本草名葈耳，俗名道人头，又名喝起草，一名胡葈，一名地葵，一名葹，一名常思，一名羊负来，《诗》谓之卷耳，《尔雅》谓之苓耳。生安陆[1]川谷及六安[2]田野，今处处有之。叶青白，类粘糊菜[3]叶。茎叶梢间结实，比桑椹短小而多刺。其实味苦、甘，性温。叶味苦、辛，性微寒，有小毒。又云无毒。

救饥：采嫩苗叶煤熟，换水浸去苦味，淘净，油盐调食。其子炒微黄，捣去皮,磨为面,作烧饼,蒸食亦可。或用子熬油点灯。

治病:文具《本草·草部》葈耳条下。

【注释】

[1] 古代县名,在今湖北安陆市一带。

[2] 古代县名,在今安徽六安市一带。

[3] 豨莶的别名,见本书第39豨莶条。

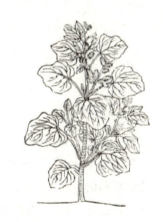

209. Cang'er [苍耳, xanthium sibiricum, Xanthium sibiricum Patrin ex Widder]

Cang'er [苍耳, xanthium sibiricum, Xanthium sibiricum Patrin ex Widder], also named Xi'er, Daorentou, Heqicao, Huxi, Dikui, Shi, Changsi, Yangfulai, Juan'er according to *Shi Jing* [《诗经》, *The Book of Songs*] and Ling'er as stated in *Er Ya* [《尔雅》, *Literary Expositor*], grows in the valleys of Anlu[1] and the fields of Liu'an[2] and presently can be seen everywhere. Its leaves are pale green like those of Nianhucai[3] [粘糊菜, siegesbeckia, Siegesbeckia orientalis L.]. Its achenes, surrounded by the barbellate phyllaries, are like mulberries but shorter and smaller. Its fruit is bitter and sweet in taste, and warm in nature. And its leaves are bitter and pungent in taste, slightly cold in nature, and slightly toxic. It is also said to be non-toxic.

For famine relief: Collect and blanch seedlings and leaves, remove the bitterness by soaking them in water, rinse them, and flavor them with oil and salt. Collect seeds, dry-fry them to yellow, pound them to remove the coats, grind them into flour to make wheaten cakes, or steam them for food. Or press oil from the seeds to light the lamps.

For disease treatment: See the clause of Xi'er [葈耳, xanthium sibiricum, Xanthium sibiricum Patrin ex Widder] in *Materia Medica · Herbaceous Plant*.

【Notes】

[1] The name of an ancient county. It is presently located in Anlu City of Hubei Province.

[2] The name of an ancient county. It is presently located in Liu'an City of Anhui Province.

[3] Another name for Xixian [豨莶, siegesbeckia, Siegesbeckia orientalis L.]. See the 39th clause of this book.

210. 姑娘菜

俗名灯笼儿，又名挂金灯，本草名酸浆，一名醋浆。生荆楚川泽及人家田园中，今处处有之。苗高一尺余。苗似水茄而小，叶似天茄儿叶窄小；又似人苋叶颇大而尖。开白花。结房如囊，似野西瓜蒴，形如撮口布袋；又类灯笼样。囊中有实，如樱桃[1]大，赤黄色，味酸，性平、寒，无毒。叶味微苦。别条又有一种三叶酸浆草，与此不同，治证亦别。

救饥：采叶煠熟，水浸淘去苦味，油盐调食。子熟摘取食之。

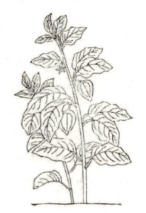

治病：文具《本草·草部》酸浆条下。

【注释】

[1] 见本书第 346 樱桃树条。

210. Guniangcai [姑娘菜, winter cherry, Physalis alkekengi L.]

Guniangcai [姑娘菜, winter cherry, Physalis alkekengi L.], also named Denglong'er, Guajindeng, Suanjiang and Cujiang, grows near the lakes and swamps of Jing and Chu Prefecture, also in common people's garden. It can be seen everywhere presently. Its plants are more than one Chi high, which are like but smaller than those of Shuiqie [水茄, eggplant, Solanum melongena L.]. Its leaves are like those of Tianqie'er [天茄儿, night shade, Solanum nigrum L.] but narrower and smaller, and like those of Renxian [人苋, velvet flower, Amaranthus caudatus] but sharper and larger. It bears white flowers. Its saccate fruit calyxes, like the capsules of Yexigua [野西瓜, hibiscus trionum, Hibiscus trionum Linn.], shape like the braced bags or lanterns. Its orange-red berries are as big as cherries[1], which are sour in taste, neutral or cold in nature and non-toxic. Its leaves taste bitter. In another clause, there is a kind of Sanye

Suanjiangcao [三叶酸浆草, creeping wood sorrel, Oxalis corniculata L.] with different shapes and indications.

For famine relief: Collect and blanch leaves, remove the bitterness by soaking and rinsing them, and flavor them with oil and salt. Collect the ripe berries to eat.

For disease treatment: See the clause of Suanjiang [酸浆, winter cherry, Physalis alkekengi L.] in *Materia Medica · Herbaceous Plant*.

【Notes】

[1] See the 346th clause of this book.

211. 土茜苗

本草[1]根名茜根，一名地血，一名茹藘，一名茅蒐，一名蒨。生乔山川谷，徐州[2]人谓之牛蔓，西土出者佳，今北土处处有之，名土茜根，可以染红。叶似枣[3]叶形，头尖下阔，纹脉竖直。茎方，茎叶俱涩，四五叶对生节间，茎蔓延附草木。开五瓣淡银褐花。结子小如绿豆粒，生青熟红。根紫赤色，味苦，性寒，无毒。一云味甘，一云味酸。畏鼠姑[4]。叶味微酸。

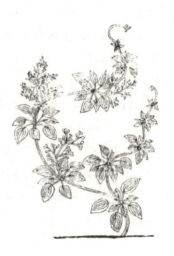

救饥：采叶煠熟，水浸作成黄色，淘净，油盐调食。其子红熟摘食。

治病：文具《本草·草部》茜根条下。

【注释】

[1] 中药的统称，下同。

[2] 古代州名，今江苏徐州市。

[3] 见本书第362枣树条。

[4] 牡丹的别名。牡丹，见本书第7石竹子条下注。

211. Tuqianmiao [土茜苗, madder, Rubia cordifolia L.]

The materia medica[1] of the root of Tuqianmiao is called Qiangen, also named Dixue, Rulv, Maosou and Qian. It grows in a valley where there is water in Qiao Hill. The people from Xuzhou[2] called it Niuman. The best Tuqianmiao is from the west of China. Nowadays, it can be seen everywhere in the north and is named Tuqiangen. It can be used to dye red. The shapes of leaves are like those of Zao[3][枣, jujube, Jujubae Fructus] with the tips sharp, the base wide, and the veins vertical. Its stems are square. Its stems and leaves are rough. Four or five leaves are opposite in the internodes. Its stems are attached and climbed on the vegetation and each of the silver-brown flowers consists of five petals. Its seeds are like the size of mung beans, green when they are raw, and red when cooked; its roots are purple, bitter in taste, cold and non-toxic. Some say sweet and some say sour in taste. It is averse to Shugu[4][鼠姑, moutan, Paeonia suffruticosa Andr]. The taste of leaves is slightly sour.

For famine relief: Collect and blanch leaves, soak them in fresh water until they turn yellow, wash and clean them, and then flavor them with oil and salt. Pluck the red ripe seeds.

For disease treatment: See the clauses of Qiangen [茜根, madder, Rubiae Radix] in *Materia Medica · Herbaceous Plant.*

【Notes】

[1] A general term for medicinals. Similarly hereinafter.

[2] The name of an ancient county. It is presently located in Xuzhou City of Jiangsu Province.

[3] See the 362th clause of this book.

[4] Another name of Mudan [牡丹, moutan, Paeonia suffruticosa Andr.]. See the 7th clause of this book

212. 王不留行

又名剪金草,一名禁宫花,一名剪金花。生太山山谷,今祥符沙堈间亦有之。苗高一尺余。其茎对节生叉。叶似石竹子叶而宽短,抪茎对生,脚叶似槐[1]叶而狭长。开粉红花。结蒴如松子大,似罂粟壳[2]样,极小。有子如葶苈子大而黑色,味苦、甘,性平,无毒。

救饥:采嫩叶煠熟,换水淘去苦味,油盐调食。子可捣为面食。

治病:文具《本草·草部》条下。

【注释】

［1］见本书第320 槐树芽条。

［2］见本书第334 御米花条。

212. Wangbuliu Xing ［王不留行, cowherb seed, Silene aprica Turcz. ex Fisch. et C. A. Mey.］

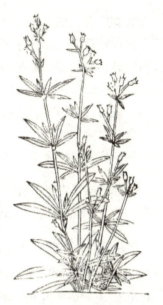

Wangbuliu Xing ［王不留行, cowherb seed, Silene aprica Turcz. ex Fisch. et C. A. Mey.］ is also named Jianjincao, Jingonghua and Jianjinhua. It grows in the valleys of Taishan and now also grows among the sandhills in Xiangfu District, Kaifeng. Its plants are more than one Chi high. Its branches are opposite on the stalk. Its leaves resemble those of Shizhuzi ［石竹子, Dianthus chinensis, Dianthus chinensis L.］ but they are relatively short and broad, and they are opposite on the stalks. Its basal leaves resemble Huaiye[1]［槐叶, sophora leaf, Sophorae Folium］, but they are narrow and long. Its flowers are pink. Its fruit is like a pine nut, shaped like a poppy shell[2], but it is small. Its seeds are like Tinglizi ［葶苈子, lepidium, Lepidii］, black, bitter and sweet in taste, neutral in nature and non-toxic.

For famine relief: Collect young leaves and blanch them, change water to get rid of the bitter taste, and flavor them with oil and salt. Its seeds can be mashed and served.

For disease treatment: See the clauses in *Materia Medica · Herbaceous Plant*.

【Notes】

［1］See the 320th clause of this book.

［2］See the 334th clause of this book.

213. 白　薇

一名白幕，一名薇草，一名春草，一名骨美。生平原川谷并陕西诸郡及滁州，今钧州密县山野中亦有之。苗高一二尺。茎叶俱青，颇类柳叶而阔短；又似女娄脚叶而长硬毛涩。开花红色,又云紫花。结角似地稍瓜而大,中有白瓤。根状如牛膝根而短,黄白色,味苦、咸,性平、大寒,无毒。恶黄耆、大黄、大戟、干姜、干漆、山茱萸、大枣。

救饥:采嫩叶煤熟,水浸,淘净,油盐调食。并取嫩角煤熟,亦可食。

治病:文具《本草·草部》条下。

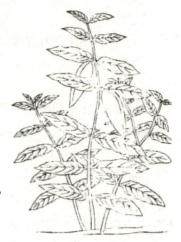

213. Baiwei [白薇, blackend swallowwort root, Cynanchum atratum Bunge]

Baiwei [白薇, blackend swallowwort root, Cynanchum atratum Bunge] is also known as Baimu, Weicao, Chuncao and Gumei. It grows in the plains and the flowing valleys. It is distributed in all the counties of Shanxi Province and Chuzhou in Anhui Province. It is now also seen in the mountains and wilderness areas of Mixian County, Chuzhou. Its plants are 1 ~ 2 Chi high. Its stems and leaves are green, like the willow leaves, but they are wider and shorter; they also resemble the basal leaves of Nvlou (女娄), but they are long, hard and rough. Its flowers are red and some say they are purple. Its follicls are like a Dishaogua, but they are larger and there are white tomenta on the seeds. Its roots are shaped like those of Niuxi [牛膝, twotoothed achyranthes root, Radix Achyranthis Bidentatae] but shorter and yellowish-white. It is bitter and salty in taste. It is neutral in nature, great cold and non-toxic. It is averse to Huangqi [黄耆, astragalus membranaceus, Astragalus membranaceus (Fisch.) Bunge], Dahuang [大黄, rhubarb, Rhei Radix et Rhizoma], Daji [大戟, euphorbia, Euphorbiae seu Knoxiae Radix], Ganjiang [干姜, dried ginger, Zingiberis Rhizoma], Ganqi [干漆, lacquer, Toxicodendri Resina], Shanzhuyu [山茱萸, cornus, Corni Fructus] and Dazao [大枣, jujube, Jujubae Fructus].

For famine relief: Collect young leaves and blanch them, soak them in water, wash and clean them, and flavor them with oil and salt. The blanched young fruit can also be eaten.

For disease treatment: See the clauses in *Materia Medica · Herbaceous Plant*.

✤ 新增
New Supplements

214. 蓬子菜

生田野中,所在处处有之。其苗嫩时,茎有红紫线楞。叶似碱蓬叶微细。苗老结子,叶则生出叉刺。其子如独扫子大。苗叶味甜。

救饥:采嫩苗叶煤熟,水浸,淘净,油盐调食,晒干煤食尤佳。及采子,捣米青色,或煮粥,或磨面作饼,蒸食皆可。

214. Pengzicai [蓬子菜, true galium, Galium verum L.]

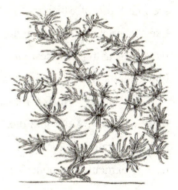

Pengzicai [蓬子菜, true galium, Galium verum L.] grows in the fields and can be seen everywhere in the areas where it is distributed. When its plants are young, there are red-purple lines on the stems. Its leaves are like those of Jianpeng [碱蓬, suaeda, Suaedae Herba] but a little thinner. When its plants are old, its seeds are solid and its leaves send forth thorns. Its fruit is as big as that of Dusaozi [独扫子, kochia, Kochiae Fructus]. Its seedlings and leaves are sweet.

For famine relief: Collect young seedlings and blanch them, soak them in water, wash and clean them, and flavor them with oil and salt. The sun-dried leaves can be blanched and the taste is good. The fruit can also be plucked and pounded, green, or used to cook congee, or you can grind it, make it cakes and eat it after steaming.

215. 胡枝子

俗亦名随军茶。生平泽中。有二种,叶形有大小。大叶者类黑豆叶,小叶者茎类蓍草,叶似苜蓿叶而长大。花色有紫白。结子如粟粒大,气味与槐相类,性温。

救饥：采子，微舂即成米，先用冷水淘净，复以滚水汤三五次，去水下锅，或作粥，或作炊饭皆可，食加野绿豆，味尤佳。及采嫩叶蒸晒为茶，煮饮亦可。

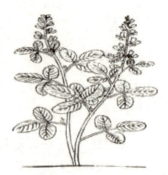

215. Huzhizi〔胡枝子，bicolor lespedeza stem and leaf，Lespedeza bicolor Tricz〕

Huzhizi〔胡枝子，bicolor lespedeza stem and leaf，Lespedeza bicolor Tricz〕is also named Suijuncha. It grows in the flat and wet grasslands. There are two types of leaf shapes. Lespedeza bicolor Tricz has bigger leaves which are similar to the black bean leaves. L. davrica (Laxm) Schindl has smaller leaves. Its stems are like those of Shicao〔蓍草，yarrow，Achillea millefolium L.〕. Its leaves are like cloverleaves, but they are longer and bigger. Its flowers are purple and white. Its seeds, as big as chestnuts, smell like Huai〔槐，flavescent sophora，Sophorae Flavescentis Radix〕and are warm in nature.

For famine relief：Collect seeds, and then gently turn them into rice. Cleanse them with cold water and then put them in the boiling water for three or five times, and then drain and make congee or meals. When eaten with wild green beans, the taste is particularly good. The young leaves can be steamed and dried to make tea.

216. 米布袋

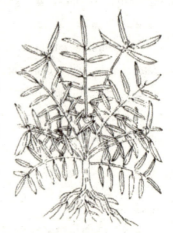

生田野中。苗揭地生。叶似泽漆叶而窄，其叶顺茎排生。梢头攒结三四角，中有子，如黍粒大，微扁，味甜。

救饥：采角取子，水淘洗净，下锅煮食。其嫩苗叶煠熟，油盐调食亦可。

216. Mibudai [米布袋, Gueldenstaedtia verna, Gueldenstaedtia verna (Georgi) Boriss.]

Mibudai [米布袋, Gueldenstaedtia verna, Gueldenstaedtia verna (Georgi) Boriss.] grows in the fields. Its plants grow on the ground. Its leaves resemble those of Zeqi [泽漆, sun euphorbia herb, Herba Euphorbiae Helioscopiae], but they are narrower. Its leaves grow along the axis of the leaves. Its flowering stalks are clustered with three or four pods, and there are seeds inside. Its seeds are as big as the grains, slightly flat and sweet.

For famine relief: Collect pods, remove the seeds, wash them with water and cook them in a pot. The young seedlings and leaves can be blanched and flavored with oil and salt.

217. 天茄儿苗

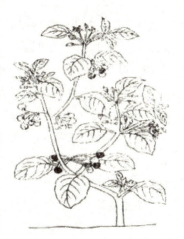

生田野中。苗高二尺许。茎有线楞。叶似姑娘草叶而大；又似和尚菜叶却小。开五瓣小白花。结子似野葡萄大，紫黑色，味甜。

救饥：采嫩叶煠熟，水浸去邪味，淘净，油盐调食。其子熟时亦可摘食。

治病：今人传说，采叶傅贴肿毒金疮[1]，拔毒。

【注释】

[1] 病名，指金属利器造成的创伤，因创伤而化脓溃烂的疮。

217. Tianqie'er Miao [天茄儿苗, solanum nigrum, Solanum nigrum L.]

Tianqie'er Miao [天茄儿苗, solanum nigrum, Solanum nigrum L.] grows in the fields, and its plants are about two Chi high. Its blades are stalked on the stems. Its leaves resemble those of Guniangcao [姑娘草, physalis alkekengi, Physalis alkekengi L.] but larger. Its leaves also resemble those of Heshangcao

[和尚草, adenocaulon himalaicum, Adenocaulon himalaicum Edgew.] but they are smaller with five white flowers. The fruit of the knot is like the size of a wild grape, purple black and sweet.

For famine relief: Collect young leaves, blanch, wash and clean them, and then flavor them with oil and salt. When the fruit is ripe, it can also be taken for food.

For disease treatment: According to the legend, the leaves can be applied to cure pyogenic infections[1] and insiced wound to draw out poison.

【Notes】

[1] It refers to the wound caused by the sharp metal weapon, and the sore that is purulent and ulcerated due to the wound.

218. 苦马豆

俗名羊尿胞。生延津县[1]郊野中,在处亦有之。苗高二尺许。茎似黄耆苗,茎上有细毛。叶似胡豆叶微小;又似蒺藜叶却大。枝叶间开红紫化。结壳如拇指顶大,中间多虚,俗呼为羊尿胞,内有子如荍子大,茶褐色。子叶俱味苦。

救饥:采叶煠熟,换水浸去苦味,淘净,油盐调食。及取子水浸淘去苦味,晒干,或磨或捣为面,作烧饼、蒸食皆可。

【注释】

[1] 今河南省延津县。

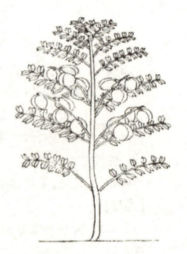

218. Kumadou [苦马豆, Sphaerophysa salsula, Sphaerophysa salsula (Pall) DC.]

Kumadou [苦马豆, Sphaerophysa salsula, Sphaerophysa salsula (Pall) DC.], commonly known as Yangniaobao, grows in the mountains and wilderness on the outskirts of Yanjin County[1], and it is distributed everywhere. Its plants are about two Chi high. Its stems are like the seedings of Huangqi [黄耆, astragalus membranaceus, Astragalus penduliflorus Lam. subsp. mongholicus (Bunge) X. Y. Zhu var. dahuricus (Fisch. ex DC.) X. Y. Zhu], with fine hairs on stems. Its leaves are like those of Hudou [胡豆, broad bean, Viciae Fabae Semen] but a little smaller, and like those of Jili [蒺藜, tribulus, Tribuli Fructus] but larger. Red and purple flowers are in the middle of branches. Its pods are as big as the top of thumbs, and its fruit is empty. The common name is Yangniaobao. Its seeds are as big as Qingmazi [苘麻子, indian mallow seed, Abutili Semen], and dark brown in color. Both seeds and leaves are bitter.

For famine relief: Collect leaves and branch them, change water to remove the bitterness by soaking them, wash and clean them, and flavor them with oil and salt. Soak the seeds in water, wash them to get rid of bitter taste, dry, grind or knead them into flour, and make Chinese style baked rolls or steam them.

【Notes】

[1] It is presently located in Yanjin County of Henan Province.

219. 猪尾把苗

一名狗脚菜。生荒野中。苗长尺余。叶似甘露儿叶而甚短小,其头颇齐,茎叶皆有细毛。每叶间顺条开小白花。结小蒴儿,中有子,小如粟粒,黑色。苗叶味甜。

救饥:采嫩叶煠熟,换水浸淘净,油盐调食。子可捣为面食。

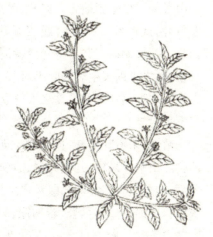

219. Zhuweiba Miao [猪尾把苗, Lysimachia, Lysimachia]

Zhuweiba Miao [猪尾把苗, Lysimachia, Lysimachia] is also named Goujiaocai. It grows in the wilderness. Its plants are more than one Chi high. Its leaves are like Ganlu'er [甘露儿, Chinese artichoke, Stachydis Sieboldii Tuber et Herba] leaves, but they are very short. The tips of its leaves are quite neat, and its stems and leaves are finely hairy. Small white flowers grow upward between the leaves. It has small fruit with seeds inside which are as small as millets, black. Both the seedlings and the leaves are sweet.

For famine relief: Collect young leaves and blanch them, change water, wash and clean them, and then flavor them with oil and salt. The fruit can be pounded into powder.

根叶可食

《本草》原有

Root and Leaf Edible
Original Ones

220. 黄精苗

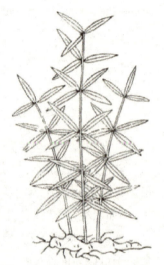

俗名笔管菜,一名重楼,一名菟竹,一名鸡格,一名救穷,一名鹿竹,一名萎蕤,一名仙人余粮,一名垂珠,一名马箭,一名白及。生山谷,南北皆有之,嵩山、茅山者佳。根生肥地者大如拳,薄地者犹如拇指。叶似竹叶,或两叶,或三叶,或四五叶,俱皆对节而生。味甘,性平,无毒。又云茎光滑者谓之太阳之草,名曰黄精,食之可以长生。其叶不对节,茎叶毛钩子者,谓之太阴之草,名曰钩吻,食之入口立死。又云茎不紫,花不黄为异。

救饥:采嫩叶煤熟,换水浸去苦味,淘洗净,油盐调食。山中人采根,九蒸九暴,食甚甘美。其蒸暴用瓮去底,安釜上,装置黄精令满,密盖蒸之,令气溜,即暴之。如此九蒸九暴,令极熟,若不熟,则刺人喉咽。久食长生辟谷。其生者,若初服,只可一寸半,渐渐增之,十日不食他食。能长服之,止三尺,服三百日后,尽见鬼神,饵必升天。又云花实极可食,罕得见,至难得。

治病:文具《本草·草部》条下。

220. Huangjingmiao [黄精苗, yellow essence, Polygonatum sibiricum Redouté]

Huangjingmiao [黄精苗, yellow essence, Polygonatum sibiricum Redouté] is also known as Biguancai, Chonglou, Tuzhu, Jige, Jiuqiong, Luzhu, Weirui, Xianren Yuliang, Chuizhu, Majian and Baiji. It grows in the valleys of the north and south of China. Its quality is better if from Song Mountain and Mao Mountain. The rhizomes that grow in the fertile land are as big as a fist, and those which grow in the barren land are as big as thumbs. Its leaves are like bamboo leaves. Some are bifoliate, some are trifoliate, and others are quadrifoliate or quinquefoliolate. All the leaves are opposite or verticillate. It is sweet, neutral in nature and non-toxic. Some say those whose stems are smooth and are the grass of the sun, called Huangjing, can make people achieve immortality. Those whose leaves are not opposite and have hairy hooks on the stems are the grass of Taiyin, called Gouwen. The person who eats it will die as soon as he or she eats it. It is said that those whose stems are not purple or the flowers are not yellow belong to different species.

For famine relief: Collect young leaves and blanch them, change water to remove the bitterness, wash and clean them, and then flavor them with oil and salt. The mountainous people dig the rhizome, and after steaming and drying nine times, it tastes very sweet. Its steaming method is to use cockroaches. Remove the bottom of the cockroach, install it on the kettle, fill it with Huangjingmiao [黄精苗, yellow essence, Polygonatum sibiricum Redouté], then cover it tightly, steam it and keep the steam, and then expose it to the sun. After steaming and drying nine times, it will be well-cooked. If it is not cooked, it will irritate the throat. Long-term taking of it can make people live longer. When you eat raw Huangjingmiao [黄精苗, yellow essence, Polygonatum sibiricum Redouté] for the first time, you can only take one and a half Cun of it and gradually increase. You can not eat other food within ten days. If you take it for a long time, no more than three Chi each time, lasting for three hundred days, you can have supernatural power. It is also said that the flowers and fruit are very suitable for consumption, but they are hard to see and even harder to obtain.

For disease treatment: See the clauses in **Materia Medica · Herbaceous Plant**.

221. 地黄苗

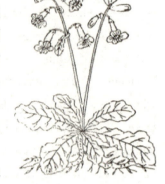

俗名婆婆奶，一名地髓，一名芐，一名芑。生咸阳川泽，今处处有之。苗初掯地生，叶如山白菜叶而毛涩，叶面深青色；又似芥菜叶而不花叉，比芥菜叶颇厚。叶中攛茎，上有细毛，茎梢开筒子花，红黄色，北人谓之牛奶子花。结实如小麦粒。根长四五寸，细如手指，皮赤黄色。味甘、苦，性寒，无毒。恶贝母，畏芜荑，得麦门冬、清酒良。忌铁器。

救饥：采叶煮羹食。或捣绞根汁，搜面作饼，及冷淘食之。或取根浸洗净，九蒸九暴，任意服食。或煎以为煎食。久服轻身不老，变白延年。

治病：文具《本草·草部》条下。

221. Dihuangmiao [地黄苗, ehmannia, Rehmannia glutinosa (Gaert.) Libosch. ex Fisch et Mey.]

Dihuangmiao [地黄苗, rehmannia, Rehmannia glutinosa (Gaert.) Libosch. ex Fisch et Mey.] is commonly named Poponai, Disui, Bian and Qi. It grows by the lakes and marshes of Xianyang, and it can be seen everywhere presently. Its plants grow on the ground when they are newly sprouted. Its leaves are like Shanbaicai [山白菜, aster, Asteris Radix] leaves, but they are rough and the surface of leaves is dark green. They are like mustard leaves, but they are not divided and a little thicker. Its flower buds are extracted from the leaves. Its stems are finely hairy, and its flowers are red-yellow at the top, and the people from the north of China call it Niunaizi Hua. Its seeds are like wheat grains. Its roots are 4 ~5 Cun long, as thick as fingers. The root bark is reddish yellow. It is sweet, bitter, cold in nature and non-toxic. It is averse to Beimu [贝母, fritillaria, Fritillariae Bulbus], and restrained by Wuyi [芜荑, elm cake, Ulmi Fructus

Praeparatio]. It is better to combine with Maimendong [麦门冬, ophiopogon, Ophiopogon japonicus] and fine rice wine. It can not be cooked in iron pot.

For famine relief: Collect leaves and cook them. Or smash the roots, remove the juice from the roots, use the juice to knead dough, make them Botuo (a kind of food made of flour) and wash them in cold water. Or take roots and soak, wash, steam and sun-dry them for nine times. Or fry them for food. The long-time taking of it can help people have white skin, lose weight and prolong life.

For disease treatment: See the clauses in *Materia Medica · Herbaceous Plant*.

222. 牛蒡子

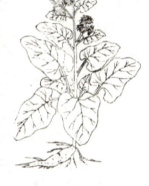

本草名恶实,未去萼名鼠粘子,俗名夜叉头,根谓之牛菜。生鲁山平泽,今处处有之。苗高二三尺。叶如芋叶,长大而涩。花淡紫色,实[1]似葡萄而褐色,外壳如栗梂而小,多刺,鼠过之则缀惹不可脱,故名。壳中有子[2],如半麦粒而扁小。根长尺余,粗如拇指,其色灰黪。味辛,性平。一云味甘,无毒。

救饥:采苗叶煠熟,水浸去邪气,淘洗净,油盐调食。及取根,水浸洗净,煮熟食之。久食甚益人,身轻耐老。

治病:文具《本草·草部》恶实条下。

【注释】

[1] 牛蒡子的瘦果。

[2] 牛蒡子的瘦果。

222. Niubangzi [牛蒡子, arctium, Arctium lappa L.]

Niubangzi [牛蒡子, arctium, Arctium lappa L.] is the materia medica of E'shi. That which has no phyllary is called Shuzhanzi. It is commonly called Yechatou. Its roots are called Niucai. It grows in the flat wetlands of Lu Mountain and presently it can be seen everywhere. Its plants are 2~3 Chi high. Its leaves are like those of Yumiao [芋苗, sweet potato, Colocasia esculenta (L.) Schoot], longer, bigger and rough. Its flowers are lavenders. Its achenes[1] are like grapes but brown in color. Its shells are like chestnuts, but they are small and spiny. When a mouse passes, they will stick and can't get rid of it, so that is why it is called Shuzhanzi (like the mouse glue). There are achenes[2] in the shells, as big as a half of grains, but they are flat and small. Its roots are more than one Chi long, like thick thumbs, and the color is gray. It is acrid in flavor, and neural in nature. It is also said to be sweet and non-toxic.

For famine relief: Collect plants and leaves, remove the strange taste by soaking them, wash and clean them, and flavor them with salt and oil. Collect roots and cook them after washing and soaking. The long-term taking of it is very beneficial to health and one can lose weight and prolong the life.

For disease treatment: See the clause of E'shi in *Materia Medica · Herbaceous Plant*.

【Notes】

[1] The achenes of Niubangzi [牛蒡子, arctium, Arctium lappa L.].

[2] The achenes of Niubangzi [牛蒡子, arctium, Arctium lappa L.].

223. 远 志

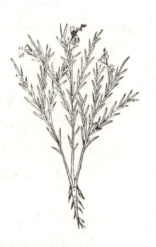

一名棘菀,一名葽绕,一名细草。生太山及冤句川谷,河、陕、商、齐、泗州亦有,俗传夷门[1]远志最佳,今密县梁家冲山谷间多有之。苗名小草,叶似石竹子叶,又极细。开小紫花,亦有开红白花者。根黄色,形如蒿根,长及一尺许,亦有根黑色者。根叶俱味苦,性温,无毒。得茯苓[2]、冬葵子、龙骨良,杀天雄、附子毒,畏珍珠、藜芦、蜚蠊、齐蛤[3]、蛴螬。

救饥:采嫩苗叶煠熟,换水浸去苦味,淘净,油盐调食。及掘取根,换水煮,浸淘去苦味,去心,再换水煮极熟,食之。不去心,令人心闷。

治病:文具《本草·草部》条下。

【注释】

[1] 古代开封的别称。

[2] 真菌。

[3] 中药马刀的别名。

223. Yuanzhi [远志, polygala, Polygala sibirica L.]

Yuanzhi [远志, polygala, Polygala sibirica L.] is also named Jiwan, Yaorao and Xicao. It grows in Tai Mountain and the valleys of Yuanju where there is flowing water. It can also be seen in He, Shan, Shang, Qi and Sizhou. It is said that Yuanzhi in Yimen[1] is the best. There are many Yuanzhi in the valleys of Liangjiachong, Mixian County. Its plants are called Xiaocao, its leaves are like those of Shizhuzi but very thin, and its flowers are small. Some are purple and some are red and white. Its roots are yellow, shaped like artemisia roots, about one Chi long. Some roots are black. Both roots and leaves are bitter, warm in nature and non-toxic. Fuling[2] [茯苓, poria cocos, Poria cocos (Schw.) Wolf.], Dongkuizi [冬葵子, cluster mallow seed, Malva verticillata L.] and Longgu [龙骨, dragon bone, Mastodi Ossis Fossilia] can enhance its efficiency. It will be toxic when used with Tianxiong [天雄, slender root of common monkshood, Aconitum carmichaeli Debx.] and Fuzi [附子, aconite, Aconiti Radix Lateralis Praeparata]. It is restrained by Zhenzhu [珍珠, pearl, Margarita], Lilu [藜芦, veratrum, Veratri Nigri Radix et Rhizoma], Feilian [蜚蠊, Pheropsophus jessoensis, Pheropsophus jessoensis (Moraw)], Qige[3] [齐蛤, saber lumps, Solen Gouldii Concha] and Qicao [蛴螬, holotrichia diomphalia, Holotrichia diomphalia Bates].

For famine relief: Collect young plants and leaves, blanch them, change water, remove the bitterness by soaking them in water, wash and clean them, and then flavor them with oil and salt. You can also dig roots, change water and cook them, remove the bitterness by soaking them in water, wash them and remove the central part, and then change water and cook them until they are well cooked. The central part of the roots, if taken, will cause chest distress.

【Notes】

[1] It refers to Kaifeng, Henan Province.

[2] It refers to fungus.

[3] The materia medica of Madao [马刀, saber lumps, Solen Gouldii Concha].

224. 杏叶沙参

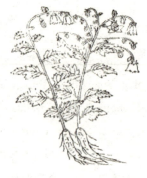

一名白面根。生密县山野中。苗高一二尺,茎色青白。叶似杏叶而小,边有叉牙;又似山小菜叶,微尖而背白。梢间开五瓣白碗子花。根形如野胡萝卜,颇肥,皮色灰黪,中间白色。味甜,性微寒。本草有沙参,苗叶根茎,其说与此形状皆不同,未敢并入条下,乃另开于此。其杏叶沙参又有开碧色花者。

救饥:采苗叶煠熟,水浸,淘净,油盐调食。掘根,换水煮食亦佳。

治病:与《本草·草部》下沙参同用。

224. Xingye Shashen [杏叶沙参, adenophora hunanensis, Adenophora petiolata Pax et Hoffm. subsp. hunanensis (Nannf.) D. Y. Hong et S. Ge]

Xingye Shashen [杏叶沙参, adenophora hunanensis, Adenophora petiolata Pax et Hoffm. subsp. hunanensis (Nannf.) D. Y. Hong et S. Ge] is also known as Baimiangen. It grows in the wilderness of the mountains in Mixian County. Its plants are 1 ~ 2 Chi high, and its stems are green and white. Its leaves are like those of Xingshu [杏树, apricot tree, Armeniaca vulgaris Lam], but they are relatively small, serrated in the margin. They are also like Shanxiaocai leaves, slightly pointed and white in the back. Its flowers are in the middle of the branches and white, five-petal and bowl-shaped. The shape of its roots is like a wild carrot which is very thick. The color of the pericarp is gray and white in the middle. It is sweet in taste and slightly cold in nature. Shashen [沙参, adenophora, Adenophorae seu Glehniae Radix] is recorded in ancient materia medica. Its plants, leaves, roots and stems are all different from those of Xingye Shashen [杏叶沙参, adenophora hunanensis, Adenophora petiolata Pax et Hoffm. subsp. hunanensis

(Nannf.) D. Y. Hong et S. Ge], so it is not recorded in the clause of Shashen [沙参, adenophora, Adenophorae seu Glehniae Radix]. This kind of Xingye Shashen [杏叶沙参, adenophora hunanensis, Adenophora petiolata Pax et Hoffm. subsp. hunanensis (Nannf.) D. Y. Hong et S. Ge] also have turquoise flowers.

For famine relief: Collect seedlings and leaves and then blanch them, wash and clean them by soaking them in water, and flavor them with oil and salt. Dig roots, change water, and then the taste is good after boiling.

For disease treatment: See the clause in *Materia Medica · Herbaceous Plant* and has the same function with Shashen [沙参, adenophora, Adenophorae seu Glehniae Radix].

225. 藤长苗

又名旋菜。生密县山坡中。拖蔓而生，苗长三四尺余。茎有细毛。叶似滴滴金叶而窄小，头颇齐。开五瓣粉红大花。根似打碗花[1]根。根叶皆味甜。

救饥：采嫩苗叶煤熟，水淘净，油盐调食。掘根，换水煮熟亦可食。

【注释】

[1] 即葍子根的别名，见本书第173 葍子根条。

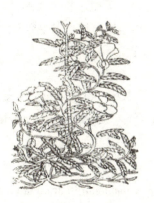

225. Tengchangmiao [藤长苗, calystegia pellita, Calystegia pellita (Ledeb.) G. Don]

Tengchangmiao [藤长苗, calystegia pellita, Calystegia pellita (Ledeb.) G. Don] is also named Xuancai. It grows on the hillsides of Mixian County. Its vines grow along branches. Its plants are 3～4 Chi long. There are fine hair on the stems. Its leaves are like those of Didijin [滴滴金, dichondra repens, Dichondra micrantha Urb.] but narrower, and the top of the leaves is not furcate. It has big pink flowers, and has five petals. Its roots are like those of Fuzigen[1] [葍子根, calystegia hederacea, Calystegia hederacea Wall. ex. Roxb.]. Its roots and leaves are sweet.

For famine relief: Collect young leaves, wash and clean them in water, and flavor them with oil and salt. Dig roots, change water and thoroughly boil them before eating.

【Notes】

[1] It refers to Fuzigen. See the 173th clause of this book.

226. 牛皮消

生密县山野中。拖蔓而生,藤蔓长四五尺。叶似马兜零叶,宽大而薄;又似何首乌叶,亦宽大。开白花,结小角儿。根类葛根而细小,皮黑肉白,味苦。

救饥:采叶煤熟,水浸去苦味,油盐调食。及取根,去黑皮,切作片,换水煮去苦味,淘洗净,再以水煮极熟食之。

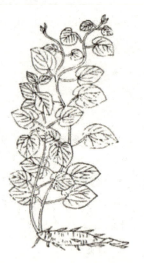

226. Niupixiao [牛皮消, cynanchum auriculatum, Cynanchum auriculatum Royle ex Wight]

Niupixiao [牛皮消, cynanchum auriculatum, Cynanchum auriculatum Royle ex Wight] grows in the mountains and wilderness of Mixian County. Its vines grow along branches, and the vines are 4~5 Chi long. Its leaves are like those of Madouling [马兜铃, aristolochia fruit, Aristolochiae Fructus]. Its leaves are wide and thin. They are also like those of Heshouwu [何首乌, flowery knotweed, Polygonum multiflorum Thunb.] but wider. Its flowers are white. Its follicles are small. Its roots are like those of Gegen [葛根, pueraria, Puerariae Radix] but smaller. Its peels are black and its flesh is white. It is bitter in taste.

For famine relief: Collect young leaves and blanch them, remove the bitterness by soaking them in water, and flavor them with salt and oil. Or take the roots and remove the black peels. Cut them into pieces, wash them to remove the bitterness, wash and clean them, and then boil them with water until they are cooked.

227. 菹 草

即水藻也。生陂塘及水泊中。茎如粗线,长三四尺。叶形似柳叶而狭长,故名柳叶菹,又有叶似蓬子叶者。根粗如钗股而色白,味微咸,性微寒。

救饥:捞取茎叶连嫩根,拣择洗淘洁净,㓡碎,煤熟,油盐调食。或加少米煮粥食,尤佳。

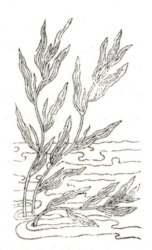

227. Zucao [菹草, algae, Potamogeton crispus]

Zucao [菹草, algae, Potamogeton crispus] is algae. It grows in ponds and moorings. Its stems are like thick lines, 3 ~ 4 Chi long. Its leaves are like willow leaves, but they are longer and narrower, so it is called Liuyezu. Another type of Zucao has the leaves which look like Pengziye [蓬子叶, utricularia vulgaris, Utricularia vulgaris L.]. Its roots are as thick as the scorpion, the color is white, the taste is slightly salty, and the nature is slightly cold.

For famine relief: Pick up their leaves together with roots, trim them for cooking, wash and clean them, then cut them up, blanch them, and flavor them with oil and salt. Or add a small amount of rice to make congee. The taste is even better.

228. 水豆儿

一名葳菜。生陂塘水泽中。其茎叶比菹草又细,状类细线,连绵不绝。根如钗股而色白,根下有豆,如退皮绿豆瓣,味甘。

救饥:采秧及根豆,择洗洁净,煮食。生腌食亦可。

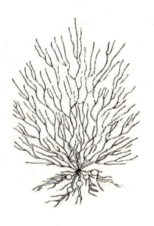

228. Shuidou'er [水豆儿, utricularia, Utricularia vulgaris L.]

Shuidou'er [水豆儿, utricularia, Utricularia vulgaris L.] is also known as Weicai and grows in the ponds. Its stems and leaves are thinner than those of Zucao [菹草, algae, Potamogeton crispus], and its shape is like a fine thread without stop. Its roots are like hairpins, and the color is white. There are beans under the roots which are like the peeled-off mung beans, and the taste is sweet.

For famine relief: Pick plants and roots, trim them, wash them clean and cook them, or pickle them when they are raw.

229. 草三奈

生密县梁家冲山谷中。苗高一尺许。叶似蘘草而狭长。开小淡红花。根[1]似鸡爪形而粗,亦香,其味甘、微辛。

救饥:采根,换水煮食。近根嫩白袴叶亦可煠食。

【注释】

[1] 根状茎。

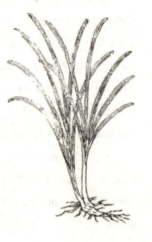

229. Caosannai [草三奈, belamcanda chinensis, Belamcanda chinensis (L.) Redouté]

Caosannai [草三奈, belamcanda chinensis, Belamcanda chinensis (L.) Redouté] grows in the valleys of Liangjiachong in Mixian County. Its plants are about one Chi high. Its leaves are like Suocao [蘘草, zingiber mioga, Zingiber mioga (Thunb.) Rosc.], but they are long and narrow. Its flowers are small and reddish. Its rhizomes[1] are like the shape of chicken feet, but they are thicker and also fragrant. It is sweet in taste and slightly spicy.

For famine relief: Dig out roots and change water to boil. The young white leaves which are near the roots can also be blanched and eaten.

【Notes】

[1] It refers to rhizomes.

230. 水　葱

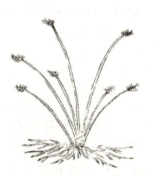

生水边及浅水中。科苗仿佛类家葱,而极细长。梢头结菁葵,仿佛类葱菁葵[1]而小,开黲白花。其根类葱根,皮色紫黑。根苗俱味甘,微咸。

救饥:采嫩苗连根,拣择洗净,煤熟,水浸淘净,油盐调食。

【注释】

[1]此处指小穗,内含多个小坚果。

230. Shuicong [水葱, robust bullrush, Scirpi Validi Caulis]

Shuicong [水葱, robust bullrush, Scirpi Validi Caulis] grows on the water front and in the shallow water. Its plants are very similar to the green onions, but they are very slender. There are follicles on the tip of branches. It looks like the follicles[1] of green onions but smaller. Its flowers are dark white. Its roots are like green onion roots, and the peels are purple and black. Both the roots and the plants are sweet and slightly salty.

For famine relief: Collect young plants and roots, trim them and then blanch, soak and wash them thoroughly, and flavor them with salt and oil.

【Notes】

[1] It refers to the spike with many nuts in it.

根笋可食

《本草》原有

Root and Shoot Edible
Original Ones

231. 蒲 笋

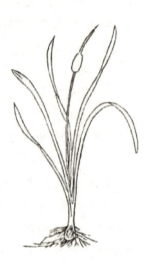

《本草》名其苗为香蒲,即甘蒲也。一名睢,一名醮,俚俗名此蒲为香蒲,谓菖蒲为臭蒲。其香蒲,水边处处有之,根比菖蒲根极肥大而少节。其叶初未出水时,叶茎红白色,采以为笋。后撺梗于丛叶中,花抱梗端,如武士棒杵,故俚俗谓蒲棒。蒲黄即花中蕊屑也,细若金粉。当欲开时,有便取之。市场间亦采之,以蜜搜作果食货卖,甚益小儿。味甘,性平,无毒。

救饥:采近根白笋,拣剥洗净,煠熟,油盐调食。蒸食亦可。或采根,刮去粗皱,晒干磨面,打饼蒸食皆可。

治病:文具《本草·草部》香蒲及蒲黄条下。

231. Pusun〔蒲笋, typha, Typha orientalis Presl.〕

In *Materia Medica*, it is called Xiangpu, Ganpu, Sui, Jiao, commonly known as Xiangpu〔香蒲, typha, Typha orientalis Presl.〕 and Changpu〔菖蒲, acorus, Acori Tatarinowii Rhizoma〕 is Choupu. Xiangpu can be seen everywhere on the water edge. Its roots are much larger than those of Changpu〔菖蒲, acorus, Acori Tatarinowii Rhizoma〕 and have less joints. When its leaves come out under water, they are red and white, which can be collected as shoots. Its scapes come from leaves, and its flowers grow on the top of scapes, like warrior's sticks, so commonly known as Pubang. Puhuang〔蒲黄, typha pollen, Typhae Pollen〕 is anther in stamen, as thin as gold powder. When its flowers are about to bloom, remove and collect the anther. Its venders also collect Puhuang〔蒲黄, typha pollen, Typhae Pollen〕, which is mixed with honey for sale. Eating this kind of fruit is very beneficial to children's health. It's sweet, neutral in nature and non-toxic.

For famine relief: Collect white bamboo shoots which are near the roots, trim, peel and clean them, blanch them, and then flavor them with oil and salt. Steamed shoots can also be eaten. Or pick the roots, scrape the rough skin, dry and grind them into powder, and make cakes for steaming.

For disease treatment: See the clauses of Xiangpu [香蒲, typha, Typha orientalis Presl.] and Puhuang [蒲黄, typha pollen, Typhae Pollen] in *Materia Medica · Herbaceous Plant*.

232. 芦笋

其苗名苇子草,本草有芦根,《尔雅》谓之葭华。生下湿陂泽中。其状都似竹,但差小,而叶抱茎生,无枝叉。花白,作穗如茅花。根如竹根,亦差小而节疏。露出浮水者不堪用。味甘,一云甘、辛,性寒。

救饥:采嫩笋煤熟,油盐调食。其根甘甜,亦可生啖食之。

治病:文具《本草·草部》芦根条下。

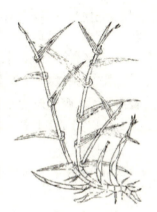

232. Lusun [芦笋, phragmites shoot, Phragmititis Surculus]

It is also named Weizicao. The materia medica of Lugen [芦根, phragmites, Phragmitis Rhizoma] is called Jiachui in *Er Ya* [《尔雅》, *Literary Expositor*]. It grows in the low-lying marshes, ponds and lakes. All parts of Lusun [芦笋, phragmites shoot, Phragmititis Surculus] are like bamboos, but they are smaller. Its leaves are stalked and grow without branches. Its flowers are white and the spikes are like the flowers of Maoyagen [茅芽根, imperata, Imperatae Rhizoma]. Its roots are like the bamboo roots but smaller, and the joints are sparser. The part which is out of the water or float in the water can not be used. It is sweet in taste, and some say it is sweet and spicy in taste, and cold in nature.

For famine relief: Collect young phragmite shoots, blanch them, and flavor them with salt and oil. Its roots are sweet and can be sucked when they are uncooked.

For disease treatment: See the clause of Lugen [芦根, phragmites, Phragmitis Rhizoma] in *Materia Medica · Herbaceous Plant*.

233. 茅芽根

本草名茅根,一名兰根,一名茹根,一名地菅,一名地筋,一名兼杜,又名白茅菅。其芽一名茅针,生楚地山谷,今田野处处有之。春初生苗,布地如针。夏生白花,茸茸然,至秋而枯。其根^[1]至洁白,亦甚甘美。根性寒,茅针性平,花性温,俱味甘、无毒。

救饥:采嫩芽,剥取嫩穰食,甚益小儿。及取根咂食甜味。久服利人,服食此可断谷。

治病:文具《本草·草部》茅根条下。

【注释】

[1] 此处指白茅的根状茎。

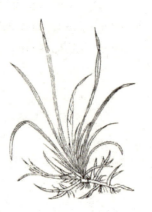

233. Maoyagen [茅芽根, imperata, Imperatae Cylindrica (L.) Beauv.]

The materia medica of Maogen [茅根, imperata, Imperatae Cylindrica (L.) Beauv.] is also known as Langen, Rugen, Dijian, Dijin, Jiandu and Baimaojian. Its buds are called Maozhen. It grows in the valleys of Chu and can be seen everywhere in the fields. In the early spring, its seedlings grow on the flat ground like needles. In the summer, its white flowers are produced and the appearance is fine. In the autumn, its flowers wither. Its rhizomes[1] are very white and sweet. Its roots are cold and neutral in nature, and the flowers are warm. All of them are sweet and non-toxic.

For famine relief: Collect young shoots, peel them off and eat the flesh. It is particularly beneficial for children. Or dig roots and suck the sweetness. The long-term use is good for health. While taking this, one may skip the meal.

For disease treatment: See the clauses of Maogen [茅根, imperata, Imperatae

Cylindrica (L.) Beauv.] in *Materia Medica · Herbaceous Plant*.

【Notes】

[1] It refers to the rhizomes of Baimao.

根及花皆可食

❋ 《本草》原有

Root and Flower Edible

Original Ones

234. 葛 根

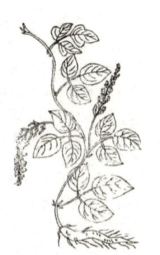

一名鸡齐根,一名鹿藿,一名黄斤。生汶山川谷,及成州、海州、浙江并澧鼎之间,今处处有之。苗引藤蔓,长二三丈,茎淡紫色。叶颇似楸叶而小,色青。开花似豌豆花,粉紫色。结实如皂荚而小。根形如手臂,味甘,性平,无毒。一云性冷。杀野葛,巴豆百药毒。

救饥:掘取根入土深者,水浸洗净,蒸食之。或以水中揉出粉,澄滤成块,蒸煮皆可食。及采花晒干煠食亦可。

治病:文具《本草·草部》条下。

234. Gegen [葛根, pueraria, Puerariae montana (Lour.) Merr.]

Gegen [葛根, pueraria, Puerariae montana (Lour.) Merr.] is also known as Jiqigen, Luhuo and Huangjin. It grows in the valleys where there are waters in Wenshan, Chengzhou, Haizhou and Zhejiang between Lizhou and Dingzhou. It can be seen everywhere presently. Its plants send forth vines which are 20~30 Chi long. Its stems are lavender. Its leaves are very similar to Chinese catalpa leaves, but they are smaller and the color is green. Its flowers are like pea flowers, pink and purple. Its fruit is like a Chinese honey locust, but it is smaller. Its roots are shaped like arms. It is sweet in taste, neutral in nature and non-toxic. Some say it is cold in nature. It is antidote to Yege [野葛, yellow jessamine, Gelsemii Herba] and Badou [巴豆, croton Fruit, Fructus Crotonis].

For famine relief: Dig the roots which are deep into soil, clean them by soaking, and eat them after steaming. Knead them in water until the starch is out, filter them into pieces, and steam and boil them. Or dry flowers in the sunshine and eat them after blanching.

For disease treatment: See the clauses in *Materia Medica · Herbaceous Plant*.

235. 何首乌

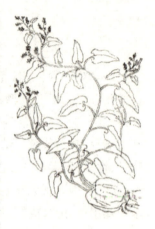

一名野苗,一名交藤,一名夜合,一名地精,一名陈知白,又名桃柳藤,亦名九真藤。出顺州南河县,其岭外江南诸州及虔州皆有,以西洛、嵩山、归德、柘城县者为胜,今钧州密县山谷中亦有之。蔓延而生,茎蔓紫色。叶似山药叶而不光。嫩叶间开黄白花,似葛勒花。结子有棱,似荞麦而极细小,如粟粒大。根大者如拳,各有五楞瓣,状似甜瓜样,中有花纹,形如鸟兽山岳之状者极珍。有赤白二种,赤者雄,白者雌。又云雄者苗叫黄白,雌者赤黄色。一云雄苗赤,生必相对,远不过三四尺,夜则苗蔓相交,或隐化不见。凡修合药,须雌雄相合服,有验。宜偶日服,二四六八日是也。其药本无名,因何首乌见藤夜交,采服有功,因以采人为名耳。又云其为仙草,五十年者如拳大,号山奴,服之一年,髭发乌黑;一百年如碗大,号山哥,服之一年,颜色红悦;百五十年如盆大,号山伯,服之一年,齿落重生;二百年如斗栲栳大,号山翁,服之一年,颜如童子,行及奔马;三百年如三斗栲栳大,号山精,服之一年,延龄、纯阳之体,久服成地仙。又云其头九数者,服之乃仙。味苦、涩,性微温,无毒。一云味甘。茯苓为之使,酒下最良。忌铁器、猪羊血及猪肉、无鳞鱼。与萝卜相恶,若并食,令人髭鬓早白、肠风多热。

救饥:掘根,洗去泥土,以苦竹刀切作片,米泔[1]浸经宿,换水煮去苦味,再以水淘洗净,或蒸或煮食之。花亦可煤食。

治病:文具《本草·草部》条下。

【注释】

[1] 即淘米水。

235. Heshouwu [何首乌, flowery knotweed, Polygonum multiflorum Thunb.]

Heshouwu [何首乌, flowery knotweed, Polygonum multiflorum Thunb] is also known as Yemiao, Jiaoteng, Yehe, Dijing, Chenzhibai, Taoliuteng and Jiuzhenteng. It grows in Nanhe County, Shunzhou Prefecture, in the counties of Jiangnan and in Qianzhou. Heshouwu [何首乌, flowery knotweed, Polygonum multiflorum Thunb] in the counties of Xiluo, Songshan, Guide and Zhecheng is of good quality. It is also seen in the valleys of Mixian County. Its climbing vines grow, and its stems are purple. Its leaves are like yam ones, but they are not shiny. Its yellow and white flowers are between young leaves, which are similar to the Gele flowers. Its fruit is angulate, like buckwheat, but very small, as small as millets. Its roots are like the size of fists, each with five lobes, shaped like a melon, with patterns inside. Those shaped like a bird or a beast are very precious. There are two kinds of Heshouwu [何首乌, flowery knotweed, Polygonum multiflorum Thunb.]. One is red and the other is white. The red one is the male plant, and the white one is the female plant. Some say that the male seedlings and leaves are yellowish white, and the female plants are reddish yellow. Others say that the male plants are red and the female plants and the male plants must be opposite. The distance between the two is only 3~4 Chi. During the night, its seedlings intersect or hide. The male and female plants must be taken together in the process or dispense of medicine, which will be very effective. Take medicine every other day. It was not named initially. A herb collector named He Shouwu found and collected it, so the herb was named after his name to praise his contribution. Others said that Heshouwu was the fairy grass. Heshouwu which has been growing for 50 years is as big as a fist. It is called Shannu. Taking it for one year will make people's beard and hair black. With the life span of a hundred years, Heshouwu is as big as a bowl. It is called Shange. Taking it for one year makes people's faces rosy. Heshouwu which has been growing for 150 years is called Shanbo. After taking it for one year, it can regenerate teeth. Heshouwu which has been growing for 200 years is called Shanweng, and taking it one year, it can make one look as young as a kid, walking like a running horse; Heshouwu which has been growing for 300 years is as big as a three-dou round-bottomed basket, and it is called Shanjing. Taking it for a year can prolong one's life, becoming a pure body. It is also said that the head of Heshouwu has nine types, which can become immortal. It is bitter, astringent, slightly warm in nature and non-toxic. One says it is sweet. Fuling [茯苓, poria cocos, Poria cocos (Schw.) Wolf] serves as its assistant herb. It is good to take it with wine and avoid iron, pig and goat blood and pork, fish without scales. It is averse to radish. Taken with radish, it will cause premature graying of the hair and intestinal wind.

For famine relief: Dig roots, wash away the soil, cut them into pieces with a bitter bamboo knife, soak them in water to wash rice[1] for a whole night, change water and remove the bitterness by boiling them, and then wash them in water, steam or boil them before their being eaten. Its flowers can also be eaten after blanching.

For disease treatment: See the clause in *Materia Medica · Herbaceous Plant*.

【Notes】

[1] It refers to the water to wash rice.

根及实皆可食

《本草》原有

Root and Fruit Edible

Original Ones

236. 瓜楼根

俗名天花粉,本草有栝楼实,一名地楼,一名果裸,一名天瓜,一名泽姑,一名黄瓜。生弘农川谷及山阴地,今处处有之。入土深者良,生卤地[1]者有毒。《诗》所谓果蓏之实是也。根亦名白药,大者细如手臂,皮黄肉白。苗引藤蔓,叶似甜瓜叶而作花叉,有细毛。开花似葫芦花,淡黄色。实在花下,大如拳,生青熟黄。根味苦,性寒,无毒。枸杞为之使,恶干姜、畏牛膝、干漆,

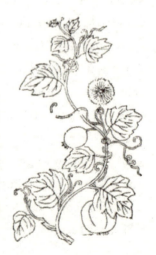

反乌头。

救饥：采根，削皮至白处，寸切之，水浸，一日一次换水，浸经四五日，取出烂捣研，以绢袋盛之，澄滤令极细如粉。或将根晒干，捣为面，水浸澄滤二十余遍，使极腻如粉。或为烧饼、或作煎饼、切细面皆可食。采栝楼穰煮粥食，极甘。取子炒干捣烂，用水熬油用亦可。

治病：文具《本草·草部》栝楼条下。

【注释】

[1]盐碱地。

236. Gualougen[瓜楼根, trichosanthes root, Trichosanthes kirlowii Maxim.]

Gualougen[瓜楼根, trichosanthes root, Trichosanthis Radix] is commonly named Tianhuafen, the materia medica of Gualoushi, and also named Dilou, Guoluo, Tiangua, Zegu and Huanggua. It grows in the valleys of Hongnong where there is flowing water and the north side of the mountain. It can be seen everywhere presently. Those with deep roots are good while those growing in the saline-alkali soil[1] are toxic. It is the fruit of Guoluo in *The Book of Songs*. Its roots are called Baiyao. The big ones are as thick as arms, with yellow bark and white flesh. Its plants are vines, and its leaves are like melon leaves, but there are divided flowers and there fine hairs on them. Its pale yellow flowers are like gourd flowers. Its fruit is under flowers, as big as fists, green when raw, and yellow after ripening. Its roots are bitter, cold in nature and non-toxic. Gouqi[枸杞, lycium chinense, Lycium chinense Mill.] is its assistance, averse to dry ginger, restrained by Niuxi[牛膝, achyranthes, Achyranthis Bidentatae Radix] and Ganqi[干漆, lac, Lacciferi Secretio], and incompatible with Wutou[乌头, aconite, Aconiti Kusnezoffii Radix].

For famine relief: Dig roots, peel straight to the white part, cut the roots into small pieces of one Cun size, soak them in water for four or five days, change water once a day, smash and grind them, and hold them in a shovel bag. Filter until they are as fine as powder. Or dry the roots, knead them into dough, soak them in water, and filter them more than twenty times to make them as fine as

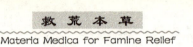

powder. Or make baked rolls, pancakes and noodles with them. Pick the flesh and cook congee, which tastes very sweet. Collect seeds and stir-fry, add water and extract oil.

For disease treatment: See the clause of Gualou in *Materia Medica · Herbaceous Plant*.

【Notes】

[1] It refers to the saline-alkali soil.

新增
New Supplements

237. 砖子苗

一名关子苗。生水边。苗似水葱而粗大、内实;又似蒲荸。梢开碎白花。结穗似水莎草穗,紫赤色。其子如黍粒大。根似蒲根而坚实,味甜,子味亦甜。

救饥:采子磨面食。及采根,择洗净,换水煮食,或晒干磨为面食亦可。

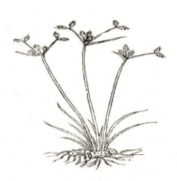

237. Zhuanzimiao [砖子苗, compact mariscus, Marisci Compacti Herba]

Zhuanzimiao [砖子苗, compact mariscus, Marisci Compacti Herba] is also known as Guanzimiao. It grows on the water's edge. Its plants are like those of Shuicong [水葱, robust bullrush, Scirpi Validi Caulis], but they are larger. Its stems are solid and like the scapes of Scirpoides holoschoenus. There are white flowers on the tip of scapes. Its spikes are like those of Shuishacao [水莎草, herb of Glomerate Galingale, Cyperus glomeratus L.], dark purple-red. Its seeds are as big as grains. Its roots are like flagroots, but they are more solid, and the taste is sweet. Its seeds are also sweet.

For famine relief: Collect seeds and dig roots, trim, wash and clean them, change water and boil them, or grind the sun-dried roots into powder.

花叶皆可食

✽ 《本草》原有

Flower and Leaf Edible
Original Ones

238. 菊　花

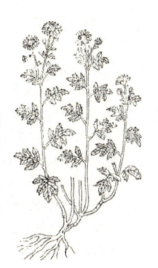

一名节华,一名日精,一名女节,一名女华,一名女茎,一名更生,一名周盈,一名傅延年,一名阴生。生雍州川泽及邓、衡、齐州田野,今处处有之。味苦、甘,性平,无毒。术、枸杞、桑根白皮为之使。

救饥:取茎紫、气香而味甘者,采叶煠食,或作羹皆可。青茎而大,气味作蒿苦者不堪食,名苦薏。其花亦可煠食,或炒茶食。

治病:文具《本草·草部》条下。

238. Juhua〔菊花, chrysanthemum, Chrysanthemum morifolium Ramat〕

Juhua〔菊花, chrysanthemum, Chrysanthemum morifolium Ramat〕is also named Jiehua, Rijing, Nvjie, Nvhua, Nvjing, Gengsheng, Zhouying, Fuyannian and Yinsheng. It grows in the lakes and swamps of Yongzhou and in the fields of Dengzhou, Hengzhou and Qizhou. It can be seen everywhere presently. It is bitter and sweet in taste and neutral in nature and non-toxic. In compatibility, Zhu〔术, rhizoma Atractylodis Macrocephalae, atractylodes macrocephala koidz〕, Gouqi〔枸杞, medlar, Lycium chinense Mill.〕and Sanggen Baipi〔桑根白皮, mulberry bark, Mori Cortex〕are its assistance.

For famine relief: Choose the plants which are purple, fragrant and sweet, and blanch them to eat. It can also be used to cook soap. Those which have big green stems and smell bitter are called Kuyi〔苦薏, wild chrysanthemum flower, Chrysanthemi Indici Flos〕and can not be eaten. Its flowers can also be eaten after blanching or being fried as tea.

For disease treatment: See the clauses in *Materia Medica · Herbaceous Plant*.

239. 金银花

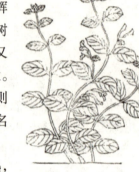

本草名忍冬,一名鹭鸶藤,一名左缠藤,一名金钗股,又名老翁须,亦名忍冬藤。旧不载所出州土,今辉县山野中亦有之。其藤凌冬不凋,故名忍冬草。附树延蔓而生,茎微紫色。对节生叶,叶似薜荔叶而青,又似水茶臼叶,头微团而软,背颇涩;又似黑豆叶而大。开花五出,微香,蒂带红色。花初开白色,经一二日则色黄,故名金银花。本草中不言善治痈疽发背,近代名人[1]用之奇效。味甘,性温,无毒。

救饥:采花煤熟,油盐调食。及采嫩叶,换水煮熟,浸去邪气,淘净,油盐调食。

治病:文具《外科精要》及《本草·草部》忍冬条下。

【注释】

[1] 指名臣高士。

239. Jinyinhua [金银花, lonicera, Lonicera japonica Thunb]

Rendong [忍冬, honeysuckle, Lonicera japonica] is also called Lusiteng, Zuochanteng, Jinchaigu, Laowengxu and Rendongteng. There was no record of its origin in ancient times, and now it can be seen in the mountains and wilderness of Huixian County. Its vines are not withered in chilly winter, and so it is named Rendongcao [忍冬草, lonicera stem, Lonicerae Caulis]. Its plants are attached to trees and grow in vines, and its stems are purple. Its leaves are opposite, like those of Bili [薜荔, creeping fig, Fici Pumilae Caulis et Folium] but greener, and like Shuichajiu but its tip is slightly round and soft, the back of the leaves is slightly rough; it is like Heidou [黑豆, black soybean, Glycinemax (L.) merr] leaves, but larger. Its flowers have five petals, slightly fragrant and lame reddish. It is white when the flowers first bloom. After one or two days, it turns yellow. So it is called Jinyinhua [金银花, lonicera, Lonicerae Flos]. It is not recorded in

Materia Medica that it is good for the treatment of effusion of the back. Famous officials and profound scholars[1] in modern times found it had a miraculous effect. It is sweet in taste, cool in nature and non-toxic.

For famine relief: Collect flowers and blanch them, and flavor them with oil and salt. Or collect young leaves, change water to cook them, remove the strange taste by soaking them, wash and clean them, and flavor them with oil and salt.

For disease treatment: See the clauses in *Essentials of External Medicine* and Rendong [忍冬, honeysuckle, Lonicera japonica] in *Materia Medica · Herbaceous Plant*.

【Notes】

[1] It refers to the famous officials and profound scholars.

※ 新增

New Supplements

240. 望江南

其花名茶花儿。人家园圃中多种。苗高二尺许。茎微淡赤色。叶似槐叶而肥大微尖；又似胡苍耳叶，颇大；及似皂角叶亦大。开五瓣金黄花。结角长三寸许。叶味微苦。

救饥：采嫩苗叶煤熟，水浸淘去苦味，油盐调食。花可炒食亦可煤食。

治病：今人多将其子作草决明子代用。

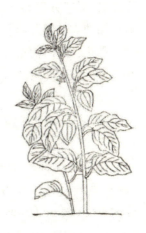

240. Wangjiangnan [望江南, coffee senna, *Senna occidentalis* (L.) Link]

The flowers of Wangjiangnan [望江南, coffee senna, *Senna occidentalis* (L.) Link] are called Chahua'er. There are many plants in the gardens of ordinary people. Its plants are about two Chi high. Its stems are slightly reddish. Its leaves are like those of Huaiye [槐叶, sophora leaf, Sophorae Folium], but they are larger and slightly sharp; they are also like those of Hucang'er [胡苍耳,

glycyrrhiza pallidiflora, Glycyrrhiza pallidiflora Maxim] but larger; they are also like those of Zaojiao [皂角, gleditsia, Gleditsiae Fructus] but larger. Its flowers have five petals, and the color is golden. Its follicles are about three Cun long. Its leaves are slightly bitter.

For famine relief: Collect young plants and leaves, blanch them and remove the bitterness by soaking them, and flavor them with oil and salt. Its flowers can be eaten after frying or blanching.

For disease treatment: Most people now use its seeds to replace Cao Juemingzi [草决明子, fetid cassia (Semen), Cassiae Semen].

241. 大 蓼

生密县梁家冲山谷中。拖藤而生。茎有线楞而颇硬,对节分生茎叉,叶亦对生。叶似山蓼叶,微短而拳曲。节间开白花。其叶味苦、微辣。

救饥:采叶煤熟,换水浸去辣味,作成黄色,淘洗净,油盐调食。花亦可煤食。

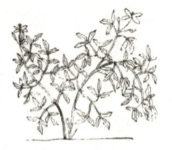

241. Daliao [大蓼, flowering clematis, Clematidis Floridae Herba]

It grows in the valleys of Liangjiachong, Mixian County. It grows along the vines. Its stems are very hard and its blades are stalked on them. Its branches are opposite, and its leaves are opposite too. Its leaves are like Shanliao leaves, but they are slightly short and curled-up. There are white flowers between the nodes. Its leaves are bitter and slightly spicy.

For famine relief: Collect leaves and blanch them, change water and remove the pungency by soaking them until the leaves turn yellow. Wash and flavor them with oil and salt. The flowers can also be eaten after blanching.

茎可食

* 《本草》原有

Stem Edible
Original Ones

242. 黑三棱

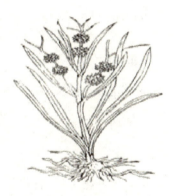

旧云河、陕、江淮、荆、襄间皆有之，今郑州贾峪山涧水边亦有。苗高三四尺。叶似菖蒲叶而厚大，背皆三棱剑脊。叶中撺葶，葶上结实，攒为刺球，状如楮桃样而大，颗瓣甚多。其颗瓣形似草决明子而大，生则青，熟则红黄色。根状如乌梅而颇大，有须蔓延相连，比京三棱体微轻，治疗并同。其葶味甜。根味苦，性平，无毒。

救饥：采嫩葶，剥去粗皮，煤熟，油盐调食。

治病：文具《本草·草部》京三棱条下。

242. Heisanleng〔黑三棱, sparganium, Sparganium stoloniferum (Buch.-Ham. ex Graebn) Buch.-Ham. ex Juz〕

It can be seen in He, Shan, Jianghuai, Jing and Xiang according to the ancient record. Presently, it can also be seen in the waters of the mountains of Jiayu, Zhengzhou. Its plants are 3 ~ 4 Chi high. Its leaves are like those of Changpu〔菖蒲, acorus, Acori Tatarinowii Rhizoma〕, but they are thicker and have a triangular back, like a sword ridge. In the middle of the leaves, the scapes are pulled out and the fruit bears on the scapes which get together like thorn balls. The shape of the fruit is like that of Chutaoshu〔楮桃树, paper mulberry, Broussonetia papyrifera (L.) L'Hér. ex Vent.〕but larger, and there is a lot of fruit. Its fruit is shaped like Cao Juemingzi〔草决明子, fetid cassia, Cassiae Semen〕, but it is larger. It is green when it is unripe, and it turns red-yellow when it is ripe. The shape of tubers is like that of Wumei〔乌梅, Armeniaca mume, Armeniaca mume Sieb.], a little larger, with rhizomes spreading in succession. It is a little lighter than Jingsanleng [京三棱, scirpus, Bolboschoenus yagara (Ohwi) Y. C. Yang et M. Zhan], and has the same therapeutic effect. Its scapes are sweet. Its roots are bitter in taste, neutral in nature and non-toxic.

For famine relief: Collect young stems, peel off the rough bark, blanch them and flavor them with oil and salt.

For disease treatment: See the clause of Jingsanleng [京三棱, scirpus, Bolboschoenus yagara (Ohwi) Y. C. Yang et M. Zhan] in *Materia Medica · Herbaceous Plant.*

新增
New Supplements

243. 荇丝菜

又名金莲儿,一名藕蔬菜。水中拖蔓而生。叶似初生小荷叶,近茎有桠劓,叶浮水上。叶中撺茎,上开金黄花。茎味甜。

救饥:采嫩茎煠熟,油盐调食。

243. Xingsicai [荇丝菜, Nymphoides peltata (S. G. Gmelin) Kuntze]

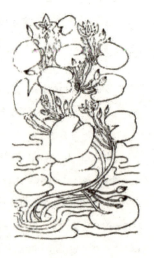

It is also known as Jinlian'er, Oushucai. Its vines grow along the branches in the water. Its leaves are like small lotus leaves, and there are cracks around the stems (heart-shaped leaves), and the leaves float on the water surface. In the middle of the leaves, the stems are pulled out and the flowers are golden. Its stems are sweet.

For famine relief: Collect young stems and blanch them, and flavor them with oil and salt.

244. 水慈菰

俗呼为剪刀草,又名箭搭草。生水中。其茎面窊背方,背有线楞。其叶三角,似剪刀形。叶中撺生茎叉,梢间开三瓣白花,黄心。结青蓇葖,如青楮桃状,颇小。根类葱根而粗大,其味甜。

救饥:采近根嫩笋茎煠熟,油盐调食。

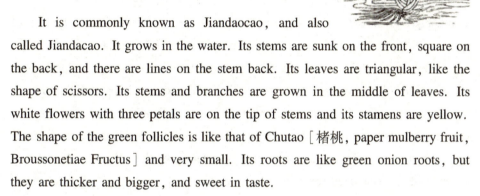

244. Shuicigu [水慈菰, savory, Clinopodii Herba]

It is commonly known as Jiandaocao, and also called Jiandacao. It grows in the water. Its stems are sunk on the front, square on the back, and there are lines on the stem back. Its leaves are triangular, like the shape of scissors. Its stems and branches are grown in the middle of leaves. Its white flowers with three petals are on the tip of stems and its stamens are yellow. The shape of the green follicles is like that of Chutao [楮桃, paper mulberry fruit, Broussonetiae Fructus] and very small. Its roots are like green onion roots, but they are thicker and bigger, and sweet in taste.

For famine relief: Collect young shoots and stems which are near the roots, blanch them, and flavor them with oil and salt.

笋及实皆可食

※ 《本草》原有

Shoot and Fruit Edible

Original Ones

245. 茭 笋

本草有菰根,又名菰蒋草,江南人呼为茭草,俗又呼为茭白。生江东池泽、水中及岸际,今在处水泽边皆有之。苗高二三尺,叶似蔗荻;又似茅叶而长大阔厚。叶间撺葶,开花如苇,结实青子。根肥,剥取嫩白笋可啖,久根盘厚生菌,细嫩,亦可啖,名菰菜。三年已上,心中生薹如藕,白软,中有黑脉,甚堪啖,名菰首。味甘,性大寒,无毒。

救饥:采茭菰笋,煤熟,油盐调食。或采子舂为米,合粟煮粥食之,甚济饥。

治病:文具《本草·草部》菰根条下。

245. Jiaosun [茭笋, infested ear of wild rice, Zizaniae Spica Infestata]

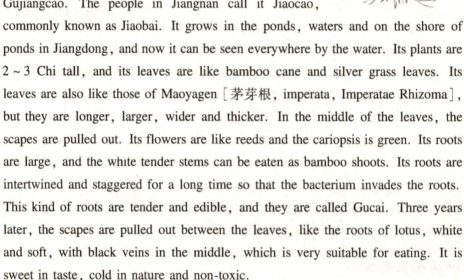

The materia medica of Gugen is also named Gujiangcao. The people in Jiangnan call it Jiaocao, commonly known as Jiaobai. It grows in the ponds, waters and on the shore of ponds in Jiangdong, and now it can be seen everywhere by the water. Its plants are 2~3 Chi tall, and its leaves are like bamboo cane and silver grass leaves. Its leaves are also like those of Maoyagen [茅芽根, imperata, Imperatae Rhizoma], but they are longer, larger, wider and thicker. In the middle of the leaves, the scapes are pulled out. Its flowers are like reeds and the cariopsis is green. Its roots are large, and the white tender stems can be eaten as bamboo shoots. Its roots are intertwined and staggered for a long time so that the bacterium invades the roots. This kind of roots are tender and edible, and they are called Gucai. Three years later, the scapes are pulled out between the leaves, like the roots of lotus, white and soft, with black veins in the middle, which is very suitable for eating. It is sweet in taste, cold in nature and non-toxic.

For famine relief: Collect young stems and blanch them, and flavor them with oil and salt. Or collect the cariopsis and pound Gumi, and make congee with millets. It is good for famine relief.

For disease treatment: See the clause of Gugen in *Materia Medica · Herbaceous Plant*.

卷下　下之前

木　部

叶可食

《本草》原有

Volume 2　The First Half
Woody Plant
Leaf Edible
Original Ones

246. 茶　树

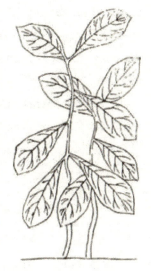

本草有茗、苦檟。《图经》云生山南汉中山谷,闽、浙、蜀、荆、江湖、淮南山中皆有之。惟建州北苑数处产者,性味独与诸方不同。今密县梁家冲山谷间亦有之。其树大小皆类栀子。春初生芽,为雀舌、麦颗。又有新芽,一发便长寸余,微粗如针,渐至环脚、软枝条之类。叶老则似水茶臼叶而长,又似初生青冈、橡叶而少光泽。又云,冬生叶可作羹饮。世呼早采者为檟,晚取者为茗,一名荈。蜀今谓之苦檟,今通谓之茶。茶、荼声近,故呼之。又有研治作饼,名为腊茶者,皆味甘、苦,性微寒,无毒。加茱萸、葱、姜等良。又别有一种,蒙山中顶上清峰茶,云春分前后,多聚人力,候雷初发声,并手齐采。若得四两,服之即为地仙。

救饥:采嫩叶或冬生叶,可煮作羹食,或蒸焙作茶,皆可。

治病:文具《本草·木部》茗、苦檟条下。

246. Chashu [茶树, tea tree, Camellia sinensis (L.) Ktze]

Chashu is the materia medica of Ming, Kucha. According to *Tu Jing* [图经, *Illustrated Pharmacopoeia*], it grows in the valleys of Hanzhong Mountain in the south of Shaanxi and are planted in the mountains of Fujian, Zhejiang, Sichuan, Jing, Jianghu and Huainan. It also grows in the valleys of Mixian County, Liangjiachong. The tea trees are all like gardenia trees, sprouting in the early spring, which is called Queshe or Maike. Then it germinates again and the new buds are longer than one Chi, and it is slightly thicker than a needle. It gradually develops into a circinate and soft branch. When its leaves are old, they are like Shuichajiu leaves, but they are longer; they are also like the newly sprouted Qinggangshu [青冈树, Quercus serrata, Quercus serrata Murray] leaves, oak leaves, but not that lucid. Some say its leaves in the winter can be made into soap. People call the early harvest Cha, and the late harvest Ming or Chuan. Grind the tea and make them into a cake, and then it is called Lacha, sweet, bitter, slightly cold in nature and non-toxic. It tastes better if Lacha is drunk with cornel, green onions, ginger, etc. In addition, there is a kind of tea, that is, Qingfeng tea produced on the top of Mengshan. It is said that before and after the spring equinox, helpers gathered. When you first hear the thunder, people will pick up the tea together. If you can get four liang of it, you can become healthy after taking it.

For famine relief: Collect young leaves or leaves grown in the winter and boil them into soap, or steam and bake them into tea.

For disease treatment: See the clauses of Ming, Kucha in *Materia Medica · Woody Plant*.

247. 夜合树

本草名合欢,一名合昏。生益州及雍、洛山谷,今钧州、郑州山野中亦有之。木似梧桐,其枝甚柔弱。叶似皂荚叶;又似槐叶,极细而密,互相交结,每一风来,辄似相解,了不相牵缀。其叶至暮而合,故名合昏。花发红白色,瓣上若丝,茸然散垂。结实作荚子，极薄细，味甘，性平，无毒。

救饥：采嫩叶煠熟，水浸淘净，油盐调食，晒干煠食尤好。

治病：文具《本草·木部》合欢条下。

247. Yeheshu［夜合树，Maackia amurensis, Albizia julibrissin Durazz. / Albizia kalkora Prain］

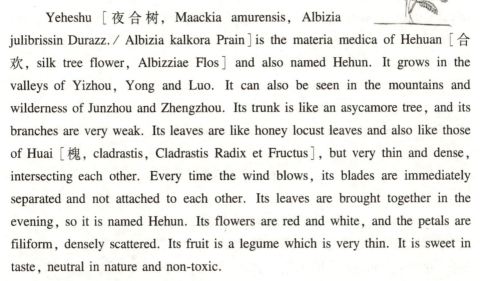

Yeheshu［夜合树，Maackia amurensis, Albizia julibrissin Durazz. / Albizia kalkora Prain］is the materia medica of Hehuan［合欢，silk tree flower, Albizziae Flos］and also named Hehun. It grows in the valleys of Yizhou, Yong and Luo. It can also be seen in the mountains and wilderness of Junzhou and Zhengzhou. Its trunk is like an asycamore tree, and its branches are very weak. Its leaves are like honey locust leaves and also like those of Huai［槐，cladrastis, Cladrastis Radix et Fructus］, but very thin and dense, intersecting each other. Every time the wind blows, its blades are immediately separated and not attached to each other. Its leaves are brought together in the evening, so it is named Hehun. Its flowers are red and white, and the petals are filiform, densely scattered. Its fruit is a legume which is very thin. It is sweet in taste, neutral in nature and non-toxic.

For famine relief：Collect young leaves and blanch them, wash and clean them by soaking, and flavor them with oil and salt. Blanch the sun-dried leaves to let them taste even better.

For disease treatment：See the clause of Hehuan in *Materia Medica · Woody Plant*.

248. 木槿树

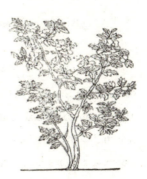

本草云木槿如小葵。花淡红色，五叶成一花。朝开暮敛，花与枝两用。湖南北人家多种植为篱障。亦有千叶者，人家园圃多栽种。性平，无毒。叶味甜。

救饥：采嫩叶煠熟，冷水淘净，油盐调食。

治病：文具《本草·木部》条下。

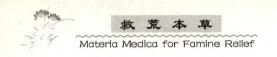

248. Mujinshu [木槿树, hibiscus syriacus, Hibiscus syriacus L.]

According to *Materia Medica*, Mujin [木槿, rose-of-Sharon root bark, Hibisci Syriaci Radicis Cortex] is like Xiaokui. Its flowers are reddish and there are five petals for each flower. Its flowers bloom in the morning and close in the evening. Its flowers and branches can be used in two ways. It is planted as barriers in the north of Hunan. Those which have multi-petal blooms are planted in the gardens of ordinary families. It is neutral in nature and non-toxic. Its leaves are sweet.

For famine relief: Collect young leaves and blanch them, wash them in cold water, and flavor them with oil and salt.

For disease treatment: See the clauses in *Materia Medica · Woody Plant.*

249. 白杨树

本草白杨树皮。旧不载所出州土,今处处有之。此木高大,皮白似杨,故名。叶圆如梨,肥大而尖,叶背甚白,叶边锯齿状,叶蒂小,无风自动也。味苦,性平,无毒。

救饥:采嫩叶煠熟,作成黄色,换水淘去苦味,洗净,油盐调食。

治病:文具《本草·木部》条下。

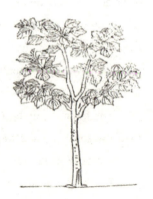

249. Baiyangshu [白杨树, white poplar, Populus alba L.]

Baiyangshu [白杨树, white poplar, Populus alba L.] is the materia medica of Baiyang Shupi [白杨树皮, David's poplar bark, Populi Davidianae Cortex]. There was no record of its origin in ancient times, and it is found everywhere now. It is tall. The tree bark is white, and it is named because it looks like a poplar. Its leaves are as round as the leaves of pears, large and sharp. The back of its leaves is white. The edge of the leaves is zigzag. Its petioles are small, and can move even there is no wind. It is bitter in taste, flat in nature and non-toxic.

For famine relief: Collect young leaves and make them yellow, change water to remove the bitterness, wash and clean them, and flavor them with oil and salt.

For disease treatment: See the clauses of *Materia Medica · Woody Plant*.

250. 黄 栌

生商洛山谷,今钧州新郑山野中亦有之。叶圆,木黄,枝茎色紫赤。叶似杏叶而圆大。味苦,性寒,无毒,木可染黄。

救饥:采嫩芽煠熟,水淘去苦味,油盐调食。

治病:文具《本草·木部》条下。

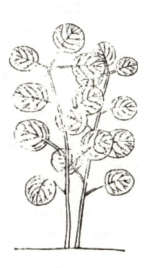

250. Huanglu [黄栌, cotinus coggygria Cotinus coggygria Scop.]

It grows in the valleys of Shangluo, and can also be seen in the mountains and plains of Junzhou and Xinzheng. Its leaves are round, and the wood is yellow. Its branches and stems are purplish red. Its leaves are like apricot leaves, but they are rounder and bigger. It is bitter in taste, cold in nature and non-toxic. The wood can be used to dye yellow.

For famine relief: Collect young leaves and blanch them. Remove the bitterness by soaking them, and flavor them with oil and salt.

For disease treatment: See the clauses of *Materia Medica · Woody Plant*.

251. 椿树芽

本草有椿木、樗木,旧不载所出州土,今处处有之。二木形干大抵相类,椿木实而叶香可啖,樗木疏而气臭,膳夫熬去其气,亦可啖。北人呼樗为山椿,江东人呼为虎目,叶脱处有痕如樗蒲子;又如眼目,故得此名。夏中生荚。樗之有花者无荚,有荚者无花。荚常生臭樗上,未见椿上有荚者,然世俗不辨椿樗之异，故俗名为椿荚，其实樗荚耳。其无花不实，木大端直为椿。有花而荚，木小干多迂矮者为樗。椿味苦，有毒。樗味苦，有小毒，性温，一云性热，无毒。

救饥：采嫩芽煤熟，水浸淘净，油盐调食。

治病：文具《本草·木部》椿木、樗木及椿荚条下。

251. Chunshuya〔椿树芽，cedrela sinensis，Toona sinensis（A. Juss.）Roem.〕

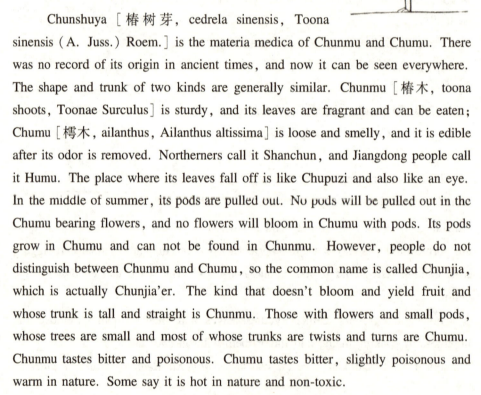

Chunshuya〔椿树芽，cedrela sinensis，Toona sinensis（A. Juss.）Roem.〕is the materia medica of Chunmu and Chumu. There was no record of its origin in ancient times, and now it can be seen everywhere. The shape and trunk of two kinds are generally similar. Chunmu〔椿木，toona shoots，Toonae Surculus〕is sturdy, and its leaves are fragrant and can be eaten; Chumu〔樗木，ailanthus，Ailanthus altissima〕is loose and smelly, and it is edible after its odor is removed. Northerners call it Shanchun, and Jiangdong people call it Humu. The place where its leaves fall off is like Chupuzi and also like an eye. In the middle of summer, its pods are pulled out. No pods will be pulled out in the Chumu bearing flowers, and no flowers will bloom in Chumu with pods. Its pods grow in Chumu and can not be found in Chunmu. However, people do not distinguish between Chunmu and Chumu, so the common name is called Chunjia, which is actually Chunjia'er. The kind that doesn't bloom and yield fruit and whose trunk is tall and straight is Chunmu. Those with flowers and small pods, whose trees are small and most of whose trunks are twists and turns are Chumu. Chunmu tastes bitter and poisonous. Chumu tastes bitter, slightly poisonous and warm in nature. Some say it is hot in nature and non-toxic.

For famine relief: Collect young buds and blanch them, soak them in water, wash and clean them, and flavor them with oil and salt.

For disease treatment: See the clauses of Chunmu, Chumu and Chunjia in *Materia Medica · Woody Plant*.

252. 椒　树

本草蜀椒,一名南椒,一名巴椒,一名蓎藙。生武都[1]川谷及巴郡、归、峡、蜀川、陕洛间,人家园圃多种之。高四五尺,似茱萸而小,有针刺,叶似刺蘗叶微小,叶坚而滑,可煮食,甚辛香。结实无花,但生于叶间,如豆颗而圆,皮紫赤。此椒江淮及北土皆有之,茎实皆相类,但不及蜀中者皮肉厚,腹里白,气味浓烈耳。又云,出金州西城者佳。味辛,性温,大热,有小毒,多食令人乏气,口闭者杀人。十月勿食椒,损气伤心,令人多忘。杏仁为之使,畏款冬花。

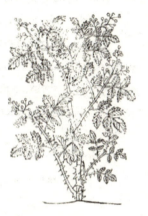

救饥:采嫩叶煠熟,换水浸淘净,油盐调食。椒颗调和百味,香美。

治病:文具《本草·木部》蜀椒条下。

【注释】

[1] 古代郡名。

252. Jiaoshu [椒树, Sichuan pepper, Zanthoxylum simulans Hance]

Jiaoshu [椒树, Sichuan pepper, Zanthoxylum simulans Hance], the materia medica of Shujiao, also named Nanjiao, Bajiao and Tangyi, grows in the valleys of Wudu County[1] with flowing water and the areas of Ba County, Gui, Xia, Shuchuan and Shanluo. People often plant it in the gardens. It is 4~5 Chi high, like the cornel, but it is relatively small and has thorns on it. Its leaves are like Cimi leaves, but a little smaller, hard and smooth. Its leaves can be cooked and eaten, and its pungent flavor is very strong. It bears fruit without blooming, and its fruit grow between the leaves like beans, but the fruit is round and purple. This kind of Jiaoshu [椒树, Sichuan pepper, Zanthoxylum simulans Hance] can be found in Jianghuai and the north. Its branches and fruit are like those of Shujiao, but Shujiao which grows in Shuzhong has thick flesh, white inner part and strong flavor. Some say Shujiao in Xicheng County, Jinzhou is of good quality. The taste is pungent. It is warm in nature, with great heat and slightly toxicity. Eating too much will cause deficiency of qi. Those with closed peels are toxic. People can not eat Shujiao in October, otherwise it will cause deficiency of qi, poor memory and heart damage. Xingren［杏仁, apricot kernel, Armeniacae Semen］ is its envoy herb. It is restrained by Kuandonghua［款冬花, coltsfoot, Farfarae Flos］.

For famine relief: Collect young leaves and blanch them, change water to soak, wash and clean them, and then flavor them with oil and salt. Its fruit can be used to flavor them, and the taste is fragrant.

For disease treatment: See the clause of Shujiao in *Materia Medica · Woody Plant*.

【Notes】

［1］ The name of a county in ancient times.

253. 椋子树

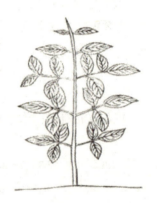

本草有椋子木,旧不载所出州土,今密县山野中亦有之。其树有大者,木则坚重,材堪为车辋。初生作科条状,类荆条,对生枝叉。叶似柿叶而薄小,两叶相当,对生。开白花,结子细圆,如牛李子,大如豌豆,生青熟黑。味甘、咸,性平,无毒,叶味苦。

救饥:采叶煤熟,水浸淘去苦味,洗净,油盐调食。

治病:文具《本草·木部》条下。

253. Liangzishu［椋子树, cornus, Cornus macrophylla Wall.］

Liangzishu［椋子树, cornus, Cornus macrophylla Wall.］ is the materia medica of Liangzimu［椋子木, large-leaved cornel wood, Corni Macrophyllae Lignum］. There was no record of its origin in ancient times. Presently it can be seen in the mountains and wilderness of Mixian County. The tall trees have hard and heavy trunks. The wood is suitable for rutting. The nascent branches are small, shaped like a wattle, and the branches are opposite. Its leaves are like persimmon leaves, but they are thinner and smaller, and the two leaves are opposite. It has white flowers, thin and round fruit, like Niulizi［牛李子, rat plum, Rhamni Davuricae Fructus], as big as peas, green when uncooked, and black when well cooked. It is sweet, salty in taste, neutral in nature and non-toxic. Its leaves are bitter.

For famine relief: Collect and blanch leaves, remove the bitterness by soaking them in water, wash and clean them, and then flavor them with oil and salt.

For disease treatment: See the clauses in Materia Medica · Woody Plant.

新增
New Supplements

254. 云 桑

生密县山野中。其树枝叶皆类桑，但其叶如云头花叉；又似木栾树叶微阔。开细青黄花。其叶味微苦。

救饥：采嫩叶煤熟，换水浸淘去苦味，油盐调食。或蒸晒作茶，尤佳。

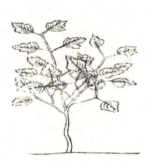

254. Yunsang [云桑, Acer ginnala, Acer tataricum L. subsp. ginnala (Maxim.) Wesmael]

It grows in the mountains and wilderness of Mixian County. Its branches and leaves all look like those of mulberry, but the leaves have uneven edges and look like clouds; its leaves are also like goldenrain tree leaves, but a little wider. Its flowers are bluish yellow. Its leaves are slightly bitter.

For famine relief: Collect young leaves and blanch them, change water and remove the bitterness by soaking them in water, and flavor them with oil and salt. It can also be steamed and dried in the sunshine, cooked and drunk as tea, and the taste is good.

255. 黄楝树

生郑州南山野中。叶似初生椿树叶而极小，又似楝叶，色微带黄。开花紫赤色，结子如豌豆大，生青，熟亦紫赤色。叶味苦。

救饥：采嫩芽叶煤熟，换水浸去苦味，油盐调食。蒸芽曝干，亦可作茶煮饮。

255. Huanglianshu〔黄楝树, pistacia chinensis bunge, Pistacia chinensis Bunge〕

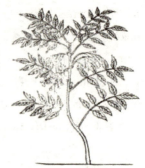

It grows in the mountains and wilderness of the south of Zhengzhou. Its leaves resemble nascent eucalyptus leaves, but they are very small, and they are also like eucalyptus leaves, slightly yellow. It blooms purple flowers, and its fruit is pea-sized, green when uncooked, and turns purple after cooking. Its leaves are bitter in taste.

For famine relief: Collect young leaves and blanch them, change water and remove the bitterness by soaking them in water, and flavor them with oil and salt. It can also be steamed and dried in the sunshine, cooked and drunk as tea.

256. 冻青树

生密县山谷间。树高丈许。枝叶似枸骨子树而极茂盛，凌冬不凋；又似樝子树叶而小；亦似稆芽叶微窄，头颇团而不尖。开白花，结子如豆粒大，青黑色，叶味苦。

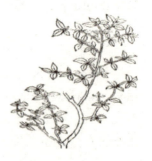

救饥：采芽叶煤熟，水浸去苦味，淘洗净，油盐调食。

256. Dongqingshu〔冻青树, ligustrum lucidum, Ligustrum lucidum Ait.〕

It grows in the valleys of Mixian County. It is about one Zhang high. Its branches and leaves are like those of Gouguzi Shu〔枸骨子树, Chinese holly fruit, Ilicis Cornutae Fructus〕, but they are very dense and don't wither in the chilly winter; its leaves are like those of Zhazishu〔樝子树, cydonia fruit, Cydoniae Fructus〕, but they are smaller; it leaves are also like those of Rongyashu

[稆芽树, yhoary willow, Fontanesia fortunei Carr.], but they are a little narrower, and the tips of the leaves are slightly round, not sharp. Its flowers are white, and its fruit is like the size of beans, black in color. The taste of its leaves is bitter.

For famine relief: Collect young leaves and blanch them, remove the bitterness by soaking them in water, wash and clean them, and flavor them with oil and salt.

257. 稆芽树

生辉县山野中。科条似槐条。叶似冬青叶微长。开白花,结青白子。其叶味甜。

救饥:采嫩叶煠熟,水淘净,油盐调食。

257. Rongyashu [稆芽树, hoary willow, Fontanesia phillyreoides Labill. subsp. fortunei (Carrière) Yalt.]

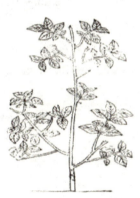

It grows in the mountains and wilderness of Huixian County. Its stems are like the branches of Huai [槐, cladrastis, Cladrastis Radix et Fructus]. Its leaves are like Dongqingye [冬青叶, Chinese ilex leaf, Ilicis Chinensis Folium] but a little longer. It has white flowers, and green and white fruit. Its leaves are slightly sweet.

For famine relief: Collect young leaves and blanch them, wash them in water, and flavor them with oil and salt.

258. 月芽树[1]

又名芴芽。生田野中。茎似槐条。叶似歪头菜叶微短,稍硬;又似稆芽叶,颇长艄,其叶两两对生,味甘、微苦。

救饥:采嫩叶煠熟,水浸淘净,油盐调食。

【注释】

[1] 似与第257稆芽树同种。

258. Yueyashu [月芽树, hoary willow, Fontanesia phillyreoides Labill. subsp. fortunei (Carrière) Yalt.][1]

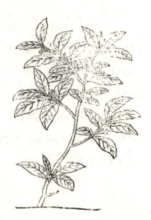

It is also called Rengya. It grows in the fields. Its stems are like the branches of Huai [槐, cladrastis, Cladrastis Radix et Fructus]. Its leaves are like those of Waitoucai, slightly shorter and harder; they are like bud leaves, a little longer and sharper. Its leaves are opposite for each other. Its leaves are sweet and bitter.

For famine relief: Collect young leaves and blanch them, wash them in water, and flavor them with oil and salt.

[Notes]

[1] The 257th clause and the 258th clause are homogeneous plants.

259. 女儿茶

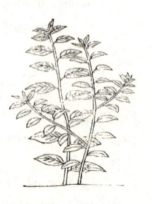

一名牛李子,一名牛筋子。生田野中。科条高五六尺。叶似郁李子叶而长大,稍尖,叶色光滑;又似白棠子叶,而色微黄绿。结子如豌豆大,生则青,熟则黑茶褐色。其叶味淡,微苦。

救饥:采嫩叶煠熟,水浸淘净,油盐调食。亦可蒸暴,作茶煮饮。

259. Nv'ercha [女儿茶, Rhamnus davurica, Rhamnus davurica Pall.]

It is also named Niulizi or Niujinzi. It grows in the fields. Its plants are 5~6 Chi high. Its leaves are like those of Yulizi [郁李子, Chinese Dwarf Cherry Seed, Semen Pruni], but they are relatively longer and bigger, slightly pointed, and its leaves are smooth; they are also like Baitangzi leaves, but slightly yellowish green. Its fruit is pea-sized, cyan when uncooked, and brown after cooking. Its leaves are light and bitter in taste.

For famine relief: Collect young leaves and blanch them, wash and clean them by soaking them in water, and flavor them with oil and salt. They can also be steamed and dried in the sun, cooked and drunk as tea.

260. 省沽油

又名珍珠花。生钧州风谷顶山谷中，科条似荆条而圆，对生枝叉，叶亦对生。叶似驴驼布袋叶而大，又似葛藤[1]叶却小，每三叶攒生一处。开白花，似珍珠色。叶味甘，微苦。

救饥：采嫩叶煤熟，水浸淘净，油盐调食。

【注释】

[1]葛的别名。见本书第234葛根条。

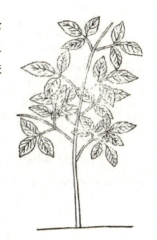

260. Shengguyou [省沽油, Staphylea bumalda, Staphylea bumalda DC.]

It is also named Zhenzhuhua. It grows on the top of Fenggu Valley in Junzhou. Its branches are like the twigs of chaste trees, and they are round. Both its branches and its leaves are opposite. Its leaves are like Lvtuo Budai leaves but larger; they are also like those of Gegen[1] [葛根, pueraria, Puerariae Radix] but smaller. Every three leaves gather together. Its flowers are white, like the color of pearls. Its leaves are sweet and slightly bitter.

For famine relief: Collect leaves and blanch them, wash and clean them by soaking them in water, and flavor them with oil and salt.

【Notes】

[1] Another name for Gegen [葛根, pueraria, Puerariae Radix]. See the 234th clause of this book.

261. 白槿树

生密县梁家冲山谷中。树高五七尺。叶似茶叶，而甚阔大光润；又似初生青冈叶而无花叉；又似山格剌树叶亦大。开白花。其叶味苦。

救饥：采嫩叶煠熟，换水浸去苦味，油盐调食。

261. Baijinshu〔白槿树, fraxinus chinensis Fraxinus chinensis Roxb.〕

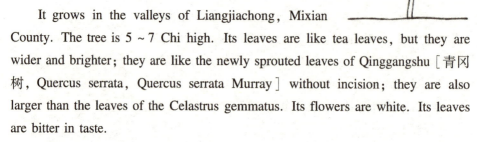

It grows in the valleys of Liangjiachong, Mixian County. The tree is 5~7 Chi high. Its leaves are like tea leaves, but they are wider and brighter; they are like the newly sprouted leaves of Qinggangshu〔青冈树, Quercus serrata, Quercus serrata Murray〕without incision; they are also larger than the leaves of the Celastrus gemmatus. Its flowers are white. Its leaves are bitter in taste.

For famine relief: Collect and blanch young plants and leaves, remove the bitterness by soaking them in fresh water, and then flavor them with oil and salt.

262. 回回醋

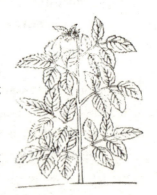

一名淋朴楸。生密县韶华山山野中。树高丈余。叶似兜栌树叶而厚大，边有大锯齿；又似厚椿叶而亦大，或三叶或五叶排生一茎。开白花，结子大如豌豆，熟则红紫色，味酸，叶味微酸。

救饥：采叶煠熟，水浸去酸味，淘净，油盐调食。其子调和汤味，如醋。

262. Huihuicu〔回回醋, rhus chinensis, Rhus chinensis Mill.〕

It is also known as Linpusu. It grows in the mountains and wilderness of Mount Shaohua in Mixian County. Its plants are more than one Zhang high. Its leaves are like those of Doulushu〔兜栌树, Platycarya strobilacea Sieb., Platycarya strobilacea Sieb. et Zucc.〕, but they are thicker and larger, and have large serrations on the edges. They are also like those of Doulushu〔兜栌树, Platycarya strobilacea Sieb., Platycarya strobilacea Sieb. et Zucc.], but they are also larger. Three or five leaves grow on one stem. Its flowers are white, and its fruit is like a pea which turns reddish purple when it is cooked. It tastes sour. Its leaves are slightly acidic.

For famine relief: Collect and blanch young plants and leaves, remove the sour by soaking them in water, and then flavor them with oil and salt. Its fruit can be used to flavor the soup, like the taste of vinegar.

263. 槭树芽

生钧州风谷顶山谷间。木高一二丈。其叶状类野葡萄叶,五花尖叉;亦似棉花叶而薄小;又似丝瓜叶却甚小,而淡黄绿色。开白花,叶味甜。

救饥:采叶煠熟,以水浸,作成黄色,换水淘净,油盐调食。

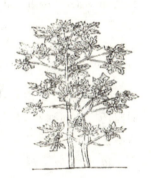

263. Seshuya [槭树芽, Acer mono, Acer pictum Thunb]

It grows in Fengguding Valley, Junzhou. Its plants are 1~2 Zhang high. Its leaves are like the shape of wild grape leaves and quinquepartite; they are like cotton leaves, but relatively thin; they are like loofah leaves but much smaller. The color is light yellow-green. Its flowers are white. Its leaves are sweet in taste.

For famine relief: Collect and blanch leaves, soak them in fresh water until they turn yellow, wash and clean them, and then flavor them with oil and salt.

264. 老叶儿树

生密县山野中。树高六七尺。叶似茶叶而窄瘦尖艄,又似李子叶而长。其叶味甘、微涩。

救饥:采叶煠熟,水浸去涩味,淘洗净,油盐调食。

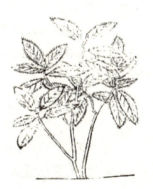

264. Laoye'er Shu [老叶儿树, Quercus variabilis, Quercus variabilis Bl.]

It grows in the mountains and wilderness of Mixian County. The tree is 6~7 Chi high. Its leaves are like tea leaves, but they are narrower and sharper; they are like plum leaves, but longer. Its leaves are sweet and slightly puckery.

For famine relief: Collect and blanch leaves, remove the astringency by soaking them in water, wash and clean them, and then flavor them with oil and salt.

265. 青杨树

在处有之，今密县山野间亦多有。其树高大。叶似白杨树叶而狭小，色青，皮亦颇青，故名青杨。其叶味微苦。

救饥：采叶煠熟，水浸，作成黄色，换水淘净，油盐调食。

265. Qingyangshu [青杨树, Cathay poplar, Populus cathayana Rehd.]

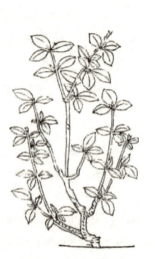

It can be seen everywhere, and there are also many in the mountains and wilderness in Mixian County. Its trunk is tall. Its leaves are like white poplar leaves, but they are narrower and smaller, green in color and slightly green in bark, so they are called Qingyang. The taste of leaves is slightly bitter.

For famine relief: Collect and blanch leaves, soak them in fresh water until they turn yellow, wash and clean them, and then flavor them with oil and salt.

266. 龙柏芽

出南阳府马鞍山中。此木久则亦大。叶似初生橡栎小叶而短，味微苦。
救饥：采芽叶煠熟，换水浸淘净，油盐调食。

266. Longboya [龙柏芽, Exochorda giraldii, Exochorda giraldii Hesse.]

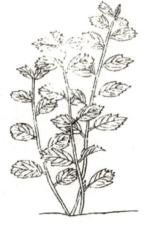

It grows in Mount Ma'an, Nanyang. This kind of trees can grow into big trees after many years. Its leaves are like those of Xiangli [橡栎, acorn, Quercus acutissima Carr.], but they are shorter. Its leaves taste slightly bitter.

For famine relief: Collect young buds and leaves, blanch them, change water to remove the bitterness by soaking them in water, wash and clean them, and flavor them with oil and salt.

267. 兜栌树

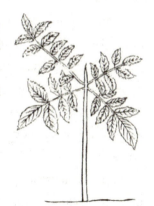

生密县梁家冲山谷中。树甚高大，其木枯朽极透，可作香焚，俗名坏香。叶似回回醋树叶而薄窄；又似花楸树叶却少花叉。叶皆对生，味苦。

救饥：采嫩芽叶煠熟，水浸去苦味，淘洗净，油盐调食。

267. Doulushu [兜栌树, Platycarya strobilacea Sieb., Platycarya strobilacea Sieb. et Zucc.]

It grows in the valleys of Liangjiachong in Mixian County. The tree is very tall, and its trunk is completely dry and rotted, it can be burned as incense. Its common name is Huaixiang. Its leaves are like those of Huihuicu [回回醋, rhus chinensis, Rhus chinensis Mill.], but they are thinner and narrower; they are like those of Huaqiushu [花楸树, Sorbus pohuashanensis, Sorbus pohuashanensis (Hance) Hedl.], but less divided on the margin of the leaves. Its leaves are opposite and bitter in taste.

For famine relief: Collect young buds and leaves, blanch them, remove the bitterness by soaking them in water, wash and clean them, and flavor them with oil and salt.

268. 青冈树

旧不载所出州土,今处处有之。其木大而结橡斗者为橡栎,小而不结橡斗者为青冈。其青冈树枝、叶、条、干皆类橡栎,但叶色颇青而少花叉。味苦,性平,无毒。

救饥:采嫩叶煠熟,以水浸渍,作成黄色,换水淘洗净,油盐调食。

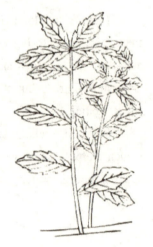

268. Qinggangshu [青冈树, Quercus serrata, Quercus serrata Murray]

Its origin was not recorded in ancient times, and now it can be seen everywhere. Those whose trunks are tall and bear oak bucks are Xiangli [橡栎, acorn, Quercus Acutissimac Fructus]; those whose trunks are small and who bear no oak bucks are Qinggang. Its branches, leaves and trunks are similar to those of Xiangli [橡栎, acorn, Quercus Acutissimae Fructus], but the leaves are green and less divided on the margin of the leaves. It is bitter in taste, neutral in nature and non-toxic.

For famine relief: Collect and blanch leaves, soak them in fresh water until they turn yellow, wash and clean them, and then flavor them with oil and salt.

269. 檀树芽

生密县山野中。树高一二丈。叶似槐叶而长大。开淡粉紫花。叶味苦。

救饥:采嫩芽叶煠熟,换水浸去苦味,淘洗净,油盐调食。

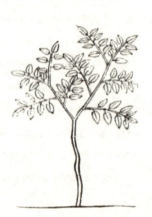

269. Tanshuya [檀树芽, Dalbergia hupeana Dalbergia hupeana Hance]

It grows in the mountains and wilderness of Mixian County. Its plants are 1~2 Zhang high. Its leaves are like those of Huai [槐, cladrastis, Cladrastis Radix et Fructus], but they are longer and bigger. Its flowers are pink purple. The taste of the leaves are bitter.

For famine relief: Collect young buds and leaves, blanch them, change water to remove the bitterness by soaking them in water, wash and clean them, and flavor them with oil and salt.

270. 山茶科

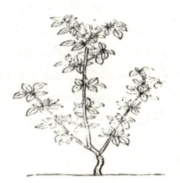

生中牟土山、田野中。科条高四五尺。枝梗灰白色。叶似皂荚叶而团；又似槐叶，亦团，四五叶攒生一处，叶甚稠密，味苦。

救饥：采嫩叶煠熟，水淘洗净，油盐调食。亦可蒸晒干，做茶煮饮。

270. Shanchake [山茶科, Rhamnus bungeana J. Vass.]

It grows in the mountains, fields and wilderness of Zhongmu. Its plants are 4~5 Chi high. Its branches are grayish white. Its leaves are like Chinese honey locust leaves, but they are more round; they are also like those of Huai [槐, cladrastis, Cladrastis Radix et Fructus] and are also rounder. Four or five leaves are clustered together. Its leaves are dense and bitter.

For famine relief: Collect leaves and blanch them, wash and clean them by soaking them in water, and flavor them with oil and salt. It can also be steamed, dried and drunk as tea.

271. 木葛

生新郑县山野中。树高丈余。枝似杏枝。叶似杏叶而团,又似葛根叶而小,味微甜。

救饥:采叶煠熟,水浸淘净,油盐调食。

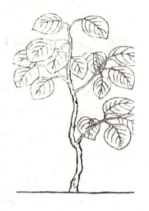

271. Muge〔木葛, pawpaw, Chaenomeles sinensis (Thouin) Koehne〕

Muge grows in the mountains and wilderness of Xinzheng County. Its plants are more than one Zhang. Its branches are like apricot branches. Its leaves are like apricot leaves, but they are round; they are like those of Gegen〔葛根, pueraria, Puerariae Radix〕, but they are smaller and the taste is slightly sweet.

For famine relief: Collect leaves and blanch them, wash and clean them by soaking them in water, and then flavor them with oil and salt.

272. 花楸树

生密县山野中。其树高大。叶似回回醋叶微薄;又似兜栌树叶,边有锯齿叉。其叶味苦。

救饥:采嫩芽叶煠熟,换水浸去苦味,淘洗净,油盐调食。

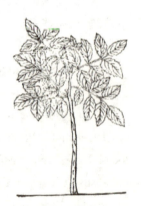

272. Huaqiushu〔花楸树, Sorbus pohuashanensis, Sorbus pohuashanensis (Hance) Hedl.〕

It grows in the mountains and wilderness of Mixian County. Its trunk is tall. Its leaves are like those of Huihuicu〔回回醋, rhus chinensis, Rhus chinensis Mill.〕, but they are slightly thin; they are like those of Doulushu〔兜栌树, Platycarya strobilacea Sieb., Platycarya strobilacea Sieb. et Zucc.〕, and serrated in the margin. Its leaves are bitter.

For famine relief: Collect young buds and leaves, blanch them, change water to remove the bitterness by soaking them in water, wash and clean them, and flavor them with oil and salt.

273. 白辛树

生荥阳塔儿山岗野间。树高丈许。叶似青檀树叶,颇长而薄,色微淡绿;又似月芽树叶而大,色亦差淡。其叶味甘、微涩。

救饥:采叶煠熟,水浸淘去涩味,油盐调食。

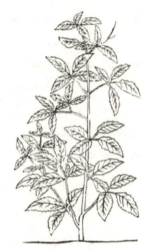

273. Baixinshu [白辛树, Pterostyrax psilophyllus, Pterostyrax psilophyllus Diels ex Perk.]

It grows in the hills and wilderness of Yingyang Ta'er. The tree is about one Zhang high. Its leaves are like Qingtan leaves, but they are a little longer and thinner, and the color is slightly greenish; they are like those of Yueyashu [月芽树, yhoary willow, Fontanesia fortunei Carr.], but they are larger and light-colored. Its leaves are sweet and slightly puckery.

For famine relief: Collect and blanch leaves, remove the astringency by soaking them in water, wash and clean them, and then flavor them with oil and salt.

274. 木栾树

生密县山谷中。树高丈余。叶似楝叶而宽大,稍薄。开淡黄花,结薄壳,中有子,大如豌豆,乌黑色,人多摘取串作数珠。叶味淡、甜。

救饥:采嫩芽叶煠熟,换水浸淘净,油盐调食。

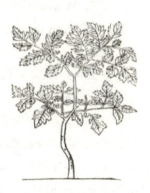

274. Muluanshu [木栾树, Koelreuteria paniculata, Koelreuteria paniculata Laxm.]

It grows in the valleys of Mixian County. The tree is more than one Zhang high. Its leaves are like those of Lian [楝, Melia azedarach, Melia azedarach L.], but they are wider and a little thinner. Its flowers are yellow, thin and shell-shaped, and its seeds in the crust are as big as peas, black. People often pick and string them into beads. Its leaves are light and sweet in taste.

For famine relief: Collect young buds and leaves, blanch them, change water, wash and clean them by soaking them in water, and then flavor them with oil and salt.

275. 乌棱树

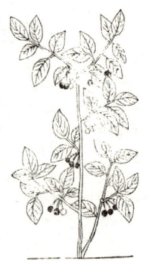

生密县梁家冲山谷中。树高丈余。叶似省沽油树叶而背白；又似老婆布鞊，微小而䔲，开白花。结子如梧桐子人，生青，熟则乌黑。其叶味苦。

救饥：采叶煠熟，换水浸去苦味，作过，淘洗净，油盐调食。

275. Wulengshu [乌棱树, lindera glauca, Lindera glauca (Sieb. et Zucc.) Bl.]

It grows in the valleys of Liangjiachong in Mixian County. The tree is more than one Zhang high. Its leaves are like those of Shengguyou [省沽油, bladdernut, Staphyleae Fructus seu Radix], but the back is white; its leaves are like those of Laopo Butie [老婆布鞊, Celastrus angulatus, Celastrus angulatus Maxim], but a little smaller and narrower. Its flowers are white. Its fruit is as big as Wutongzi [梧桐子, firmiana seed, Firmianae Semen], which is blue when it is uncooked, and black after being cooked. Its leaves are bitter.

For famine relief: Collect leaves, branch them, change water to remove the bitterness by soaking them in water, wash and clean them, and flavor them with oil and salt.

276. 刺楸树

生密县山谷中。其树高大。皮色苍白,上有黄白斑点。其枝梗间多有大刺。叶似楸叶而薄,味甘。

救饥:采嫩芽叶煤熟,水浸淘净,油盐调食。

276. Ciqiushu [刺楸树, Kalopanax septemlobus, Kalopanax septemlobus (Thunb.) Koidz.]

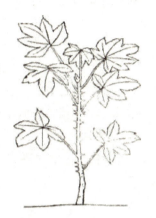

It grows in the valleys of Mixian County. Its trunk is tall. Its bark is pale in color with yellow and white spots. There are many big thorns on its branches. Its leaves are like those of Qiushu [楸树, Catalpa bungei, Catalpa bungei C. A. Mey.], but they are thinner and sweet in taste.

For famine relief: Collect young leaves, blanch them, soak them in water, wash and clean them, and then flavor them with oil and salt.

277. 黄丝藤

生辉县太行山山谷中。条类葛条。叶似山格刺叶而小;又似婆婆枕头叶颇硬,背微白,边有细锯齿,味甜。

救饥:采叶煤熟,水浸淘净,油盐调食。

277. Huangsiteng [黄丝藤, Dodder seed, Semen Cuscutae]

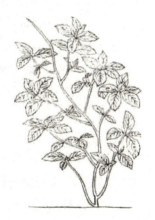

It grows in the valleys of Taihang Mountain, Hui County. Its branches are like the branches of pueraria. Its leaves are like Shangela leaves but smaller; they are also like Popo Zhentou leaves but harder, the back is slightly white and serrulate in the margin. It is sweet in taste.

For famine relief: Collect leaves, blanch them, wash and clean them by soaking them in water, and then flavor them with oil and salt.

278. 山格剌树

生密县韶华山山野中。作科条生。叶似白槿树叶，颇短而尖艄，又似茶树叶而阔大；及似老婆布鞊叶亦大，味甘。

救饥：采叶煠熟，水浸作成黄色，淘洗净，油盐调食。

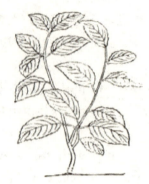

278. Shangela Shu［山格剌树，Celastrus gemmatus，Celastrus gemmatus Loes.］

It grows in the mountains and wilderness of Mount Shaohua in Mixian County. Its plants have branches. Its leaves are like those of Baijinshu［白槿树，fraxinus chinensis Fraxinus chinensis Roxb.］, but they are shorter and thinner; they are like tea leaves, but they are larger; they are like Laopo Butie leaves but they are also larger and sweet in taste.

For famine relief: Collect and blanch leaves, soak them in fresh water until they turn yellow, wash and clean them, and then flavor them with oil and salt.

279. 筭 树

生辉县太行山山谷中。其树高丈余。叶似槐叶而大，却颇软薄；又似檀树叶而薄小。开淡红色花。结子如绿豆大，熟则黄茶褐色。其叶味甜。

救饥：采叶煠熟，水浸淘净，油盐调食。

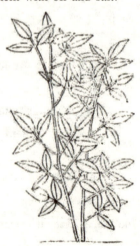

279. Hangshu [杭树, Euonymus verrucosoides, Euonymus verrucosoides Loes.]

It grows in the valleys of Taihang Mountain in Huixian County. The tree is more than one Zhang high. Its leaves are like those of Huai [槐, cladrastis, Cladrastis Radix et Fructus], but they are larger, quite soft and thin; they are also like those of Tanshu [檀树, Dalbergia hupeanaDalbergia hupeana Hance], but they are relatively thin. Its flowers are light red. Its fruit is as big as mung beans, and turns yellowish-brown after cooking. Its leaves are sweet.

For famine relief: Collect leaves and blanch them, wash and clean them by soaking them in water, and flavor them with oil and salt.

280. 报马树

生辉县太行山山谷间。枝条似桑[1]条色。叶似青檀叶而大,边有花叉;又似白辛[2]叶,颇大而长硬。叶味甜。

救饥:采嫩叶煠熟,水淘净,油盐调食。硬叶煠熟,水浸作成黄色,淘去涎沫,油盐调食。

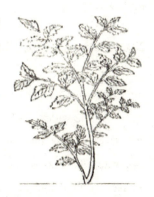

【注释】

[1]见本书第323桑椹树条。

[2]即白辛树。见本书第273白辛树条。

280. Baomashu [报马树, Celtis koraiensis, Celtis koraiensis Nakai]

It grows in the valleys of Taihang Mountain in Huixian County. The color of its branches is like that of the stripes[1]. Its leaves are like those of Qingtanshu [青檀树, wingceltis, Pteroceltis tatarinowii Maxim.], but larger and divided on the margin; they are also like those of Baixinshu[2] [白辛树, Pterostyrax psilophyllus, Pterostyrax psilophyllus Diels ex Perk.], but bigger, longer and harder. Its leaves are sweet.

For famine relief: Collect young leaves, blanch them, wash them in water, and flavor them with oil and salt. Blanch the hard leaves until they turn yellow, elutriate the foam and flavor them with oil and salt.

[Notes]

[1] See the 323th clause of this book.

[2] It is Baixinshu [白辛树, Pterostyrax psilophyllus, Pterostyrax psilophyllus Diels ex Perk.]. See the 273th clause of this book.

281. 椴 树

生辉县太行山山谷间。树甚高大,其木细腻,可为桌器。枝叉对生。叶似木槿叶而长大微薄,色颇淡绿,皆作五花桠叉,边有锯齿。开黄花。结子如豆粒大,色青白。叶味苦。

救饥:采嫩叶煤熟,水浸去苦味,淘洗净,油盐调食。

281. Duanshu [椴树, linden, Tilia mongolica Maxim]

Duanshu [椴树, linden, Tilia mongolica Maxim] grows in the valleys of Taihang Mountain in Huixian County. The tree is very tall, and the wood is delicate which can be used to make a table. Its branches are opposite. Its leaves are like those of Mujinshu [木槿树, hibiscus, Hibiscus syriacus Linn], but they are longer, bigger and thinner. Its leaves are light green, quinquefid and serrated. Its flowers are yellow. Its fruit is as big as beans, green white. Its Leaves taste bitter.

For famine relief: Collect young leaves, blanch them, remove the bitterness by soaking them in water, wash and clean them, and flavor them with oil and salt.

282. 臭 萩

生密县杨家冲山谷中。科条高四五尺。叶似柞瓜[1]叶而尖䏶;又似金银花叶亦尖䏶,五叶攒生如一叶。开花白色。其叶味甜。

救饥：采叶煤熟，水浸淘净，油盐调食。

【注释】

［1］野木瓜的别名。

282. Chouhong［臭荄, Eleutherococcus nodiflorus, Eleutherococcus nodiflorus（Dunn）S. Y. Hu］

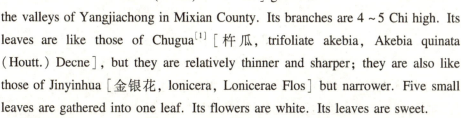

Chouhong［臭荄, Eleutherococcus nodiflorus, Eleutherococcus nodiflorus（Dunn）S. Y. Hu］grows in the valleys of Yangjiachong in Mixian County. Its branches are 4～5 Chi high. Its leaves are like those of Chugua[1]［杵瓜, trifoliate akebia, Akebia quinata（Houtt.）Decne］, but they are relatively thinner and sharper; they are also like those of Jinyinhua［金银花, lonicera, Lonicerae Flos］but narrower. Five small leaves are gathered into one leaf. Its flowers are white. Its leaves are sweet.

For famine relief: Collect leaves, blanch them, wash and clean them by soaking them in water, and flavor them with oil and salt.

【Notes】

［1］Another name for Yemugua［野木瓜, trifoliate akebia, Akebia quinata（Houtt.）Decne］.

283. 坚荚树

生辉县太行山山谷中。其树枝干坚劲，可以作棒。皮色乌黑，对分枝叉，叶亦对生。叶似拐枣叶而大，微薄，其色淡绿；又似土栾叶，极大而光润。开黄花。结小红子。其叶味苦。

救饥：采嫩叶煤熟，水浸去苦味，淘洗净，油盐调食。

283. Jianjiashu［坚荚树, Viburnum schensianum Maxim］

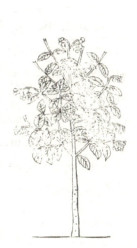

It grows in the valleys of Taihang Mountain in Huixian County. Its branches and trunks are tough and can be used to make sticks. The bark is black in color. Its branches are opposite, and its leaves are also opposite. Its leaves are like those of Guaizao [拐枣, honey raisin tree, Hovenia dulcis Thunb.], but bigger, a little thinner, and the color is light green; they are like those of Tuluanshu [土栾树, Viburnum schensianum, Viburnum schensianum Maxim], but they are bigger and shiny. Its flowers are yellow. Its fruit is red. Its leaves are bitter.

For famine relief: Collect young buds and leaves, blanch them, remove the bitterness by soaking them in water, wash and clean them, and flavor them with oil and salt.

284. 臭竹树

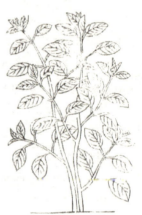

生辉县太行山山野中。树甚高大。叶似楸叶而厚，颇艄，却少花叉；又似拐枣叶亦大。其叶面青背白，味甜。

救饥：采叶煤熟，水浸去邪臭气味，油盐调食。

284. Chouzhushu [臭竹树, Clerodendrum trichotomum, Clerodendrum trichotomum Thunb.]

Chouzhushu [臭竹树, Clerodendrum trichotomum, Clerodendrum trichotomum Thunb.] grows in the mountains and wilderness of Taihang Mountain in Huixian County. Its trunk is very tall. Its leaves are like Chinese catalpa leaves, but they are thicker, a little narrower, fairly pointed, and with less leaf division; they are like those of Guaizao [拐枣, honey raisin tree, Hovenia dulcis Thunb.], but they are larger. Its leaves are green on the surface and white on the back, and the taste is sweet.

For famine relief: Collect young buds and leaves, blanch them, remove the stink by soaking them in water, and flavor them with oil and salt.

285. 马鱼儿条

俗名山皂角。生荒野中。叶似初生刺蘼花叶而小。枝梗色红,有刺似棘针微小。叶味甘、微酸。

救饥：采叶煤熟，水浸淘净，油盐调食。

285. Mayu'er Tiao [马鱼儿条, Gleditsia microphylla, Gleditsia microphylla D. A. Gordon ex Isely]

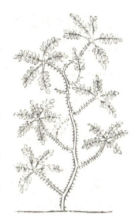

It is also named Shanzaojiao. It grows in the wilderness. Its leaves are like those of Cimihua [刺蘼花, multiflora rose, Rosa multiflora Thunb.], but smaller. Its branches are red, and there are calthrop-like thorns on them. Its leaves are sweet and slightly sour.

For famine relief: Collect leaves, blanch them, wash and clean them by soaking them in water, and flavor them with oil and salt.

286. 老婆布靴

生钧州风谷顶山野间。科条淡苍黄色。叶似匙头样，色嫩绿而光俊；又似山格剌叶却小。味甘，性平。

救饥：采叶煤熟，水浸作过，淘净，油盐调食。

286. Laopo Butie [老婆布靴, Celastrus angulatus, Celastrus angulatus Maxim]

It grows in the mountains and wilderness of Fengguding of Junzhou. Its branches are pale yellow. The shape of leaves is like a spoon, and the color is green and bright; its leaves are like Shangela leaves, but smaller. It is sweet in taste and neutral in nature.

For famine relief: Collect leaves, blanch them, wash and clean them by soaking them in water, and flavor them with oil and salt.

实可食

✱ 《本草》原有

Fruit Edible

Original Ones

287. 蕤核树

俗名蕤李子。生函谷川谷,及巴西、河东皆有,今古崤关西茶店山谷间亦有之。其木高四五尺。枝条有刺。叶细似枸杞叶而尖长,又似桃叶而狭小,亦薄。花开白色。结子红紫色,附枝茎而生,状类五味子。其核仁味甘,性温、微寒,无毒。其果味甘、酸。

救饥:摘取其果红紫色熟者,食之。

治病:文具《本草·木部》条下。

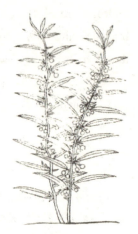

287. Ruiheshu [蕤核树, Prinsepia uniflora Batal, Prinsepia uniflora Batal]

Ruiheshu is commonly known as Ruilizi. It grows in the valleys of Hangu where there is flowing water. It can also be seen in Baxi and Hedong. Presently it can be seen in the valleys of Xichadian, Xiaoguan. The trunk is 4~5 Chi high. There are thorns on the branches. Its leaves are as thin as those of Gouqi [枸杞, medlar, Lycium chinense Mill.], but they are more pointed and longer; its leaves are also like peach leaves, but they are narrower and thinner. Its flowers are white. The fruit is reddish purple, growing on the stems of branches, and it is shaped like Wuweizi [五味子, northern schisandra, Schisandrae Chinensis Fructus]. Its nuts are sweet, cool in nature, slightly cold and non-toxic. Its fruit is sweet and sour.

For famine relief: Pick the red purple fruit and eat it.

For disease treatment: See the clauses in *Materia Medica · Woody Plant*.

288. 酸枣树

《尔雅》谓之樲枣。出河东川泽,今城垒、坡野间多有之。其木似枣而皮细,茎多棘刺。叶似枣叶微小。花似枣花。结实紫红色,似枣而圆小。核中仁微扁,名酸枣仁,入药用,味酸,性平。一云性微热,恶防己。

救饥:采取其枣,为果食之。亦可酿酒,熬作烧酒饮。未红熟时采取煮食亦可。

治病:文具《本草·木部》条下。

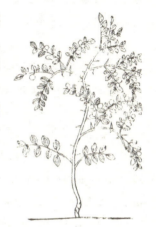

288. Suanzaoshu [酸枣树, crataegus, Ziziphus jujuba var. spinosa (Bunge) Hu ex H. F. Chow]

Suanzaoshu [酸枣树, crataegus, Ziziphus jujuba var. spinosa (Bunge) Hu ex H. F. Chow] is called Er'zao in *Er Ya* [《尔雅》, *Literary Expositor*]. It grows by the lakes and swamps in Hedong, and presently there are many in cities and ramps in the wilderness. It is like a jujube tree, but the bark is fine and its stems are thorny. Its leaves are like jujube leaves, but a little smaller. Its flowers are like jujube flowers, and its fruit is purple-red, like jujubes, but rounder and smaller. The kernel which is called Suanzaoren [酸枣仁, spiny jujube, Ziziphi Spinosi Semen] can be used as medicine. It is sour in taste and neutral in nature. Some say it is slightly hot. It is averse to Fangji [防己, Stephaniae Tetrandrae, Stephaniae Tetrandrae Radix].

For famine relief: Pick the jujube and eat a fruit. It can also be used to make wine. When the fruit is not red and ripe, it can be collected and cooked for eating.

For disease treatment: See the clauses in *Materia Medica · Woody Plant*.

289. 橡子树

本草橡实,栎木子也,其壳一名杼斗。所在山谷有之。木高二三丈,叶似栗叶而大。开黄花。其实橡也,有梂彙,自裹其壳,即橡斗也。橡实味苦、涩,性微温,无毒。其壳斗可染皂。

救饥:取子,换水浸煮十五次,淘去涩味,蒸极熟,食之。厚肠胃,肥健人,不饥。

治病:文具《本草·木部》橡实条下。

289. Xiangzishu [橡子树, acorn, Quercus acutissima Carr.]

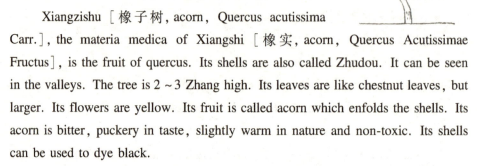

Xiangzishu [橡子树, acorn, Quercus acutissima Carr.], the materia medica of Xiangshi [橡实, acorn, Quercus Acutissimae Fructus], is the fruit of quercus. Its shells are also called Zhudou. It can be seen in the valleys. The tree is 2~3 Zhang high. Its leaves are like chestnut leaves, but larger. Its flowers are yellow. Its fruit is called acorn which enfolds the shells. Its acorn is bitter, puckery in taste, slightly warm in nature and non-toxic. Its shells can be used to dye black.

For famine relief: Take acorns, dip them in water for 15 times, remove the astringency and steam until cooked. It invigorates stomach and small intestine, and it is good for health. It can help people feel less hungry.

For disease treatment: See the clause of Xiangshi in *Materia Medica · Woody Plant*.

290. 荆子

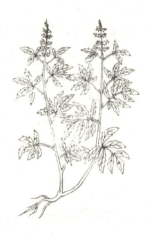

本草有牡荆实,一名小荆实,俗名黄荆。生河间、南阳、冤句山谷,并眉州、蜀州、平寿、都乡高岸及田野中,今处处有之,即作棰杖者。作科条生,枝茎坚劲,对生枝叉。叶似麻叶而疏短;又有叶似楝叶而短小,却多花叉者。开花作穗,花色粉红,微带紫。结实大如黍粒而黄黑色。味苦,性温,无毒。防风为之使,恶石膏、乌头。陶隐居《登真隐诀》云:荆木之华叶,通神见鬼精。

救饥:采子,换水浸淘去苦味,晒干,捣磨为面食之。

治病:文具《本草·木部》牡荆实条下。

290. Jingzi [荆子, negundo vitex, Vitex negundo L.]

Jingzi [荆子, negundo vitex, Vitex negundo L.], the materia medica of Mujingshi and Xiaojingshi, has the common name "Huangjing". It grows in the valleys of Hejian, Nanyang and Yuanju, and in the high shores and fields of Meizhou, Shuzhou, Pingshou and Duxiang. It can be seen everywhere presently, and it can be used as a cane. Its plants have branches, and both of them are tough. Its branches are opposite. Its leaves are like cannabis leaves, but they are sparse and short; its leaves are also like eucalyptus leaves, but they are shorter and more lobed. Its flowers are spiked. The color of the flowers is pink and slightly purple. Its fruit is as big as grains, but the color is yellowish black. It is bitter in taste, warm in nature and non-toxic. Fangfeng [防风, saposhnikovia, Saposhnikoviae Radix] is its envoy herb. Shigao [石膏, gypsum, Gypsum Fibrosum] and Wutou [乌头, aconite, Aconiti Kusnezoffii Radix] are averse to it.

For famine relief: Collect seeds, change water, remove the bitterness by soaking them in water, dry them, mash and grind them into powder.

For disease treatment: See the clause of Mujingshi in *Materia Medica · Woody Plant*.

291. 实枣儿树

本草名山茱萸，一名蜀枣，一名鸡足，一名魁实，一名鼠矢。生汉中川谷及琅琊、冤句、东海承县、海州，今钧州密县山谷中亦有之。木高丈余。叶似榆叶而宽，稍团，纹脉微粗。开淡黄白花。结实似酸枣大，微长，两头尖䏶，色赤，既干则皮薄。味酸，性平，微温，无毒。一云味咸、辛，大热，蓼实为之使，恶桔梗、防风、防己。

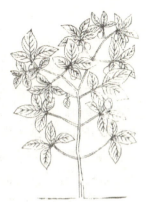

救饥：摘取实枣红熟者食之。

治病：文具《本草·木部》山茱萸条下。

291. Shizao'er Shu [实枣儿树, cornus, Cornus officinalis Sieb. et Zucc]

Shizao'er Shu [实枣儿树, cornus, Cornus officinalis Sieb. et Zucc], the materia medica of Shanzhuyu, is also named Shuzao, Jizu, Jishi and Shushi. It grows in the valleys where there is flowing water in Hanzhong, Langya, Yuanju, Donghaicheng County and Haizhou, and presently it can be seen in the valleys of Mixian County, Junzhou. Its plants are more than one Zhang high. Its leaves are like those of Yuqianshu [榆钱树, siberian elm, Ulmus pumila L.], but wider, slightly round, and veins slightly thicker. Its flowers are yellowish white. Its fruit is as big as jujube, but it is slightly longer, and the two ends are long and thin, red in color, and will be thinner after drying. It is sour in taste, neutral in nature, slightly warm and non-toxic. One says that it is salty, spicy and with great heat. Liaoshi [蓼实, water pepper fruit, Polygoni Hydropiperis Fructus] is its envoy herb. It is averse to Jiegeng [桔梗, platycodon, Platycodonis Radix], Fangfeng [防风, saposhnikovia, Saposhnikoviae Radix] and Fangji [防己, fangji, Stephaniae Tetrandrae Radix].

For famine relief: Take the red ripe dates and eat them.

For disease treatment: See the clause of Shanzhuyu in *Materia Medica · Woody Plant*.

292. 孩儿拳头

本草名荚蒾，一名击蒾，一名羿先。旧不著所出州土，但云所在山谷多有之。今辉县太行山山野中亦有。其木作小树。叶似木槿而薄，又似杏叶颇大，亦薄涩。枝叶间开黄花。结子似溲疏，两两切并，四四相对，数对共为一攒。生则青，熟则赤色。味甘、苦，性平，无毒。盖檀[1]榆[2]之类也。其皮堪为索。

救饥：采子红熟者食之。又煮枝汁，少加米作粥，甚美。

治病：文具《本草·木部》荚蒾条下。

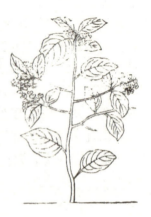

【注释】

[1] 见本书第269檀树芽条。

[2] 见本书第324榆钱树条。

292. Hai'er Quantou [孩儿拳头, Viburnum dilatatum, Grewia biloba G. Don var. parviflora (Bge.) Hand.-Mazz.]

Hai'er Quantou [孩儿拳头, Viburnum dilatatum, Grewia biloba G. Don var. parviflora (Bge.) Hand.-Mazz.], the materia medica of Jiami, is also named Jimi and Yixian. There was no record of its origin in the ancient times. It is said that it can be seen in valleys. It can also be found in the mountains and wilderness of Taihang Mountain in Huixian County. Its plants are small trees. Its leaves are like those of Mujinshu [木槿树, hibiscus, Hibiscus syriacus Linn], but thinner; they are also like apricot leaves, but a little larger, thinner and rough. There are yellow flowers between branches and leaves. Its fruit seems to be sparse. Every two of them is connivent, and every four of them is opposite. Its fruit is green when it is unripe, and turns red when it is ripe. It is sweet, bitter in taste, neutral in nature and non-toxic. It belongs to the species of Tanshuya[1] [檀树芽, Dalbergia hupeanaDalbergia hupeana Hance] and Yuqianshu[2] [榆钱树, siberian elm, Ulmus pumila L.].

For famine relief: Collect the fruit which is red and ripe. Boil the branches and add a small amount of rice in the soup to make congee which tastes good.

For disease treatment: See the clause of Jiami in *Materia Medica · Woody Plant*.

【Notes】

[1] See the 269th clause of this book.

[2] See the 324th clause of this book.

新增
New Supplements

293. 山棃儿

一名金刚树,又名铁刷子。生钧州山野中。科条高三四尺,枝条上有小刺。叶似杏叶,颇团小。开白花。结实如葡萄颗大,熟则红黄色,味甘酸。

救饥:采果食之。

293. Shanli'er [山棃儿, Smilax china, Smilax china L.]

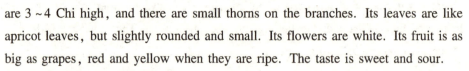

It is also named Jingangshu and Tieshuazi. It grows in the mountains and wilderness of Junzhou. Its plants are 3~4 Chi high, and there are small thorns on the branches. Its leaves are like apricot leaves, but slightly rounded and small. Its flowers are white. Its fruit is as big as grapes, red and yellow when they are ripe. The taste is sweet and sour.

For famine relief: Collect and eat the fruit.

294. 山里果儿

一名山里红,又名映山红果。生新郑县山野中。枝茎似初生桑条,上多小刺。叶似菊花叶稍团;又似花桑叶,亦团。开白花。结红果,大如樱桃,味甜。

救饥:采树熟果食之。

294. Shanli Guo'er [山里果儿, Crataegus pinnatifida Bunge, Crataegus pinnatifida Bunge var. pinnatifida]

It is also named Shanlihong and Yingshan Hongguo. It grows in the mountains and wilderness of Xinzheng County. Its branches and stems are like nascent mulberry trees with many small thorns on them. Its leaves are like chrysanthemum leaves, but slightly rounded; they are also like Huasang leaves, but they are also round. Its flowers are white. Its fruit is red, as big as cherries, and it tastes sweet.

For famine relief: Collect and eat the ripe fruit on the tree.

295. 无花果

生山野中,今人家园圃中亦栽。叶形如葡萄叶,颇长硬而厚,梢作三叉。枝叶间生果,初则青小,熟大,状如李子,色似紫茄色,味甜。

救饥:采果食之。

治病:今人传说,治心痛,用叶煎汤服,甚效。

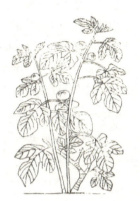

295. Wuhuaguo [无花果, fig, Ficus carica L.]

Wuhuaguo [无花果, fig, Ficus carica L.] grows in the mountains and wilderness, and it is now in the gardens of ordinary people. Its leaves are like grape leaves, but they are long, hard and thick. Its leaves are trifid on the top. Its fruit is in the middle of branches and leaves. They are small and green when new-sprung and become big after maturing. It is shaped like plums, the color is like the color of purple eggplants, and it tastes sweet.

For famine relief: Collect and eat the fruits.

For disease treatment: It is said that it can treat chest pain, and it is very effective to decort the leaves.

296. 青舍子条

生密县山谷间。科条微带柿黄色。叶似胡枝子叶而光俊微尖。枝条梢间开淡粉紫花。结子似枸杞子[1],微小,生则青,而后变红,熟则紫黑色,味甜。

救饥:采摘其子紫熟者食之。

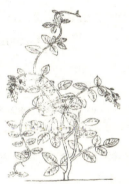

【注释】

[1]见本书第307枸杞条。

296. Qingshe Zitiao [青舍子条, Berchemia floribunda, Berchemia floribunda (Wall.) Brongn]

It grows in the valleys of Mixian County. Its branches are slightly persimmon yellow. Its leaves are like those of Huzhizi [胡枝子, bicolor lespedeza stem and leaf, Lespedezae Bicoloris Caulis et Folium], but they are brighter and slightly pointed. Its pink purple flowers are on the top of branches. Its fruit is like Gouqizi[1] [枸杞子, lycium, Lycii Fructus], but smaller. Its fruit green when unripe and then turns red and purple black when ripe. They taste sweet.

For famine relief: Collect the purple ripe fruits to eat.

【Notes】

[1] See the 307th clause of this book.

297. 白棠子树

一名沙棠梨儿,一名羊奶子树,又名剪子果。生荒野中。枝梗似棠梨[1]树枝而细,其色微白。叶似棠梨叶而窄小,色亦颇白;又似女儿茶叶却大而背白。结子如豌豆大,味酸甜。

救饥:其子甜熟时,摘取食之。

【注释】

[1]见本书第321棠梨树条。

297. Baitang Zishu [白棠子树, Elaeagnus multiflora, Elaeagnus multiflora Thunb.]

Baitang Zishu [白棠子树, Elaeagnus multiflora, Elaeagnus multiflora Thunb.] is also named Shatang Li'er, Yangnai Zishu and Jianziguo. It grows in the wilderness. Its branches are like those of Tanglishu[1] [棠梨树, Callery Pear tree, Pyrus calleryana Decne.], but they are thinner and slightly white in color. Its leaves are like those of Tanglishu [棠梨树, Callery Pear tree, Pyrus calleryana Decne.], but they are narrower and the color is white; they are also like those of Nv'ercha [女儿茶, rat plum, Rhamni Davuricae Fructus], but they are bigger, and the back of the leaves is white. Its fruit is pea-sized, sweet and sour.

For famine relief: When the fruit is sweet and ripe, pick and eat it.

【Notes】

[1] See the 321th clause of this book.

298. 拐枣

生密县梁家冲山谷中。叶似楮叶而无花叉,却更尖䂕,面多纹脉,边有细锯齿。开淡黄花。结实状似生姜拐叉而细短,深茶褐色,故名拐枣,味甜。

救饥:摘取拐枣成熟者食之。

298. Guaizao [拐枣, honey raisin tree, Hovenia dulcis Thunb.]

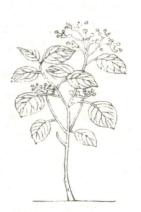

It grows in the valleys of Liangjiachong in Mixian County. Its leaves are like Chuye [楮叶, paper mulberry leaf, Broussonetiae Folium], but they are not divided and sharper. There are many veins on the leaves, and they are serrulated. Its flowers are light yellow. Its fruit is like a ginger's gibbosity, but it is thinner and shorter. The color is dark brown, so it is called Guaizao. It tastes sweet.

For famine relief: Collect the ripe fruit to eat.

299. 木桃儿树

生中牟土山间。树高五尺余。枝条上气脉积聚为疙瘩,状类小桃儿,极坚实,故名木桃。其叶似楮叶而狭小,无花叉,却有细锯齿;又似青檀叶。梢间另又开淡紫花。结子似梧桐子而大,熟则淡银褐色,味甜可食。

救饥:采取其子熟者食之。

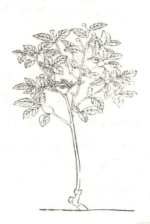

299. Mutao'er Shu [木桃儿树, Celtis bungeana, Celtis bungeana Bl.]

Mutao'er Shu [木桃儿树, Celtis bungeana, Celtis bungeana Bl.] grows in the dirt hills of Zhongmu. The tree is more than five Chi high. The accumulation of qi on the branches becomes a tree gall which shapes like a small peach. It is very solid, so it is called Mutao. Its leaves are like paper mulberry leaves (Broussonetiae Folium), but they are narrower and smaller. Its leaves are not divided, but they have fine serrations; they are also like those of Qingtanshu [青檀树, wingceltis, Pteroceltis tatarinowii Maxim.]. There are light purple flowers on the top of branches. Its fruit is like Wutongzi [梧桐子, firmiana seed, Firmianae Semen], but it is bigger. After ripening, it becomes light silver brown. The taste is sweet.

For famine relief: Pick the ripe fruit to eat.

300. 石冈橡

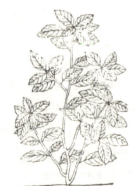

生汜水西茶店山谷中。其木高丈许。叶似橡栎叶，极小而薄，边有锯齿而少花叉。开黄花。结实如橡斗而极小，味涩、微苦。

救饥：采实，换水煮五七水，令极熟，食之。

300. Shigangxiang [石冈橡, Quercus baronii, Quercus baronii Skan]

Shigangxiang [石冈橡, Quercus baronii, Quercus baronii Skan] grows in the valleys of Xichadian, Sishui. The trunk is about one Zhang high. Its leaves are like those of Xiangli [橡栎, acorn, Quercus acutissima Carr.], but they are very small and thin, with serration and less divided. Its flowers are yellow. Its fruit is like an oak buck, but it is very small, astringent and slightly bitter.

For famine relief: Pick the fruit and boil it for five to seven times until it is well cooked.

301. 水茶臼

生密县山谷中。科条高四五尺。茎上有小刺。叶似大叶胡枝子叶而有尖；又似黑豆叶而光厚，亦尖。开黄白花。结果如杏大，状似甜瓜瓣而色红，味甜酸。

救饥：果熟红时，摘取食之。

301. Shuichajiu〔水茶臼, Rosaceae, Rosaceae〕

It grows in the valleys of Mixian County. Its plants are 4~5 Chi high. There are small thorns on the stems. Its leaves are like those of Huzhizi〔胡枝子, bicolor lespedeza stem and leaf, Lespedezae Bicoloris Caulis et Folium〕, but they are sharper; they are also like black bean leaves, but they are thicker, shiny and sharper. Its flowers are yellow and white. Its fruit is like an apricot, shaped like a melon blade, but the color is red, and the taste is sweet and sour.

For famine relief: When the fruit is ripe and turns red, pick it to eat.

302. 野木瓜

一名八月楂，又名杵瓜。出新郑县山野中。蔓延而生，妥附草木上。叶似黑豆叶微小，光泽，四五叶攒生一处。结瓜如肥皂大，味甜。

救饥：采嫩瓜换水煮食，树熟者亦可摘食。

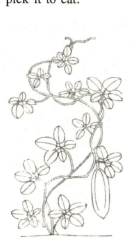

302. Yemugua〔野木瓜, trifoliate akebia, Akebia quinata (Houtt.) Decne〕

Yemugua〔野木瓜, trifoliate akebia, Akebia quinata (Houtt.) Decne〕 is also named Bayuezha and Chugua. It grows in the mountains and wilderness of Xinzheng County. It grows along the vines and attaches itself to grass and wood.

Its leaves are like black bean leaves, but a little smaller and shiny. The four or five (small) leaves gather together. Its fruit is like Feizaojia [肥皂荚, gymnocladus fruit, Gymnocladus chinensis Baill] and sweet in taste.

For famine relief: Pick young melons, change water to cook them. The naturally ripe fruit of the tree can also be eaten.

303. 土栾树

生汜水西茶店山谷中。其木高大坚劲,人常采斫以为秤杆。叶似木葛叶,微狭而厚,背颇白,微毛;又似青杨叶亦窄。开淡黄花。结子小如豌豆而扁,生则青色,熟则紫黑色,味甘。

救饥:摘取其实紫熟者食之。

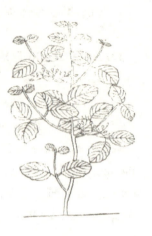

303. Tuluanshu [土栾树, Viburnum schensianum, Viburnum schensianum Maxim]

It grows in the valleys of Xichadian, Sishui. Its trunk is tall and tough, and people often cut it to make scales. Its leaves are like those of Muge [木葛, pawpaw, Chaenomeles sinensis (Thouin) Koehne], but slightly narrow and thick. Its leaves are slightly white on the back and slightly hairy; they are also like the leaves of Qingyangshu [青杨树, Cathay poplar, Populus cathayana Rehd.], but they are also narrower. Its flowers are yellow. Its fruit is as big as a pea, but it is oblate, green when it is unripe, and purple black after cooking. It is sweet.

For famine relief: Pick the purple ripe fruit to eat.

304. 驴驼布袋

生郑州沙岗间。科条高四五尺,枝梗微带赤黄色。叶似郁李子叶,颇大而光;又似省沽油叶而尖,颇齐,其叶对生。开花色白。结子如绿豆大,两两并生,熟则色红,味甜。

救饥:采红熟子食之。

304. Lvtuo Budai [驴驼布袋, Lonicera fragrantissima, Lonicera fragrantissima Lindl. et Paxt.]

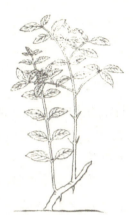

It grows in Shagang, Zhengzhou. Its plants are 4~5 Chi high, and its branches are reddish yellow. Its leaves are like those of Yulizi [郁李子, Chinese Dwarf Cherry Seed, Semen Pruni], large and shiny; they are also like those of Shengguyou [省沽油, bladdernut (fruit or root), Staphyleae Fructus seu Radix], but they are pointed and regular arranged, and they are opposite. Its flowers are white. Its fruit is as big as a mung bean and coalesced. When the fruit is ripe, it turns red, and it is sweet in taste.

For famine relief: Pick the red ripe fruit to eat.

305. 婆婆枕头

生钧州密县山坡中。科条高三四尺。叶似樱桃叶而长艄。开黄花。结子如绿豆大，生则青，熟红色。味甜。

救饥：采熟红子食之。

305. Popo Zhentou [婆婆枕头, Bilobed Grewia, Grewia biloba G. Don]

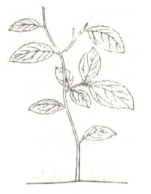

It grows on the hillsides of Mixian County, Junzhou. Its plants are 3~4 Chi high. Its leaves are like cherry leaves, but they are longer and narrower. Its flowers are yellow. Its fruit is as big as mung beans. It is green when it is unripe, and red after cooking, and it is sweet in taste.

For famine relief: Pick the ripe red fruit to eat.

306. 吉利子树

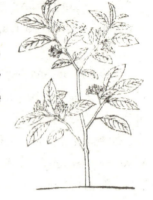

一名急藨子科。荒野处处有之。科条高五六尺。叶似野桑叶而小；又似樱桃叶亦小。枝叶间开五瓣小尖花，碧玉色，其心黄色。结子如椒粒大，两两并生，熟则红色。味甜。

救饥：其子熟时，采摘食之。

306. Jilizi Shu [吉利子树, Root of Bilobed Grewia, Grewia biloba G. Don var. parviflora (Bge.) Hand. -Mazz.]

It is also named Jimizi Ke. It can be seen everywhere in the wilderness. Its branches are 5 ~ 6 Chi high. Its leaves are like those of Sangshenshu [桑椹树, mulberry, Fructus Moriz], but they are smaller; they are also like cherry leaves, but smaller. On the top of branches there are five-petal jade flowers with yellow flower hearts. Its fruit is as big as peppers and coalesced. The ripe ones are red. The taste is sweet.

For famine relief: When the fruit is ripe, pick and eat.

叶及实皆可食

《本草》原有

Leaf and Fruit Edible

Original Ones

307. 枸 杞

一名杞根，一名枸忌，一名地辅，一名羊乳，一名却暑，一名仙人杖，一名西王母杖，一名地仙苗，一名托卢，或名天精，或名却老，一名枸，一名苦杞，俗呼为甜菜子，根名地骨。生常山平泽，今处处有之。其茎干高三五尺，上有小刺。春生苗，叶如石榴叶而软薄。茎叶间开小红紫花。随便结实，形如枣核，熟则红色,味微苦,性寒。根大寒。子微寒,无毒。一云味甘,平。白色无刺者良。陕西枸杞长一二丈,围数寸,无刺,根皮如厚朴,甘美异于诸处。生子如樱桃,全少核,暴干如饼,极烂有味。

救饥:采叶煤熟,水淘净,油盐调食、作羹食皆可。子红熟时亦可食。若渴煮叶作饮,以代茶饮之。

治病:文具《本草·木部》条下。

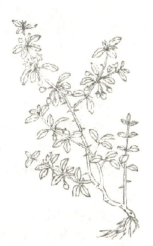

307. Gouqi [枸杞, medlar, Lycium chinense Mill.]

It is named Qigen, Gouji, Difu, Yangru, Queshu, Xianrenzhang, Xiwang Muzhang, Dixianmiao, Tuolu, Tianjing, Quelao, Gou and Kuqi, and it is commonly called Tiancaizi. Its roots are called Digu. It grows in the flat and watery wetlands of Changshan Mountain, and now can be seen everywhere. Its plants are 3~5 Chi high and have small thorns on the stems. Its seedlings grow in spring. Its leaves are like pomegranate leaves, but softer and thinner. Red and purple flowers are between stems and leaves. Its blooms and fruit grow at the same time. The shape of the fruit is like jujube nucleus. It turns red when it is ripe, and it is bitter in taste and cold in nature. Its roots are great cold. Its seeds are slightly cold and non-toxic. Some say it is sweet in flavor and neutral in nature. Those which are white and have no thorns are of good quality. Gouqi in Shaanxi is 1~2 Zhang long, and its stems are several Cun thick and have no thorns. Its root bark is like Houpu [厚朴, officinal magnolia bark, Magnoliae Officinalis Cortex], and the sweetness is different from that of other places. Its fruit is like a cherry lacking the kernel, and the sun dried Gouqi can make a cake. After cooking it turns soft, and it is delicious in taste.

For famine relief: Collect leaves, blunch them, wash them in water, and flavor them with oil and salt. The fruit can also be eaten when it turns red and mature. If you are thirsty, you can boil the leaves to drink and use it as tea.

For disease treatment: See the clause in *Materia Medica · Woody Plant*.

308. 柏 树

本草有柏实。生太山山谷及陕州、宜州,其乾州者最佳,密州侧栢叶尤佳,今处处有之。味甘。一云味甘、辛,性平,无毒。叶味苦。一云味苦、辛,微温,无毒。牡蛎及桂、瓜子为之使,畏菊花、羊蹄草,诸石及面曲。

救饥:《列仙传》云,赤松子食柏子,齿落更生。采栢叶新生并嫩者,换水浸其苦味,初食苦涩,入蜜或枣肉和食尤好,后稍易吃,遂不复饥,冬不寒,夏不热。

治病:文具《本草·木部》柏实条下。

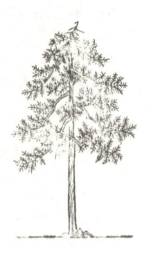

308. Baishu [柏树, cypress tree, Platycladus orientalis (L.) Franco]

Baishu [柏树, cypress tree, Platycladus orientalis (L.) Franco] grows in Taishan Valley, Shanzhou and Yizhou. That growing in Qianzhou is of good quality. Cebai [侧柏, Platycladus orientalis (L.) Franco] produced in Mixian County is especially good, and presently it can be seen everywhere. The taste is sweet. It is also said that it is sweet, spicy in taste, neutral in nature and non-toxic. Its leaves taste bitter. Some say bitter, spicy in taste, slightly warm in nature and non-toxic. Oysters, laurel and melon seeds are its envoy herbs. It is restrained by Juhua [菊花, chrysanthemum, Chrysanthemi Flos Chuzhouensis], Yangticao [羊蹄草, emilia, Emiliae Herba cum Radice], Mianqu [面曲, medicated leaven, Massa Medicata Fermentata] and various minerals.

For famine relief: *Lie Xian Zhuan* [《列仙传》, *The Biography of Many Supernatural Beings*] records that Chisongzi eats Baizi [柏子, arborvitae seed, Platycladi Semen] and the teeth regenerate. Collect new and young leaves, dip them in water, and remove the bitterness by soaking them in water. It is bitter and sorrowful at the beginning. It is especially good when the honey or jujube is added. It is a little easier to eat and then one no longer feels hungry. After eating, one does not feel cold in winter and does not feel hot in summer.

For disease treatment: See the clause of Baishi in *Materia Medica · Woody Plant*.

309. 皂荚树

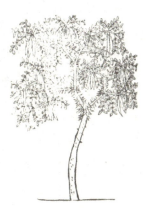

生雍州川谷及鲁之邹县，怀、孟产者为胜，今处处有之。其木极有高大者。叶似槐叶，瘦长而尖，枝间多刺。结实有三种，形小者为猪牙皂荚，良；又有长六寸及尺二者。用之当以肥厚者为佳。味辛、咸，性温，有小毒。枯实为之使，恶麦门冬，畏空青、人参、苦参。可作沐药，不入汤。

救饥：采嫩芽煠熟，换水浸洗淘净，油盐调食。又以子不拘多少炒，春去赤皮，浸软煮熟，以糖渍之，可食。

治病：文具《本草·木部》条下。

309. Zaojiashu [皂荚树, soap-bark tree, Gleditsia sinensis Lam.]

It grows in the valleys where there is flowing water in Yongzhou and Zouxian of Shandong. It is good in Huai and Meng, and now it can be seen everywhere. Its trunk is very tall. Its leaves are like those of Huaiye [槐叶, sophora leaf, Sophorae Folium], elongated and pointed, with many thorns between branches. There are three types of fruit: The small fruit is named Zhuya Zaojia, and its quality is good; the other two types are six Cun long and 1~2 Chi long respectively. It is better to use the thick one in the medicine. It is spicy, salty in taste, warm in nature and slightly poisonous. Baishi [柏实, arborvitae seed, Platycladi Semen] is its envoy herb. It is averse to Maimendong and restrained by Kongqing, Renshen and Kushen. It can be used for bathing and it can not be used in decoction.

For famine relief: Collect tender buds and blanch them. Wash them after soaking them in water, and then flavor them with oil and salt. The seeds can be cooked and pounded to get rid of the red huskhull. Soak them until they become soft and then boil them. Then use sugar to pickle them.

For disease treatment: See the clauses in *Materia Medica · Woody Plant*.

310. 楮桃树

本草名楮实,一名榖实。生少室山,今所在有之。树有二种,一种皮有班花纹,谓之班榖,人多用皮为冠。一种皮无花纹,枝叶大相类,其叶似葡萄叶,作瓣叉。上多毛涩而有子者为佳。其桃如弹大,青绿色,后渐变深红色乃成熟。浸洗去穰,取中子入药。一云皮斑者是楮皮,白者是榖皮,可作纸。实味甘,性寒。叶味甘,性凉。俱无毒。

救饥:采叶并楮桃带花,煠烂,水浸过,握干作饼,焙熟食之。或取树熟楮桃红蕊食之,甘美,不可久食,令人骨软。

治病:文具《本草·木部》楮实条下。

310. Chutaoshu [楮桃树, paper mulberry, Broussonetia papyrifera (L.) L'Hér. ex Vent.]

Chutaoshu [楮桃树, paper mulberry, Broussonetia papyrifera (L.) L'Hér. ex Vent.], the materia medica of Chushi [楮实, paper mulberry fruit, Broussonetiae Fructus], is also named Goushi. It grows in Shaoshi Mountain and now can be seen everywhere. There are two types of paper mulberries: The one that has a speckled pattern is called Bangou. People usually use its bark to make a hat. The other type has no speckle patterns. The two types of paper mulberries have similar branches and leaves. Its leaves are like grape leaves and there are lobes on them. Those which have rough hair on the leaves and fruit are good. Its fruit is the same size as the projectile, blue-green, and then gradually becomes dark red. Soak them in water, wash the flesh and take the seeds into medicine. One said that those which have speckled barks are Chupi and the white ones are named Goupi. It can be made of paper. Its fruit is sweet in taste and cold in nature. Its leaves are sweet and cool in nature. Its seeds, fruit and leaves are non-toxic.

For famine relief: Collect leaves and unripe fruit, blanch them and soak them in water, dry them to make a cake and then bake. Or take the ripe achene and it tastes sweet. Do not eat it for a long time or it will make people weak.

For disease treatment: See the clause of Chushi in *Materia Medica · Woody Plant*.

311. 柘 树

本草有柘木。旧不载所出州土,今北土处处有之。其木坚劲,皮纹细密,上多白点,枝条多有刺。叶比桑叶甚小而薄,色颇黄淡,叶稍皆三叉,亦堪饲蚕。绵柘刺少,叶似柿[1]叶微小。枝叶间结实,状如楮桃而小,熟则亦有红蕊,味甘、酸。叶味甘、微苦。柘木味甘,性温,无毒。

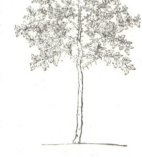

救饥:采嫩叶煠熟,以水浸渍,作成黄色,换水浸去邪味,再以水淘净,油盐调食。其实红熟,甘酸可食。

治病:文具《本草·木部》条下。

【注释】

[1] 见本书第348 柿树条。

311. Zheshu [柘树, cudrania, Cudraniae Lignum]

Zheshu [柘树, cudrania, Cudraniae Lignum] is the materia medica of Zhemu [柘木, cudrania, Cudraniae Lignum]. There was no record of its origin in ancient times, and it now can be seen everywhere in the north. Its wood is tough, its bark is finely textured with white spots on it, and its branches are mostly thorny. Its leaves are smaller and thinner than the mulberry leaves. The color of its leaves is slightly yellowish, and the upper part of its leaves is trifid. Its leaves can also be used to feed silkworms. Maclura tricuspidata Carr. has less thorns, and its leaves are like persimmon[1] leaves, but a little smaller. Its fruit is between branches and leaves and shaped like Chutao [楮桃, paper mulberry fruit, Broussonetiae Fructus]. Its stamens are red after ripening. It is sweet and sour. Its leaves are sweet and slightly bitter. Zhemu [柘木, cudrania, Cudraniae Lignum] is sweet in taste, warm in nature and non-toxic.

For famine relief: Collect young leaves and blanch them, soak them in water until they turn yellow, change water to remove the peculiar smell, wash and clean them in water, and then flavor them with oil and salt. It can be eaten when the fruit turns red and ripe, and the taste is sweet and sour.

For disease treatment: See the clauses in *Materia Medica · Woody Plant*.

[Notes]

[1] See the 348th clause of this book.

New Supplements

312. 木羊角科

又名羊桃科，一名小桃花。生荒野中。紫茎。叶似初生桃叶，光俊，色微带黄。枝间开红白花。结角似豇豆角[1]，甚细而尖艄，每两角并生一处，味微苦酸。

救饥：采嫩梢叶煠熟，水浸淘净，油盐调食。嫩角亦可煠食。

【注释】

[1] 见本书第343豇豆苗条。

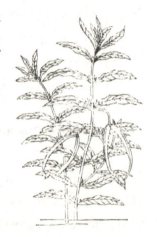

312. Muyangjiao Ke〔木羊角科, periploca, Periploca sepium Bunge〕

Muyangjiao Ke〔木羊角科, periploca, Periploca sepium Bunge〕, also named Yangtaoke and Xiaotaohua, grows in the wilderness. Its stems are purple. Its leaves are like the nascent leaves of peaches, bright, beautiful and slightly yellow. Its red and white flowers stand in the middle of branches. Its fruit that looks like cowpea[1] is very thin and sharp, and each two legumes grows together. It is slightly bitter and sour in taste.

For famine relief: Collect young leaves, blanch and elutriate them in hot water, and then flavor them with oil and salt. The tender legumes can also be eaten after blanching.

[Notes]

[1] See the 343th clause of this book.

313. 青檀树

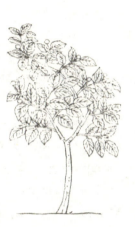

生中牟南沙岗间。其树枝条有纹,细薄。叶形类枣叶,微尖艄,背白而涩;又似白辛树叶微小。开白花。结青子,如梧桐子大。叶味酸涩,实味甘酸。

救饥:采叶煠熟,水浸淘去酸味,油盐调食。其实成熟,亦可摘食。

313. Qingtanshu [青檀树, celtis, Celtis bungeana Bl.]

Qingtanshu [青檀树, celtis, Celtis bungeana Bl.] grows in the sandhills of the south of Zhongmu. There are veins in its twigs, slender and thin. Its leaves are like those of jujube, slightly sharp. The back of its leaves is white and rough. Besides, they are also like those of Baixinshu [白辛树, pterostyrax, Pterostyrax psilophyllus Diels ex Perk], but slightly smaller. Its flowers are white, and its fruit is green, as big as the seeds of Wutong [梧桐, firmiana, Firmiana platanifolia (L. f.) Marsili]. Its leaves are sour and bitter in taste, and its fruit is sweet and sour.

For famine relief: Collect young leaves, blanch and elutriate them in hot water so as to get rid of the sour taste, and then flavor them with oil and salt. The ripe fruit can also be eaten.

314. 山苘树

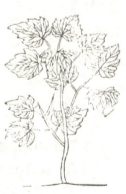

生密县梁家冲山谷中。树高丈余。叶似初生苘[1]叶;又似芙蓉叶而小;又似牵牛花叶,叶肩两傍却又有角叉。开白花。结子如枸杞子大,熟则紫黑色,味甘酸。叶味苦。

救济:采叶煠熟,水浸去苦味,淘洗净,油盐调食。其子熟时,摘取食之。

【注释】

[1] 即苘麻。见本书第191苘子条。

314. Shanqingshu [山茼树, alangium platanifolium, Alangium platanifolium (Sieb. et Zucc.) Harms, var. trilobum (Miq.) Ohwi]

Shanqingshu [山茼树, alangium platanifolium, Alangium platanifolium (Sieb. et Zucc.) Harms, var. trilobum (Miq.) Ohwi] grows in the valleys of Liangjiachong in Mixian County. The tree is more than one Zhang high. Its leaves are like the incipient leaves of Qingma[1] [苘麻, abutilon, Abutilon theophrasti Medicus], and they are like those of Furong [芙蓉, hibiscus mutabilis, Hibiscus mutabilis Linn.], but smaller. They are like the Morning Glory leaves, and there are lobes on both sides of leaves. Its flowers are white. Its fruit is as big as that of Gouqizi [枸杞子, lycium, Lycii Fructus], and the ripe fruit is purple and black. It is sweet in taste. Its leaves are bitter in taste.

For famine relief: Collect young leaves, blanch and elutriate them in hot water so as to get rid of the bitter taste, and then flavor them with oil and salt. The ripe fruit can also be eaten.

【Notes】

[1] See the 191th clause of this book.

花可食

※ 新增

Flower Edible
New Supplements

315. 藤花菜

生荒野中沙岗间。科条丛生。叶似皂角叶而大;又似嫩椿叶而小,浅黄绿色。枝间开淡紫花,味甘。

救饥:采花煠熟,水浸淘净,油盐调食。微焯过,晒干煠食,尤佳。

315. Tenghuacai [藤花菜, wisteria villosa, Wisteria villosa Rehd.]

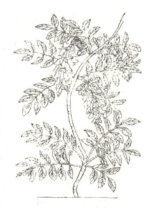

Tenghuacai [藤花菜, wisteria villosa, Wisteria villosa Rehd.] grows in the wilderness of sandhills. Its branches and strips grow together. Its leaves look like those of Zaojiao [皂角, gleditsia, Gleditsiae Fructus], but larger than them, and like the young leaves of Chun [椿, toona sinensis, Toona sinensis (A. Juss.) Roem.], but smaller than them. It is light yellow and green in color. The pale purple flowers bloom between branches, and they taste sweet.

For famine relief: Collect young leaves, blanch and elutriate them in hot water, and then flavor them with oil and salt. It is especially delicious after their elutricating in hot water and being dried in the sunshine.

316. 把齿花

本名锦鸡儿,又名酱瓣子。生山野间,人家园宅间亦多栽。叶似枸杞子叶而小,每四叶攒生一处。枝梗亦似枸杞,有小刺。开黄花,状类鸡形。结小角儿。味甜。

救饥:采花煤熟,油盐调食,炒熟吃茶亦可。

316. Bachihua [把齿花, caragana, Caragana sinica (Buc'hoz) Rehd.]

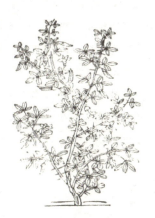

Bachihua [把齿花, caragana, Caragana sinica (Buc'hoz) Rehd.], also called Jinji'er and Jiangbanzi, grows in the mountains and wilderness, and in the nursery gardens of common people. The leaflets are like those of Gouqizi [枸杞子, lycium, Lycii Fructus], but much smaller, and every four leaves gathers together. Its branches are also like those of Gouqi [枸杞, wolfberry, Lycium chinense Mill.], and there are small thorns. The yellow-colored flowers are in the shape of chicken. Its legumes are small, and it is sweet in taste.

For famine relief: Collect flowers, elutriate them in hot water, and then flavor them with oil and salt. Besides, it can be used as tea after being cooked.

317. 楸 树

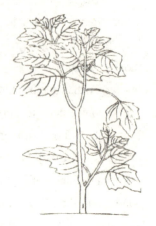

所在有之，今密县梁家冲山谷中多有。树甚高大，其木可作琴瑟。叶类梧桐叶而薄小，叶梢作三角尖叉。开白花，味甘。

救饥：采花煠熟，油盐调食。及将花晒干，或煠或炒，皆可食。

317. Qiushu [楸树, catalpa bungei, Catalpa bungei C. A. Mey.]

Qiushu [楸树, catalpa bungei, Catalpa bungei C. A. Mey.] is distributed everywhere, mostly in the valleys of Liangjiachong in Mixian County. The tree is so big that its wood can be used as a harp. Its leaves look like those of Wutong [梧桐, Chinese parasol, Sterculiaceae], but relatively thin and small. The front of the leaves has triangular pointed forks. Its white flowers taste sweet.

For famine relief: Collect flowers and elutriate them in hot water, and then flavor them with oil and salt. Or being dried in the sunshine, the flowers can be eaten after being blanched and elutriated in hot water or stir-fried.

318. 腊梅花

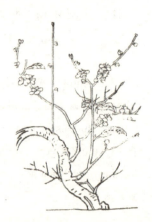

多生南方，今北土亦有之。其树枝条颇类李[1]。其叶似桃[2]叶而宽大，纹脉微粗。开淡黄花，味甘、微苦。

救饥：采花煠熟，水浸淘净，油盐调食。

【注释】

[1] 见本书第 351 李子树条。

[2] 见本书第 363 桃树条。

318. Lameihua [腊梅花, Winter sweet, Chimonanthus praecox (L.) Link]

Lameihua [腊梅花, Winter sweet, Chimonanthus praecox (L.) Link] mostly grows in the south, and nowadays it can also be seen in the north. Its branches look like those of Lizi[1] [李子, Plum, Prunus salicina Lindl.]. Its leaves are like those of Tao[2] [桃, Peach, Amygdalus persica L.], but relatively wide and slightly rough in texture. Its yellow flowers taste sweet but slightly bitter.

For famine relief: Collect flowers, blanch and elutriate them in hot water, and then flavor them with oil and salt.

【Notes】

[1] See the 351th clause of this book.

[2] See the 363th clause of this book.

319. 马 棘

生荥阳岗野间。科条高四五尺。叶似夜合树叶而小；又似蒺藜叶而硬；又似新生皂荚科叶，亦小。梢间开粉紫花，形状似锦鸡儿[1]花，微小，味甜。

救饥：采花煤熟，水浸淘净，油盐调食。

【注释】

[1] 把齿花的本名，见本书第 316 把齿花条。

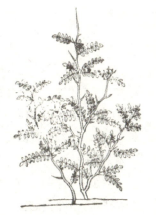

319. Maji [马棘, sophora davidii, Sophora davidii (Franch.) Skeels]

Maji [马棘, sophora davidii, Sophora davidii (Franch.) Skeels] grows in the hills and the wilderness in Xingyang, a county in Henan Province. Its seedlings are 4~5 Chi high, and its leaves are like those of Yeheshu [夜合树, albizia julibrissin, Albizia julibrissin Durazz.], but a little smaller. Besides, its leaves are also like those of Jili [蒺藜, Tribulus terrestris, Fructus Tribuli], however relatively hard. And its leaves are like those of Zaojia [皂荚, soap pod, Gleditsia sinensis Lam.] as well, but smaller. The pink and purple flowers bloom in the middle of branches, the shape which is like that of Jinji'er[1] [锦鸡儿, caragana, Caragana sinica (Buc'hoz) Rehd] is also slightly small, and they are sweet in taste.

For famine relief: Collect flowers, blanch and elutriate them in hot water, and then flavor them with oil and salt.

【Notes】

[1] See the 316th clause of this book.

花叶皆可食

✳ 《本草》原有

Flower and Leaf Edible

Original Ones

320. 槐树芽

本草有槐实。生河南平泽,今处处有之。其木有极高大者。《尔雅》云槐有数种,叶大而黑者名欀槐,昼合夜开者名守宫槐,叶细而青绿者但谓之槐。其功用不言有别。开黄花。结实似豆角状,味苦、酸、咸,性寒,无毒。景天为之使。

救饥:采嫩芽煠熟,换水浸淘,洗去苦味,油盐调食。或采槐花,炒熟食之。

治病:文具《本草·木部》槐实条下。

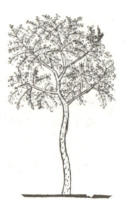

320. Huaishuya [槐树芽, sophora japonica, Sophora japonica L.]

Huaishuya [槐树芽, sophora japonica, Sophora japonica L.], recorded in materia medica, grows in the flat and grassy wetlands in Henan Province.

Presently, it can be seen everywhere. The trunk of some kind is high. It is recorded in *Er Ya* [《尔雅》, *Literary Expositor*] that there are several kinds of Huai, among of them, Chahuai is characterized by big and black leaves, and the flowers of Shougonghuai are usually closed in the morning and in bloom at night. Its leaves which are small and green are called Huai. But there is no record explaining their differences in the function. Its flowers are yellow and its fruit which is shaped as beans tastes bitter, sour and salty. It is cold in nature, but non-toxic. In compatibility, Jingtian [景天, herb of Common Stonecrop, *Sedum erythrostictum* Miq. (*S. alboroseum* Baker; *S. spectabile* Boreau)] is its assistance.

For famine relief: Collect young leaves, blanch them, remove the bitterness by elutriating them in water, and then flavor them with oil and salt. Flowers can be collected and eaten after being stir-fried.

For disease treatment: See the clause of Huaishi [槐实, sophora japonica, *Sophora japonica* L.] in the part of *Materia Medica · Woody Plant*.

花叶实皆可食

* 新增

Flower, Leaf and Fruit Edible
New Supplements

321. 棠梨树

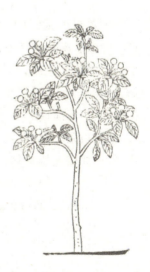

今处处有之,生荒野中。叶似苍术叶,亦有团叶者,有三叉叶者,叶边皆有锯齿;又似女儿茶叶,其叶色颇黪白。开白花。结棠梨如小楝子大,味甘、酸。花、叶味微苦。

救饥:采花煠熟食,或晒干磨面,作烧饼食亦可。及采嫩叶煠熟,水浸淘净,油盐调食,或蒸晒作茶亦可。其棠梨经霜熟时摘食,甚美。

321. Tanglishu [棠梨树, pyrus betulifolia, Pyrus betulifolia Bunge]

Tanglishu [棠梨树, pyrus betulifolia, Pyrus betulifolia Bunge] can be seen everywhere in the wilderness presently. Its leaves are like those of Cangzhu [苍术, Atractylodes, Atractylodes Lancea (Thunb.) DC.]. Some are round, and others are trilobated. The edges of the leaves are serrated. Besides, they are like those of Nv'ercha [女儿茶, diversifolious buckthorn root or leaf, Rhamnus davurica Pall.]. Its leaves are dark white. Its white flowers are in bloom. Its fruit is as small as that of Xiaolianzi [小楝子, melia azedarach, Melia azedarach L.], which tastes sweet and sour. Its flowers and leaves are a bit bitter in taste.

For famine relief: Collect flowers, blanch and elutriate them in hot water, or grind them to flour after they are dried in the sunshine and then make them Shaobing, a Chinese-style baked roll, and it tastes better. Or collect young leaves, blanch and soak them in water, and flavor them with oil and salt. Steam and dry them to make tea. The ripe fruit is delicious after frosting.

322. 文冠花

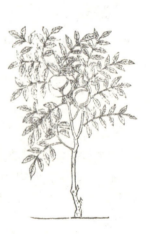

生郑州南荒野间。陕西人呼为崖木瓜。树高丈许。叶似榆树叶而狭小；又似山茱萸叶,亦细短。开花仿佛似藤花而色白,穗长四五寸。结实状似枳壳而三瓣,中有子二十余颗,如肥皂角子。子中瓤如栗子,味微淡,又似米面,味甘可食。其花味甜,其叶味苦。

救饥：采花煤熟,油盐调食。或采叶煤熟,水浸淘去苦味,亦用油盐调食。及摘实取子,煮熟食瓤。

322. Wenguanhua [文冠花, Xanthoceras sorbifolium, Xanthoceras sorbifolium Bunge]

Wenguanhua [文冠花, Xanthoceras sorbifolium, Xanthoceras sorbifolium

Bunge] grows in the wilderness in the south of Zhengzhou. People in Shaanxi Province call it Yamugua. Its plants are about one Zhang high. Its leaves are like those of Yushu [榆树, Ulmus pumila, Ulmus pumila L.], but relatively small. And they are also like those of Shanzhuyu [山茱萸, asiatic cornelian cherry fruit, Fructus Corni.], but slender and short. Its white flowers are like those of Ziteng [紫藤, wisteria, Wisteria sinensis], but the spica can be about 4~5 Chi long. The shape of its fruit is like that of Zhiqiao [枳壳, ruta graveolens, Ruta graveolens L.], but the fruit cracks into three lobes, and each has about 20 seeds, like that of Zaojiao [皂角, gleditsia, Gleditsiae Fructus]. Its flesh which is like that of Lizi [栗子, castanea, Castanea mollissima Bl.], light in taste, and like that of Millet flour, sweet in taste, can be eaten. Its flowers taste sweet, but the leaves taste bitter.

For famine relief: Collect flowers, blanch and elutriate them in hot water. Collect young leaves, blanch them and remove the bitterness by soaking them in water, and then flavor them with oil and salt. Or collect its fruit to get the seeds, and then eat the flesh after cooking.

叶皮及实皆可食

* 《本草》原有

Leaf, Peel and Fruit Edible
Original Ones

323. 桑椹树

本草有桑根白皮。旧不载所出州土,今处处有之。其叶饲蚕,结实为桑椹,有黑白二种,桑之精英尽在于椹。桑根白皮,东行根益佳,肥白者良,出土者不可用,杀人。味甘,性寒,无毒。制造忌铁器及铅。叶桠者名鸡桑,最堪入药。续断、麻子、桂心为之使。桑椹味甘,性暖。或云木白皮亦可用。

救饥:采桑椹熟者食之。或熬成膏,摊于桑叶上晒干,捣作饼收藏。或直取椹子晒干,可藏经年。及取椹子清汁置瓶中,封三二日即成酒,其色味似葡萄[1]酒,

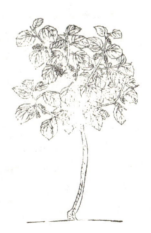

甚佳。亦可熬烧酒，可藏经年，味力愈佳。其叶嫩老，皆可煤食。皮炒干磨面，可食。

治病：文具《本草·木部》桑根白皮条下。

【注释】

［1］见本书第350葡萄条。

323. Sangshenshu ［桑椹树，mulberry，Morus alba L.］

Sangshenshu ［桑椹树，mulberry，Morus alba L.］ is also named Sanggen Baipi ［桑根白皮，white mulberry root-bark，Morus alba L.］. There was no record about its origin in the ancient times. Presently it can be found everywhere. Its leaves can be used for raising silkworms, and its fruit is named Sangshen, divided into white and black kinds. The essence is concentrated in its fruit.

The roots in the east row, by removing the outer epithelium and phloem, is particularly good. The quality of fat and white roots is good, but those exposed to soil surface can not be used and may cause death. It is sweet in taste, cold in nature and non-toxic. Avoid iron ware and lead when processing the roots. The lobated leaves are called Jisang ［鸡桑，morus australis，Morus australis Poir.］, which is appropriate to be used for making medicine. In compatibility, Xuduan ［续断，Phlomis umbrosa，Phlomis umbrosa Turcz.］, Mazi ［麻子，cannabis sativa，Cannabis sativa L.］ and Guixin ［桂心，cinnamomum cassia，Cinnamomum cassia Presl］ are its assistance. The taste is sweet, and it is warm in nature. It is said that the white bark on a tree trunk can also be used.

For famine relief: Collect ripe mulberries, boil them and put them on the leaves to dry in the sunshine, and then make them pancakes. Or dry the mulberries to store. Extract its juice to store in the jar so as to make wine in two or three days. The flavor and aroma are like those of Putao[1] ［葡萄，grape，Vitis vinifera L.］. It is also used to make Chinese distillate spirits, which can be preserved for many years.

For disease treatment: See the clause of Sanggen Baipi ［桑根白皮，white mulberry root-bark，Morus alba L.］ of *Materia Medica · Woody plant*.

【Notes】

[1] See the 350th clause of this book.

324. 榆钱树

本草有榆皮,一名零榆。生颍川[1]山谷、秦州,今处处有之。其木高大。春时未生叶,其枝条间先生榆荚。形状似钱而薄小,色白,俗呼为榆钱。后方生叶,似山茱萸叶而长,尖艄润泽。榆皮味甘,性平,无毒。

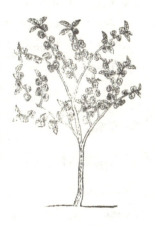

救饥:采肥嫩榆叶煤熟,水浸淘净,油盐调食。其榆钱煮糜羹食佳,但令人多睡。或焯过,晒干备用,或为酱,皆可食。榆皮刮去其上干燥皱裂者,取中间软嫩皮剉碎,晒干,炒焙极干,捣磨为面,拌糠麸、草末蒸食,取其滑泽易食。又云,榆皮与檀皮为末,服之令人不饥。根皮亦可捣磨为面食。

治病:文具《本草·木部》榆皮条下。

【注释】

[1]古代郡名。

324. Yuqianshu [榆钱树, ulmus pumila, Ulmus pumila L.]

Yuqianshu [榆钱树, ulmus pumila, Ulmus pumila L.], also named Yupi and Lingyu, growing in the valleys of Yingchuan[1] and Qinzhou, can be seen everywhere presently. Its trunk is high and big. Its pods come before the leaves come into buds in spring, just like copper coins, but comparatively thin and small. It is white, and it is generally named Yuqian. Then it produces its leaves, which are like those of Shanzhuyu [山茱萸, asiatic cornelian cherry fruit, Fructus Corni], but quite long and sharp, lustrous. Its skin is sweet in taste, neutral in nature and non-toxic.

For famine relief: Collect young leaves, blanch and soak them in fresh water, and then flavor them with oil and salt. It can be made congee which will make people sleep too much. Dry them in the sunshine after elutriating them in water or make them paste. Collect the interior young bark after scratching the exterior bark and dry it in the sunshine, and then bake it until it is very dry and crush it into dough. Mix the dough with some chaff grass, and then steam them. It is also said if the skin of Yushu and Tanshu is ground into powder, people will not feel hungry after eating the powder. The bark of its roots can also be made into flour.

For disease treatment: See the clause of Yupi [榆皮, elm bark, Ulmus pumila L.] in *Materia Medica · Woody Plant*.

【Notes】

[1] The name of an ancient county.

笋可食

《本草》原有

Shoot Edible

Original Ones

325. 竹 笋

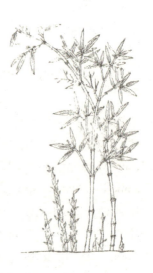

本草竹叶有簜竹叶、苦竹叶、淡竹叶。《本经》并不载所出州土，今处处有之。竹之类甚多，而入药者惟此三种，人多不能尽别。簜竹坚而促节，体圆而质劲，皮白如霜，作笛者有一种，亦不名簜竹。苦竹亦有二种，一种出江西及闽中，本极粗大，笋味甚苦，不可啖；一种出江浙，近地亦时有之，肉厚而叶长阔，笋微苦味，俗呼甜苦笋，食所最贵者，亦不闻入药用。淡竹肉薄，节间有粉，南人以烧竹沥者，医家只用此一品。又有一种薄壳者，名甘竹叶，最胜。又有实中竹、篁竹，并以笋为佳，于药无用。凡取竹沥，惟用淡竹、苦竹、簜竹尔。陶隐居云："竹实出蓝田[1]，江东乃有花而无实，而顷来斑斑有实，状如小麦，堪可为饭。"《图经》云："竹笋味甘，无毒。"又云寒。

救饥：采竹嫩笋煤熟，油盐调食。焯过晒干，煤食尤好。

治病：文具《本草·木部》竹叶条下。

【注释】

[1] 古县名。

325. Zhusun [竹笋, bamboo shoot, Bambusoideae]

Zhuye [竹叶, folium phyllostachytis, Phyllostachys nigra (Lodd.) Munro var. henonis (Mitf.) Stapf ex Rendle] is also named Jinzhuye, Kuzhuye and Danzhuye. There is no record about its place of origin in *Shennong Bencaojing* [《神农本草经》, *Shennong's Classics of Materia Medica*], but it is commonly seen everywhere. There are many types of bamboos, and only three of them are used as medicine, and most of them can not be identified. Jinzhu is hard and its joint is short, it is round in shape and tough in texture. Its skin is white. There is a kind of bamboos that can be used as a flute, but not Jinzhu. There are also two kinds of bitter bamboos, one of which is produced in Jiangxi and Minzhong. The bamboo rafts are very thick; the bamboo shoots are very bitter and cannot be eaten. The other one is produced in Jiangsu and Zhejiang, and occasionally there are such bamboos nearby. This kind of bamboos is thick, and their leaves are long and wide. This kind of bamboo shoots is slightly bitter in taste. So it is called Tiankusun. It is the most precious of the edible bamboo shoots, and it is not heard that it can be used for medicinal purposes. The bamboo wall of Lophatherum herb is thinner, and there is powder in the joints. This kind of bamboos is used by the southern doctors to burn to extract succus bambusae. There is also a thin wall called Ganzhuye, the best kind among them. There are also other kinds of bamboos called Shizhongzhu and Huangzhu, and the bamboo shoots produced by them are of good quality. It is useless to make medicine. Only Danzhu, Kuzhu and Jinzhu can be used to extract succus bambusae. Tao Hujing, a famous pharmacist in ancient China, said that the fruit of bamboos was produced from Lantian[1], the bamboos in Jiangdong could be flowering but not strong, but sometimes it suddenly yielded streaky fruit, shaped like wheat, which could be used for cooking. According to *Tu Jing Ben Cao* [《图经本草》, *Illustrated Classics of Materia Meddica*], the bamboo shoots are sweet in taste and non-toxic. It is also recorded to be cold in nature.

For famine relief: Collect and blanch young bamboo shoots, and then flavor them with oil and salt. It is more delicious after they are dried and blanched.

For disease treatment: See the clause of Zhuye [竹叶, folia bambosae, Phyllostachys nigra (Lodd.) Munro var. henonis (Mitf.) Stapf ex Rendle] in *Materia Medica · Woody Plant*.

【Notes】

[1] The name of an ancient county.

米谷部

实可食

新增

Herbaceous Cereal
Fruit Edible
New Supplements

326. 野豌豆

生田野中。苗初就地拖秧而生,后分生茎叉,苗长二尺余。叶似胡豆[1]叶稍大;又似苜蓿[2]叶亦大。开淡粉紫花。结角似家豌豆角,但秕小,味苦。

救饥:采角煮食,或收取豆煮食,或磨面,制造食用,与家豆同。

【注释】

[1] 见本书第330胡豆条。

[2] 见本书第379苜蓿条。

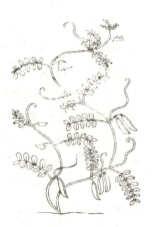

326. Yewandou [野豌豆, vicia sepium, Vicia sativa L.]

Yewandou [野豌豆, vicia sepium, Vicia sativa L.] grows in the fields. The seedlings creep on the ground, and then many branches will grow. The plant is more than two Chi long. Its leaves are like those of Hudou[1][胡豆, lima bean, Vicia faba L.], but a little bigger. And they are also like those of Muxu[2][苜蓿, herb of Alfalfa, Medicago Sativa Linn], but bigger as well. Its flowers are light pink purple. Its fruit, like that of Wandou [豌豆, pea, Pisum sativum Linn], more wizened and smaller, is bitter in taste.

For famine relief: Collect and cook its beans, or grind them into flour just like peas.

【Notes】

[1] See the 330th clause of this book.

[2] See the 379th clause of this book.

327. 䝁豆

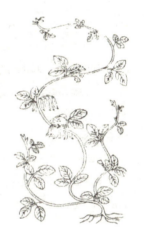

生平野中,北土处处有之。茎蔓延附草木上。叶似黑豆叶而窄小,微尖。开淡粉紫花。结小角,其豆似黑豆形,极小,味甘。

救饥:打取豆,淘洗净,煮食。或磨为面,打饼蒸食,皆可。

327. Laodou [䝁豆, wild soybean, Glycine soja Sieb. et Zucc.]

Laodou [䝁豆, wild soybean, Glycine soja Sieb. et Zucc.], growing in the wide and flat plains, can be seen everywhere in the north. Its stems and vines cling to the grass and trees. Being small and slightly sharp, its leaves are like those of Heidou [黑豆, black soy beans, Glycinemax (L.) merr], and its flowers are light pink purple. Its beans, which are like those of Heidou [黑豆, black soy beans, Glycinemax (L.) merr], are small in size and sweet in taste.

For famine relief: Collect beans, elutriate them in water, and then cook them. They can be ground into flour or made a steamed Chinese cookie.

328. 山扁豆

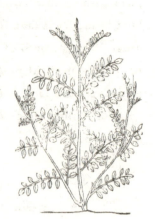

生田野中。小科苗高一尺许。梢叶似蒺藜叶微大,根叶比苜蓿叶颇长;又似初生豌豆叶。开黄花。结小扁角儿,味甜。

救饥:采嫩角煤食,其豆熟时,收取豆煮食。

328. Shanbiandou〔山扁豆, senna, Senna nomame(Makino)T. C. Chen〕

Shanbiandou〔山扁豆, senna, Senna nomame(Makino)T. C. Chen〕grows in the fields. Its plants are so small that they are only about one Chi high. Its apical lobules are like those of Jili〔蒺藜, tribulus terrestris, Fructus Tribuli〕, but a little bigger. The basal lobules are a bit longer than those of Muxu〔苜蓿, herb of Alfalfa, Medicago Sativa Linn〕. It is also like that of Wandou〔豌豆, pea, Pisum sativum Linn〕, and its flowers are yellow. Its small and oblate pods taste sweet.

For famine relief: Collect young pods, blanch and elutriate them in hot water. The ripe beans can be cooked and taken as food.

329. 回回豆

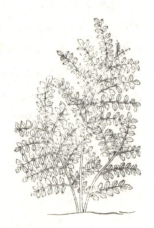

又名那合豆。生田野中。茎青。叶似蒺藜叶;又似初生嫩皂荚叶,而有细锯齿。开五瓣淡紫花,如蒺藜花样。结角如杏人[1]样而肥,有豆如牵牛子,微大,味甜。

救饥:采豆煮食。

【注释】

[1]见本书第361杏树条。

329. Huihuidou [回回豆, chickpea, Cicer arietinum L.]

Huihuidou [回回豆, chickpea, Cicer arietinum L.], also named Nahedou, grows in the fields, with green stems. Its leaves, finely serrulated, are like those of Jili [蒺藜, tribulus terrestris, Fructus Tribuli], and like those of the tender soap pods. Each of its lavender flowers has five petals, and they are also like those of Jili [蒺藜, tribulus terrestris, Fructus Tribuli]. Its pods are like those of Xingren[1] [杏仁, bitter apricot kernel, Amygdalus Communis Vas], but quite thick. There are beans in the pods, just like the seeds of Qianniu [牵牛, morning glory, Pharbitis nil (L.) Choisy], but a bit bigger than the latter. It is sweet in taste.

For famine relief: Collect beans and cook them.

【Notes】

[1] See the 361th clause of this book.

330. 胡 豆

生田野间。其苗初揭地生，后分茎叉。叶似苜蓿叶而细。茎叶梢间开淡葱白褐花。结小角，有豆如豌豆状，味甜。

救饥：采取豆煮食，或磨面食，皆可。

330. Hudou [胡豆, indigofera decora, Indigofera decora Lindl.]

Hudou [胡豆, indigofera decora, Indigofera decora Lindl.] grows in the fields. Initially its plants creep on the ground, and then produce a lot of branches. Its leaves are like those of Muxu [苜蓿, herb of Alfalfa, Medicago Sativa Linn], but a bit slender. Its flowers bloom in the twigs between stems and branches. Its pods are like those of Laodou [豌豆, wild soybean, Glycine soja Sieb. et

Zucc.], and it is sweet in taste.

For famine relief: Collect beans, elutriate them in water and cook, or grind them into flour.

331. 蚕 豆

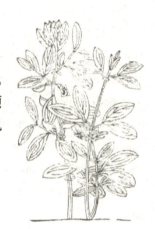

今处处有之,生田园中。科苗高二尺许。茎方。其叶状类黑豆叶而团长光泽,纹脉竖直,色似豌豆,颇白。茎叶梢间开白花。结短角,其豆如豇豆[1]而小,色赤,味甜。

救饥:采豆煮食,炒食亦可。

【注释】

[1] 见本书第343豇豆苗条。

331. Candou [蚕豆, broad bean, Vicia faba L.]

Candou [蚕豆, broad bean, Vicia faba L.], growing in the fields and gardens, can be seen everywhere presently. Its plants are about two Chi high with squarish stems. Its leaves, with flat veins, are like those of Heidou [黑豆, black Bean, Glycinemax (L.) merr], but sharper, rounder and shiny. Its color is like that of peas, slightly white. Its white flowers grow in the middle of stems and leaves. Its pods are small, and its red beans are like those of Jiangdou[1] [豇豆, cowpea, Vigna unguiculata (Linn.) Walp.], but smaller than the latter. It is sweet in taste.

For famine relief: Collect beans to cook or stir-fry.

【Notes】

[1] See the 343th clause of this book.

332. 山绿豆

生辉县太行山车箱冲山野中。苗茎似家绿豆[1]茎微细。叶比家绿豆叶狭窄尖艄。开白花。结角亦瘦小,其豆黪绿色,味甘。

救饥：采取其豆煮食，或磨面摊煎饼食，亦可。

【注释】

［1］即绿豆。

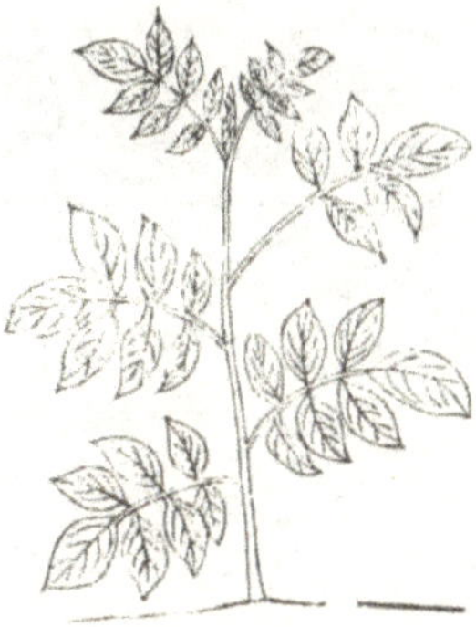

332. Shanlvdou ［山绿豆，indigofera kirilowii，Indigofera kirilowii Maxim. ex Palibin］

Shanlvdou ［山绿豆，indigofera kirilowii, Indigofera kirilowii Maxim. ex Palibin］ grows in the mountains and wilderness of Mount Taihang in Huixian County. Its stems are like those of Lvdou[1]［绿豆，mung bean，Vigna radiata (Linn.) Wilczek］, slightly thin, but its leaves are narrower and sharper than the latter. Its flowers are white and pods are small. Its beans are dark green and sweet in taste.

For famine relief: Collect beans from the pods to cook, or grind them into flour to make Shaobing, a Chinese style of a steamed pancake.

【Notes】

［1］It refers to Lvdou ［绿豆，mung bean，Vigna radiata (Linn.) Wilczek］.

卷下 下之后

米谷部

叶及实皆可食

《本草》原有

Volume 2　The Second Half
Herbaceous Cereal
Leaf and Fruit Edible
Original Ones

333. 荞麦苗

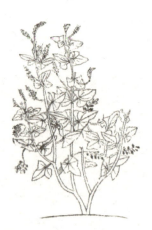

处处种之。苗高二三尺许,就地科叉生。其茎色红,叶似杏叶而软,微觥。开小白花。结实作三棱蒴儿,味甘、平、寒,无毒。

救饥:采苗叶煠熟,油盐调食。多食微泻。其麦,或蒸使气馏,于烈日中晒,令口开,舂取仁煮作饭食,或磨为面,作饼蒸食皆可。

治病:文具《本草·米谷部》条下。

333. Qiaomaimiao［荞麦苗, fagopyrum esculentum, Fagopyrum esculentum］

Qiaomaimiao［荞麦苗, fagopyrum esculentum, Fagopyrum esculentum］is planted everywhere. Its plants are about 2～3 Chi high, and they will produce branches near the ground. With red stems, its leaves are like those of Xing［杏,

apricot, Armeniaca vulgaris Lam], but very soft and slightly sharp. Its flowers are white, and its fruit is triangular achene. It is sweet in taste, neutral and cold in nature and non toxic.

For famine relief: Collect young leaves and plants, blanch and elutriate them in hot water, and then flavor them with oil and salt. It may cause diarrhea after people eat too much. Steam or dry the fruit to make it rupture to get rid of buckwheat husk to obtain the kernel for making congee. Or it is edible when ground into flour to make Shaobing, a Chinese style of a steamed pancake.

For disease treatment: See the relevant clause in *Materia Medica · Herbaceous Cereal*.

334. 御米花

本草名罂子粟,一名象谷,一名米囊,一名囊子。处处有之。苗高一二尺。叶似靛叶色而大,边皱,多有花叉。开四瓣红白花,亦有千叶花者。结壳似骲箭头,壳中有米数千粒,似葶苈子,色白,隔年种则佳。米味甘,性平,无毒。

救饥:采嫩叶煠熟,油盐调食。取米作粥,或与面作饼,皆可食。其米和竹沥煮粥,食之极美。

治病:文具《本草·米谷部》罂子粟条下。

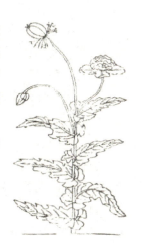

334. Yumihua [御米花, papaver somniferum, Papaver somniferum L.]

Yumihua [御米花, papaver somniferum, Papaver somniferum L.], also named Yinzisu, Xianggu, Minang and Nangzi, can be commonly seen everywhere presently. Its plants are 1~2 Chi high, and the color of its leaves is like that of Dian [靛, polygonum tinctoriu, Polygonum tinctorium Ait.], but a little bigger. With rugose leaves and flower lobus, there are double or four petals in flowers which are red or white. The husk of its fruit is like that of the bone-made arrow. There are thousands of white seeds in the fruit husk, just like the seeds of draba nemorosa, it is better to be planted every two years. The seeds are sweet in taste, neutral in nature and non-toxic.

For famine relief: Collect young leaves, blanch and elutriate them in hot water, and then flavor them with oil and salt. Pick seeds, make them congee, and mix them with flour to make Shaobing, a Chinese style of baked pancake. It is delicious to make congee with seeds and Zhuli [竹沥, henon bamboo juice, Phyllostachyl nigra (Lodd. ex Lindl.) Munro var. henonis (Mitf.) Stapf et Rendle].

For disease treatment: See the clause of Yinzisu [罂子粟, papaver somniferum, Papaver somniferum L.] in *Materia Medica · Herbaceous Cereal*.

335. 赤小豆

《本草》旧云江淮间多种莳，今北土亦多有之。苗高一二尺。叶似豇豆叶微团艄。开花似豇豆花微小，淡银褐色，有腐气，人故亦呼为腐婢。结角比绿豆角颇大，角之皮色微白带红。其豆有赤、白、䵟色三种，味甘、酸，性平，无毒。合鲊食成消渴，为酱合鲊食成口疮，人食则体重。

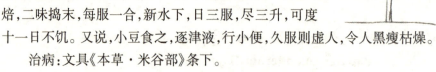

救饥：采嫩叶煠熟，水淘洗净，油盐调食，明目。豆角亦可煮食。又法，赤小豆一升半，炒大豆黄一升半，焙，二味捣末，每服一合，新水下，日三服，尽三升，可度十一日不饥。又说，小豆食之，逐津液，行小便，久服则虚人，令人黑瘦枯燥。

治病：文具《本草·米谷部》条下。

335. Chixiaodou [赤小豆, azuki Bean, Vigna angularis (Willd.) Ohwi et Ohashi]

Chixiaodou [赤小豆, azuki Bean, Vigna angularis (Willd.) Ohwi et Ohashi] is mostly planted in the area of Yangtze River and Huaihe River according to *Materia Medica*, and it is also planted in the north. Its plants are 1~2 Chi high. Its leaves are like those of cowpea, but slightly round and sharp. Its light silver brownish flowers are like those of cowpeas, but a bit smaller, with the rotten flavor, so it is also named Fubi. Its pods are a little bigger than those of Lvdou [绿豆, mung bean, Vigna radiata (Linn.) Wilczek], and the husk of pods is slight white and red. Its pods are red, white or black and yellow. It is sweet and sour in taste, neutral in nature and non-toxic. Being eaten with Zha, a kind of fermented food made by some meat and vegetables mixing with rice noodle, it can be used to treat the Xiaoke syndrome which refers to a common disease in clinic with the typical syndrome of polyphagia, polydispia, polyuria, weariness and emaciation, or to treat the aphtha when it is cooked into sauce. However, people will gain weight if eating too much of them.

For famine relief: Collect young leaves, blanch and elutriate them in hot water, and then flavor them with oil and salt. It can improve the eyesight. The pods can be cooked. Or bake a liter and a half of them and a liter and a half of stir-fried Dadouhuang, a kind of steamed Heidadou, pound them into powder, and take them three times a day. People will not feel hungry in eleven days after eating them. It is also said to make people feeble, black and thin, fluid exhaustion with blood dryness after taking them for a long time.

For disease treatment: See the clause of Chixiaodou [赤小豆, azuki Bean, Vigna angularis (Willd.) Ohwi et Ohashi] in *Materia Medica · Herbaceous Cereal*.

336. 山丝苗

本草有麻蕡,一名麻勃,一名苧,一名麻母。生太山川谷,今皆处处有之,人家园圃中多种莳,绩其皮以为布。苗高四五尺,茎有细线楞。叶形似柳叶,而边皆有叉牙锯齿,每八九叶攒生一处;又似荆叶而狭,色深青。开淡黄白花,结实小如绿豆颗而扁。《图经》云:麻蕡,此麻上花勃勃者,味辛,性平,有毒。麻子味甘,性平、微寒,滑利,无毒。入土者损人。畏牡蛎、白薇,恶茯苓。

救饥:采嫩叶煠熟,换水浸去邪恶气味。再以水淘洗净,油盐调食。不可多食,亦不可久食,动风。子可

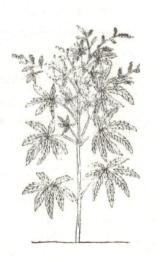

炒食，亦可打油用。

治病：文具《本草·米谷部》麻蕡条下。

336. Shansimiao ［山丝苗，cannabis sativa，Cannabis sativa L.］

Shansimiao ［山丝苗，cannabis sativa，Cannabis sativa L.］, also named Mafen, Mabo, Yu and Mamu, grows in the valleys where there is flowing water in Mount Tai, and it can be seen everywhere presently. It is also cultivated in the nursery gardens of common people. Besides, its peels can be rubbed and twisted as the twine to make clothes. Its plants are 4~5 Chi high with thin-ridged stems. Its leaves are like those of willow trees with dentate margin. Every eight or nine leaves grows together. Its leaves are like the twigs of chaste trees, but very narrow and dark green. Its flowers are light yellow. Its fruit is like that of Lvdou ［绿豆, mung bean, Vigna radiata (Linn.) Wilczek］, but quite flat. According to *Tu Jing Ben Cao* ［《图经本草》, *Illustrated Classics of Materia Meddica*］, Mafen, the fruit of Dama ［大麻, cannabis sativa, Cannabis sativa L.］, is pungent in taste, neutral in nature and toxic. Mazi, the seed of Dama, is sweet in taste, neutral and slightly cold in nature, non-stagnant and non-toxic. The seeds in the soil do harm to human body. They will be restrained by Muli ［牡蛎, ostreae testa, Concha Ostreae］ and Baiwei ［白薇, blackend swallowwort root, Radix Cynanchi Atrati］, and they are averse to Fuling ［茯苓, poria cocos, Poria］ in compatibility.

For famine relief: Collect young leaves, blanch and soak them in fresh water, remove the foul smell by elutriating them in water, and flavor them with oil and salt. They may cause wind syndrome after being eaten too much or for long time. The seeds can be stir-fried or pressed for oil.

For disease treatment: See the clause of Mafen ［麻蕡, cannabis sativa, Cannabis sativa L.］ in *Materia Medica · Herbaceous Cereal*.

337. 油子苗

本草有白油麻,俗名脂麻。旧不著所出州土,今处处有之,人家园圃中多种。苗高三四尺。茎方,笏面四楞,对节分生枝叉。叶类苏子^[1]叶而长,尖艄,边多花叉。叶间开白花,结四棱蒴儿,每蒴中有子四五十余粒。其子味甘、微苦,生则性大寒,无毒,炒熟则性热,压笮为油,大寒。

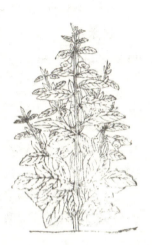

救饥:采嫩叶煠熟,水浸淘洗净,油盐调食。其子亦可炒熟食,或煮食及笮为油食,皆可。

治病:文具《本草·米谷部》白油麻条下。

【注释】

[1]见本书第342苏子苗条。

337. Youzimiao [油子苗, sesamum indicum, Sesamum indicum Linn.]

Youzimiao [油子苗, sesamum indicum, Sesamum indicum Linn.] is also named Baiyouma and Zhima. There is no record about its origin in ancient books, but now it can be seen everywhere, especially in the courtyards of common people. Its plants are about 3~4 Chi high. Its stems are squarish with quadruple rims and opposite branches. Its leaves are like those of Suzi[1] [苏子, perillaseed, Perilla frutescens (L.) Britt.], but quite long and sharp. There are some lobes in the leaf margin. Its flowers are white. The capsule that is tetragonal has forty or fifty seeds which taste sweet and a bit bitter. It is cold in nature but non-toxic when it is raw. It is warm in nature after being stir-fried. Its fruit can be used to extract oil, and it is cold in nature.

For famine relief: Collect young leaves, blanch and soak them in fresh water, and then flavor them with oil and salt. The seeds can be stir-fried or boiled. They can be used to extract oil.

For disease treatment: See the clause of Baiyouma [白油麻, sesame indicum, Sesamum indicum L.] in *Materia Medica · Herbaceous Cereal*.

【Notes】

〔1〕See the 342th clause of this book.

新增

New Supplements

338. 黄豆苗

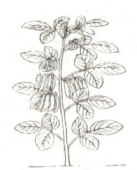

今处处有之，人家田园中多种。苗高一二尺。叶似黑豆叶而大。结角比黑豆角稍肥大。其叶味甘。

救饥：采嫩苗叶煠熟，水浸淘净，油盐调食。或采角煮食，或收豆煮食，及磨为面食，皆可。

338. Huangdoumiao〔黄豆苗, soybean, Glycine max (L.) Merr.〕

Huangdoumiao〔黄豆苗, soybean, Glycine max (L.) Merr.〕can be seen everywhere presently. It is often planted in the fields or courtyards of common people. Its plants are 1~2 Chi high. Its leaves are like those of Heidou〔黑豆, black soy beans, Glycinemax (L.) merr〕, but a little bigger. Its beans are stronger than those of Heidou. Its leaves are sweet in taste.

For famine relief: Collect young leaves and plants, blanch and soak them in fresh water, and then flavor them with oil and salt. Its beans can be boiled or crushed into flour.

339. 刀豆苗

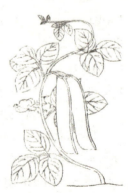

处处有之，人家园篱边多种之。苗叶似豇豆叶肥大。开淡粉红花。结角如皂角状而长，其形似屠刀样，故以名之，味甜、微淡。

救饥：采嫩苗叶煠熟，水浸淘净，油盐调食。豆角嫩时煮食。豆熟之时，收豆煮食，或磨面食亦可。

339. Daodoumiao [刀豆苗, sword bean, Canavalia gladiata Dc. Merr.]

Daodoumiao [刀豆苗, sword bean, Canavalia gladiata Dc. Merr.] can be seen everywhere presently. It is often planted in the courtyards with fences or hedges of common people. Its leaves are like the lobules of Jiangdou [豇豆, cowpea, Vigna unguiculata (Linn.) Walp], but a little stronger. Its flowers are light pink. Its beans are like those of Zaojiao [皂角, gleditsia, Gleditsiae Fructus], but longer. It is named after Daodou, because the shape of the beans is like the butcher's hacking knife. It is sweet in taste and slightly bland.

For famine relief: Collect young leaves and plants, blanch and soak them in fresh water, and then flavor them with oil and salt. The young peas are edible after being boiled. The ripe peas are edible after being boiled or being ground into flour.

340. 眉儿豆苗

人家园圃中种之。妥蔓而生。叶似绿豆叶而肥大阔厚,润泽光俊,每三叶攒生一处。开淡粉紫花,结扁角,每角有豆止三四颗。其豆色黑扁而皆白眉,故名。味微甜。

救饥:采嫩苗叶煠食。豆角嫩时,采角煮食。豆成熟时,打取豆食。

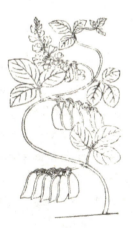

340. Mei'erdou Miao [眉儿豆苗, lablab purpureus, Lablab purpureus (L.) sweet]

Mei'erdou Miao [眉儿豆苗, lablab purpureus, Lablab purpureus (L.) sweet], cultivated in the nursery gardens of common people, creeps on the ground. Its leaves are like those of Lvdou [绿豆, mung bean, Vigna radiata (Linn.) Wilczek], but a little stronger, wider, thicker and lustrous. Having compound leaves with three leaflets, its flowers are pinkish purple, and its beans are flat. There are three or four peas in each bean, black and flat. It is named after

Mei'erdou Miao because its hilum is like the white eyebrows. It is sweet in taste.

For famine relief: Collect and blanch young leaves and seedlings, blanch them by elutriating them in water. The young peas are edible after boiling. The ripe peas are edible after being threshed and peeled.

341. 紫豇豆苗^[1]

人家园圃中种之。茎叶与豇豆同，但结角色紫，长尺许，味微甜。

救饥：采嫩苗叶煠熟，油盐调食。角嫩时采角煮食，亦可做菜食。豆成熟时打取豆食之。

【注释】

［1］现代植物分类学认为豇豆和紫豇豆是同一种，见本书第343豇豆苗条。

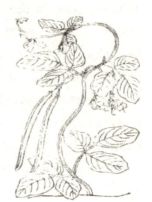

341. Zijiangdou Miao[1]［紫豇豆苗, cowpea, Vigna unguiculata（Linn.）Walp.］

Zijiangdou Miao［紫豇豆苗, vigna unguiculata, Vigna unguiculata（Linn.）Walp.］is cultivated in the courtyards of common people. Its stems and leaves are like those of Jiangdou［豇豆, cowpea, Vigna unguiculata（Linn.）Walp.］, but its peas are purple, one Chi long, and sweet in taste.

For famine relief: Collect and blanch young leaves and plants, and then flavor them with oil and salt. The young peas are edible after boiling. The ripe peas are edible after being threshed and peeled.

【Notes】

［1］According to the modern plant taxonomy, Zijiangdou Miao and Jiangdoumiao are considered to be the same species, and see the 343th clause of this book.

342. 苏子苗

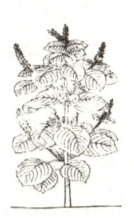

人家园圃中多种之。苗高二三尺。茎方,笊面,四楞,上有涩毛。叶皆对生,似紫苏叶而大。开淡紫花。结子比紫苏子亦大,味微辛,性温。

救饥:采嫩叶煠熟,换水淘洗净,油盐调食。子可炒食,亦可笮油用。

342. Suzimiao［苏子苗, perilla frutescens, Perilla frutescens（L.）Britt.］

Suzimiao［苏子苗, perilla frutescens, Perilla frutescens（L.）Britt.］is widely cultivated in the courtyards of common people. Its plants are 2～3 Chi high. Its stems are squarish, concave, strigose and tetragonal. Its leaves are decussate, just like those of Zisu［紫苏, perilla frutescens, Perilla frutescens（L.）Britt. Var］, but a little bigger. Its flowers are light purple. Its seeds are larger than the latter. It is a bit pungent in taste and warm in nature.

For famine relief: Collect young leaves, blanch and soak them in fresh water, and then flavor them with oil and salt. Its seeds can be cooked or used to extract oil.

343. 豇豆苗

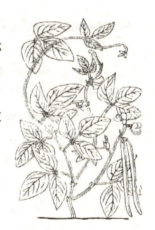

今处处有之,人家田园中多种。就地拖秧而生,亦延篱落。叶似赤小豆叶而极长艄。开淡粉紫花。结角长五七寸,其豆味甘。

救饥:采嫩叶煠熟,水浸淘净,油盐调食。及采嫩角煠食亦可。其豆成熟时,打取豆食。

343. Jiangdoumiao [豇豆苗, cowpea, Vigna unguiculata (Linn.) Walp.]

Jiangdoumiao [豇豆苗, cowpea, Vigna unguiculata (Linn.) Walp.], widely planted in the courtyards of common people or in the fields, can be seen everywhere presently. It creeps on the ground and grows along the vines. Its leaves are like those of Chixiaodou [赤小豆, azuki Bean, Vigna angularis (Willd.) Ohwi et Ohashi], but very long and sharp. Its flowers are pinkish purple. Its pods are 5 ~7 Chi high and sweet in taste.

For famine relief: Collect young leaves and pods, blanch and soak them in fresh water, and then flavor them with oil and salt. The ripe pods are edible after being threshed and peeled.

344. 山黑豆

生密县山野中。苗似家黑豆每三叶攒生一处, 居中人叶如绿豆叶, 傍两叶似黑豆叶, 微圆。开小粉红花, 结角比家黑豆角极瘦小, 其豆亦极细小, 味微苦。

救饥: 苗叶嫩时, 采取煠熟, 水淘去苦味, 油盐调食。结角时采角煮食或打取豆食皆可。

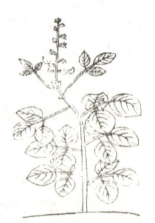

344. Shanheidou [山黑豆, wild black soybean, Glycine soja Sieb. et Zucc.]

Shanheidou [山黑豆, wild black soybean, Glycine soja Sieb. et Zucc.] grows in the mountainous regions and the wilderness of Mixian County. Its plants are like those of Heidou [黑豆, black soy bean, Glycinemax (L.) merr], and grow with three leaves together. The lager ones in the middle are like those of Lvdou [绿豆, mung bean, Vigna radiata (Linn.) Wilczek], and the others on each side are like those of Heidou [黑豆, black soy bean, Glycine soja Sieb. et Zucc.], but slightly round. Its pink flowers are small. Its pods are much thinner and smaller than black soybeans. And its beans are much smaller and a little bitter in taste.

For famine relief: Collect young leaves and seedlings, blanch them and remove the bitterness by elutriating them in water, and then flavor them with oil and salt. Its beans are edible after being cooked or threshed and peeled.

345. 舜芒谷

俗名红落藜。生田野及人家旧庄窠上多有之。苗高五尺余。叶似灰菜[1]叶而大，微带红色。茎亦高粗，可为拄杖。其中心叶甚红。叶间出穗。结子如粟米颗，灰青色，味甜。

救饥：采嫩苗叶晒干，揉去灰，煠熟，油盐调食。子可磨面，做烧饼蒸食。

【注释】

[1] 见本书第 412 灰菜条。

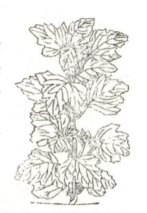

345. Shunmanggu [舜芒谷, chenopodium giganteum, Chenopodium giganteum D. Don.]

Shunmanggu [舜芒谷, chenopodium giganteum, Chenopodium giganteum D. Don.], also named Hongluoli, grows in the fields or the old courtyards of common people. Its plants are more than five Chi high. Its reddish leaves are like those of Huicai[1] [灰菜, chenopodium album, Chenopodium album L.], but a little larger. Its stems are also taller and thicker than Huicai, which can be made a scepter. Its leaves in the middle are very red. The spica grows out of its leaves. Its seeds are like those of Sumi [粟米, millet, Setaria italica (L.) Beauv.], dark bluish grey, and sweet in taste.

For famine relief: Collect and dry leaves and young seedlings in the sunshine, make them clean and blanch them in hot water, and then flavor them with oil and salt. Its seeds can be ground into flour and made dough to steam.

【Notes】

[1] See the 412th clause of this book.

果 部

实可食

《本草》原有

Herbaceous Fruit
Fruit Edible
Original Ones

346. 樱桃树

处处有之。古谓之含桃。叶似桑叶而狭窄，微软。开粉红花，结桃似郁李子[1]而小，红色鲜明，味甘，性热。

救饥：采果红熟者食之。

治病：文具《本草·果部》条下。

【注释】

[1] 见本书第354郁李子条。

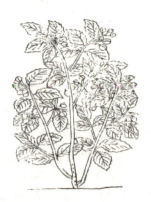

346. Yingtaoshu［樱桃树, cherry tree, Cerasus pseudocerasus（Lindl.）G. Don］

Yingtaoshu［樱桃树, cherry tree, Cerasus pseudocerasus（Lindl.）G. Don］can be seen everywhere presently. It used to be called Hantao in ancient times. Its leaves are like those of Sangshu［桑树, mulberry, Morus alba L.］, but slightly narrow and soft. Its flowers are pink and red. Its fruit is like that of Yuli[1]［郁李, prunus japonica, Cerasus japonica（Thunb.）Lois］, but relatively small and bright red. It is sweet in taste and hot in nature.

For famine relief: The ripe cherries are edible.

For disease treatment: See the relevant clause in *Materia Medica · Herbaceous Fruit*.

【Notes】

[1] See the 354th clause of this book.

347. 胡桃树

一名核桃。生北土,旧云张骞从西域将来,陕[1]洛[2]间多有之,今钧郑间亦有。其树大株,叶厚而多阴。开花成穗,花色苍黄。结实外有青皮包之,状似梨,大熟时沤去青皮,取其核是胡桃,味甘,性平。一云性热,无毒。

救饥:采核桃沤去青皮,取瓤食之,令人肥健。

治病:文具《本草·果部》条下。

【注释】

[1] 古代地名,见《图经本草》。又称"陕陌",在今河南陕县西南。

[2] 水名,见《图经本草》。即今河南洛河,发源于陕西,流入河南。

347. Hutaoshu [胡桃树, walnut tree, Juglans regia L.]

Hutaoshu [胡桃树, walnut tree, Juglans regia L.], also named Hetao, grows in the north. It was brought back by Zhang Qian, a famous Ambassador of Han Dynasty who was sent to visit the Western regions according to the ancient legend. It is widely cultivated in Shaanxian[1] and Luo River[2] in Henan Province. And now it is also planted in Junzhou and Zhengzhou. Its plants are tall, and its leaves are thick, which cast shade. Its spica is greenish yellow. The outside of the fruit is covered with green peels. The hard core inside is a walnut. It is sweet in taste and neutral in nature. It is also said to be hot in nature and non-toxic.

For famine relief: Collect and soak walnut in water to strip off the green peels outside. The core is edible, and it makes people strong and healthy.

For disease treatment: See the relevant clause in *Materia Medica ·*

Herbaceous Fruit.

【Notes】

[1] The name of an ancient county. Presently it refers to the southwest of Shaanxian in Henan Province.

[2] The name of a river. Presently it refers to Luo River in Henan Province.

348. 柿 树

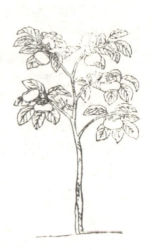

旧不载所出州土,今南北皆有之,然华山者皮薄而味甘珍,宣[1]、歙[2]、荆、襄、闽、广诸州,但生啖,不堪为干。椑柿,压丹石毒。乌柿,宣越者性温。诸柿食之皆善而益人。其树高一二丈。叶似软枣[3]叶,颇小而头微团。结实种数甚多,有牛心柿、蒸饼柿、盖柿、塔柿、蒲楪红柿、黄柿、朱柿、椑柿。其干柿,火干者谓之乌柿。诸柿味甘,性寒,无毒。

救饥:摘取软熟柿食之。其柿未软者,摘取以温水醃熟食之。粗心柿不可多食,令人腹痛。生柿弥冷,尤不可多食。

治病:文具《本草·果部》条下。

【注释】

[1] 古代州名,见《图经本草》。

[2] 古代州名,见《图经本草》。辖境相当于今安徽新安江流域、祁门县及江西婺源等地。

[3] 见本书第356软枣条。

348. Shishu〔柿树, persimmon tree, Diospyros kaki Thunb.〕

There was no record about its origin in ancient times. Presently, it can be seen in the north and south. But those growing in Mount Hua are thin-skinned and sweet in taste. Those produced in Xuanzhou[1] and Xizhou[2] in Anhui Province, Jingzhou and Xiangyang in Hubei Province, the south of Fujian Province and Guangxi Province can be eaten rather than made dried persimmon, but Beishi〔椑

柿, diospyros oleifer, Diospyros oleifera Cheng] can be used to treat mineral intoxication. Wushi growing in Xuanzhou and Yuezhou is warm in nature. All kinds of persimmon are edible and beneficial. The persimmon tree is 1~2 Zhang high. Its leaves are like those of Ruanzao[3] [软枣, diospyros lotus, Diospyros lotus L.], but slightly small. And the top of leaves is slightly round. There is a variety of fruits such as Niuxinshi, Zhengbingshi, Gaishi, Tashi, Pudiehong Shi, Huangshi, Zhushi and Baishi. Those dried persimmon made from roasted fruits are called Wushi. They are sweet in taste, cold in nature and non-toxic.

For famine relief: The ripe and softened persimmon is edible. The unsoftened persimmon can be edible after being soaked in hot water to remove the bitterness. The persimmon with rough core can not be eaten too much, otherwise it may cause stomachache, especially the unripe persimmon, and it can not be eaten too much because it is cold in nature.

For disease treatment: See the relevant clause in *Materia Medica · Herbaceous Fruit*.

【Notes】

[1] The name of an ancient county. Presently it refers to the city of Xuanzhou in Anhui Province.

[2] The name of an ancient county. Presently it refers to the regions in the Xin'anjiang areas of Anhui Province, and Qimen County and Wuyuan in Jiangxi Province.

[3] See the 356th clause of this book.

349. 梨 树

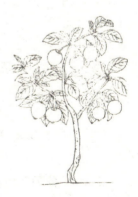

出郑州及宣城,今处处有。其树叶似棠叶而大,色青,开花白色,结实形样甚多。鹅梨出郑州,极大,味香美而浆多。乳梨出宣城,皮厚而肉实,味极长。水梨出北都,皮薄而浆多,味差短。又有消梨、紫煤梨、赤梨、甘棠、御儿梨、紫花梨、青梨、茅梨、桑梨之类,不能尽具其名。梨实味甘、微酸,性寒,无毒。

救饥:其梨结硬未熟时,摘取煮食。已经霜熟,摘取生食。或蒸食亦佳。或削其皮，晒作梨糁，收而备用，亦可。

349. Lishu［梨树，pear tree，Pyrus pyrifolia（Burm.）Nakai］

Lishu［梨树，pear tree，Pyrus pyrifolia（Burm.）Nakai］grows in Zhengzhou and Xuancheng. Presently, it can be seen everywhere. Its green leaves are like those of Tanglishu［棠梨树，pyrus betulifolia，Pyrus betulifolia Bunge］, but a little larger. Its flowers are white, and there is a variety of fruits. E'li, produced from Zhengzhou, is big, sweet and succulent. Ruli comes from Xuancheng, its peel is thick, its flesh is firm, and it is delicious. Shuili originates from Beidu, an ancient capital, with thin peels, succulent flesh and distasteful flavor. There are different kinds of pear trees, such as Xiaoli, Zimeili, Chili, Gantang, Yu'erli, Zihuali, Qingli, Maoli, Sangli, etc. Its fruit is sweet but slightly sour in taste, cold in nature and non-toxic.

For famine relief: Collect the hard and unripe fruit to boil in hot water. The ripe fruit can be eaten or steamed. Dry peeled pears into food for reservation.

350. 葡　萄

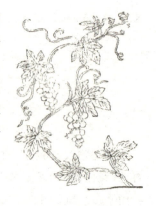

生陇西、五原、敦煌山谷及河东，旧云汉张骞使西域得其种，还而种之，中国始有。盖北果之最珍者，今处处有之。苗作藤蔓而极长大，盛者一二本绵被山谷。叶类丝瓜叶，颇壮而边多花叉。开花极细而黄白色。其实有紫白二色，形之圆锐亦二种；又有无核者。味甘，性平，无毒。又有一种蘡薁，真相似，然蘡薁乃是千岁藥，但山人一概收而酿酒。

救饥：采葡萄为果食之，又熟时取汁以酿酒饮。

治病：文具《本草·果部》条下。

350. Putao［葡萄，grape，Vitis vinifera L.］

Putao［葡萄，grape，Vitis vinifera L.］grows in the valleys of the west of

Mount Long and other places like Wuyuan, Dunhuang, and in the east of the Yellow River. According to the legend, Zhang Qian, an Ambassador of Han Dynasty who paid a visit to the Western territories, brought back the grape seeds and then planted them in the central plains. Grapes used to be regarded as the most valuable fruit in the north, and can be seen everywhere presently. The grapes belong to a kind of liana, and the vines are very long and big. One or two thriving plants can stretch across the valleys. With some lobes at the fringe, its leaves are like those of Sigua［丝瓜, loofa, Luffa cylindrica (L.) Roem.］, very large. Its flowers are small and yellowish white. There are purple and white kinds of fruit. The shape is round or oval, and some are seedless. It is sweet in taste, neutral in nature and non-toxic. Yingyu［蘡薁, wild grape, Vitis bryoniifolia Bunge］, a kind of grape ivy, is indeed similar to grapes, and is used to make wine by residents in the mountains.

For famine relief: The grape is edible as a kind of fruit, and it can be made wine by extracting its juice when it is ripe.

For disease treatment: See the relevant clause in *Materia Medica · Herbaceous Fruit*.

351. 李子树

本草有李核人。旧不载所出州土，今处处有之。其树大，高丈余。叶似郁李子叶，微尖䔲，而润泽光俊。开白花，结实种类甚多，见《尔雅》者有：休，无实李，李之无实者，一名赵李李。痤，接虑李，即今之麦李，细实有沟道，与麦同熟，故名之。驳，赤李，其子赤者是也。又有青李、绿李、赤李、房陵李、朱仲李、马肝李、黄李、紫李、水李、散见书传，美其味之可食，皆不入药。今有穿条红、御黄子。其李实味甘、微苦，一云味酸。核人味苦，性平，俱无毒。

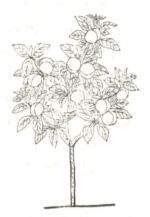

救饥：摘取李实色熟者食之。不可临水上食，亦不可和蜜食，损五脏。及与雀肉同食，和浆水食，令人霍乱、涩气。多食，令人虚热。

治病：文具《本草·果部》李核人[1]条下。

【注释】

[1] 现指李核仁。

351. Lizishu [李子树, plum tree, Prunus salicina Lindl.]

Lizishu [李子树, plum tree, Prunus salicina Lindl.] is also named Liheren. There was no record about its origin in ancient times, but it can be seen everywhere presently. The plum tree is about one Zhang high. Its leaves are like those of Yulizi [郁李子, cerasus japonica, Cerasus japonica (Thunb.) Lois.], slightly sharp, nourishing and lustrous. Its flowers are white, and there are many kinds of fruits. According to *Er Ya* [《尔雅》, *Literary Expositor*], for instance, among all kinds of plums, there is one kind without its fruit called Zhaolili. With small fruit, it is known as "Maili", because it ripens with wheat. Chili is known for its red fruit. Others are Qingli, Lvli, Shuili, etc., described in different kinds of books or bibliographies. Plums are delicious and edible, but they can not be used as medicine. Chuantiaohong and Yuhuangzi are two species among the plums, and they are sweet and slightly bitter in taste. It is also said to be sour in taste. The kernel is bitter in taste, neutral in nature and non-toxic.

For famine relief: The ripe plum is edible. It is not edible if it floats on the water. It may do harm to five-zang organs if eaten with honey. Besides, it may cause cholera and astringent qi with sparrow meat and berry soup. Eating too many plums will cause spleen deficiency and dampness-heat syndrome.

For disease treatment: See the clause of Liheren[1] [李核仁, plum, Prunus salicina lindl.] in *Materia Medica · Herbaceous Fruit*.

[Notes]

[1] Presently it refers to Liheren [李核仁, plum, Prunus salicina lindl.].

352. 木　瓜

生蜀中并山阴兰亭，其宣州者佳，今处处有之。其树枝状似柰。花深红色。叶又似柿叶，微小而厚，《尔雅》谓之楙。其实形如小瓜；又似栝楼而小，两头尖长，淡黄色。味酸，性温，无毒。

救饥:采成熟木瓜食之,多食亦不益人。

治病:文具《本草·果部》条下。

352. Mugua［木瓜, pawpaw, Chaenomeles sinensis（Thouin）Koehne］

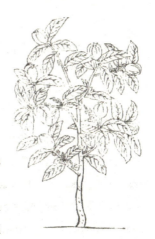

Mugua［木瓜, pawpaw, Chaenomeles sinensis（Thouin）Koehne］, growing in the middle of Sichuan Province and Lanting of Zhejiang Province, can be seen everywhere presently. Especially, the breed from Xuanzhou is of good quality. Its trees and branches are like those of Nai［柰, apple, Malmpumila Mill.］. Its flowers are crimson. Its leaves are like those of persimmon tree, but a little smaller and thicker than the latter. In *Er Ya*［《尔雅》, *Literary Expositor*］, it is called Mao. The shape of its fruit is like that of Xiaogua［小瓜, zucchini, Cucurbita pepo L］, besides it is also like Gualou［栝楼, trichosanthes, Trichosanthes kirilowii Maxim.］but a little smaller. It is sharp and long at both ends, light yellow. It is sour in taste, warm in nature and non-toxic.

For famine relief: The ripe pawpaw is edible, but eating too much is not beneficial.

For disease treatment: See the relevant clause in *Materia Medica · Herbaceous Fruit*.

353. 楂子树

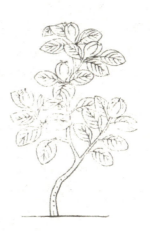

旧不著所出州土,今巩县[1]赵峰山野中多有之。树高丈许。叶似冬青树叶稍阔厚,背色微黄,叶形又类棠梨叶,但厚。结果似木瓜,稍团,味酸甜、微涩,性平。

救饥:果熟时采摘食之,多食损齿及筋。

治病:文具《本草·果部》木瓜条下。

【注释】

[1] 明代县名,属河南府,1991年改设巩义市。

353. Zhazishu [楂子树, cydonia oblonga, Cydonia oblonga Mill.]

There was no record about its origin in ancient times. Zhazishu [楂子树, cydonia oblonga, Cydonia oblonga Mill.] grows in the mountainous regions or fields of Mount Zhaofeng, Gongxian County[1]. The tree is one Zhang high. Its leaves are like those of Dongqing [冬青, holly tree, Ilex chinensis Sims], but a little wider and thicker than the latter. The leaves at the back are light yellow. Its leaves are like those of Tangli [棠梨, Birchleaf pear Pyrus betulaefolia], but a little thicker. Its fruit is like that of Mugua [木瓜, pawpaw, Chaenomeles sinensis (Thouin) Koehne], but slightly round. It is sour, sweet and a little bitter in taste, and neutral in nature.

For famine relief: Its ripe fruit is edible, but eating too much will do harm to teeth and muscle tendon.

For disease treatment: See the clause of Mugua [木瓜, pawpaw, Chaenomeles sinensis (Thouin) Koehne] in *Materia Medica · Herbaceous Fruit*.

【Notes】

[1] The name of an ancient county. Presently it refers to Gongyi City in Henan Province.

354. 郁李子

本草郁李人，一名爵李，一名车下李，一名雀梅，即奥李也，俗名櫍梨儿。生隰州[1]高山川谷丘陵上，今处处有之。木高四五尺。枝条花叶皆似李，惟子小。其花或白或赤，结实似樱桃，赤色。其人味酸，性平；一云味苦、辛。其实味甘、酸。根性凉。俱无毒。

救饥：其实红熟时摘取食之，酸甜味美。

治病：文具《本草·木部》郁李人[2]条下。

【注释】

[1] 现指郁李仁。

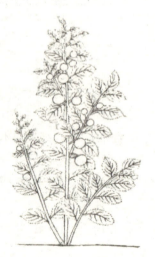

354. Yulizi [郁李子, cerasus japonica, Cerasus japonica (Thunb.) Lois.]

Yulizi [郁李子, cerasus japonica, Cerasus japonica (Thunb.) Lois.] is also named Yuliren, Jueli, Chexiali, Quemei and Aoli, and Ouli'er is its trivial name. Growing the valleys where there is flowing water in the mountains in Xizhou[1], it can be seen everywhere presently. The tree is 4~5 Chi high, its twigs, flowers and leaves are like those of Lizi [李子, plum, Prunus salicina lindl.], and only its fruit is smaller than the latter. Its flowers are white or red, and its red fruit is like that of Yingtao [樱桃, cherry, Cerasus pseudocerasus Lindl.]. Its kernel is sour in taste and neutral in nature. It is also said to be bitter and pungent in taste. Its fruit is sweet and sour in taste. Its roots are cool in nature; all the kernel, fruit and roots are non-toxic.

For famine relief: It tastes sweet and sour when the fruit turns red and ripe.

For disease treatment: See the clause of Yuliren [郁李仁, cerasus japonica, Cerasus japonica (Thunb.) Lois.] in *Materia Medica · Herbaceous Fruit*.

【Notes】

[1] The name of an ancient county.

[2] Presently it refers to Yuliren [郁李仁, cerasus japonica, Cerasus japonica (Thunb.) Loisel.].

355. 菱 角

本草名芰实,一名菱。处处有之。水中拖蔓生,叶浮水上,三尖锯齿叶。开黄白花,花落而实生。实有二种,一种四角,一种两角,两角中又有嫩皮而紫色者,谓之浮菱,食之尤美。味甘。性平,无毒。一云性冷。

救饥:采菱角鲜大者,去壳生食。壳老及杂小者,煮熟食。或晒其实,火燔以为米充粮。作粉极白润,宜人。服食家蒸暴,蜜和饵之,断谷长生。又云,杂白蜜食,令人生虫。一云多食脏冷,损阳气,痿茎,腹胀满。暖姜酒饮,或含吴茱萸,咽津液即消。

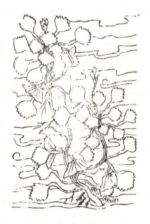

治病:文具《本草·果部》芰实条下。

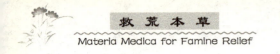

355. Lingjiao [菱角, water chestnut, Trapa natans L.]

Lingjiao [菱角, water chestnut, Trapa natans L.], also named Jishi and Ling, can be seen everywhere presently. It is decumbent in water, and its triangular leaves with serrate fringe are floating on the water. Its flowers are yellowish white. The fruit comes after flowering. There are two kinds of fruits: one has four horns, and the other has two horns. The kind of Fuling that is known for its tender and purple peels is especially delicious. It is sweet in taste, neutral in nature and non-toxic. It is also said to be cold in nature.

For famine relief: Collect and remove the husk of freshwater chestnut, and then the husk can be cooked after it turns cluttered and small. Or dry the fruit in the sunshine and then roast them into rice as the food. They can be eaten after their being made powder. Steam the water chestnut and then dry them in the sunshine, and flavor them with honey. It will make people live without food for a long time. It is also said that it will make people have parasites in the stomach after their being flavored with jaggery. Another saying goes like that eating them too much will make people cold in five-zang organs and do harm to yang qi, and cause abdominal distension or flaccid paralysis. The syndrome will disappear after drinking ginger wine or swallowing Wuzhuyu [吴茱萸, medicinal evodia fruit, ruticarpum (A. Juss.) T. G. Hartley] with fluid.

For disease treatment: See the clause of Jishi [菱实, water chestnut, Trapa natans L.] in *Materia Medica · Herbaceous Fruit*.

新增
New Supplements

356. 软 枣

一名丁香柿，又名牛乳柿，又呼羊矢枣，《尔雅》谓之梬。旧不载所出州土，今北土多有之。其树枝叶条干皆类柿，而结实甚小，干熟则紫黑色，味甘，性温。一云微寒，无毒。多食动风，发冷风咳嗽。

救饥:采取软枣成熟者食之,其未熟结硬时摘取,以温水渍养,酭去涩味。另以水煮熟食之。

356. Ruanzao〔软枣, diospyros lotus, Diospyros lotus L.〕

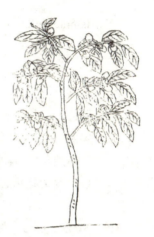

Ruanzao〔软枣, diospyros lotus, Diospyros lotus L.〕is also named Dingxiangshi, Niurushi, Yangshizao and Ying in *Er Ya*〔《尔雅》, *Literary Expositor*〕. There was no record of its origin in ancient times, and nowadays it is widely planted in the north. The sticks, branches and twigs, leaves and trunks are like those of Shishu〔柿树, persimmon tree, Diospyros kaki Thunb.〕, but its fruit is small, which will turn purple and black when it is ripe. It is sweet in taste and warm in nature. It is also said to be slightly cold in nature and non-toxic. Eating too much will cause wind stiring, such as cough.

For famine relief: Eat the ripe fruit or collect the unripe fruit to soak in water to remove the bitterness. Or cook the fruit in water for food.

357. 野葡萄

俗名烟黑。生荒野中,今处处有之。茎叶及实俱似家葡萄,但皆细小。实亦稀疏,味酸。

救饥:采葡萄颗紫熟者食之,亦中酿酒饮。

357. Yeputao〔野葡萄, wild grape, Vitis bryoniifolia Bunge〕

Yeputao〔野葡萄, wild grape, Vitis bryoniifolia Bunge〕, also named Yanhei, grows in the wilderness, and presently it can be seen everywhere. Its stems, leaves and fruit are like those of Putao〔葡萄, grape, Vitis vinifera L.〕, but small and thin. The fruit is also sparse, and tastes sour.

For famine relief: Collect the purple and ripe fruit to eat or to make wine.

358. 梅杏树

生辉县太行山山谷中。树高丈余。叶似杏叶而小,又颇尖艄,微涩,边有细锯齿。开白花。结实如杏实大,生青熟则黄色,味微酸。

救饥:摘取黄熟梅杏果食之。

358. Meixingshu [梅杏树, plum apricot tree, Armeniaca limeixing J. Y. Zhang et Z. M. Wang]

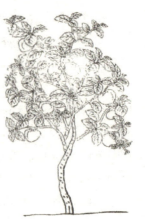

Meixingshu [梅杏树, plum apricot tree, Armeniaca limeixing J. Y. Zhang et Z. M. Wang] grows in the valleys of Mount Taihang in Huixian County. The tree is more than one Zhang high. Its leaves, with fine serrations on the edge, are like those of Xing [杏, apricot, Armeniaca vulgaris Lam.], but much smaller, slightly sharp and rough. Its flowers are white. Its fruit is as big as an apricot. The raw fruit is green, but it will turn yellow when it becomes ripe. It is sour in taste.

For famine relief: Collect the ripe fruit to eat.

359. 野樱桃

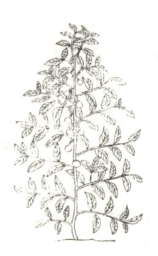

生钧州山谷中。树高五六尺。叶似李叶更尖。开白花,似李子花。结实比樱桃又小,熟则色鲜红,味甘、微酸。

救饥:摘取其果红熟者食之。

359. Yeyingtao [野樱桃, nanking cherry, Cerasus tomentosa (Thunb.) Wall.]

Yeyingtao [野樱桃, nanking cherry, Cerasus tomentosa (Thunb.) Wall.] grows in the valleys of Junzhou. The tree is 5～6 Chi high. Its leaves are like those of Lishu [李树, plum tree, Prunus salicina Lindl.], but sharper than the latter. So are its flowers. Its flowers are white. Its fruit is as small as a cherry. It will become bright red as soon as it becomes ripe. It is sweet and slightly sour in taste.

For famine relief: Collect the ripe fruit to eat.

叶及实皆可食

《本草》原有

Leaf and Fruit Edible
Original Ones

360. 石 榴

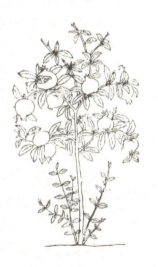

本草名安石榴,一名丹若,《广雅》谓之若榴。旧云汉张骞使西域得其种还,今处处有之。木不甚高大,枝柯附干,自地便生作丛,种极易成,折其枝条,盘土中便生。其叶似枸杞叶而长,微尖,叶绿,微带红色。花有黄赤二色。实亦有甘酸二种,甘者可食,酸者入药。味甘、酸,性温,无毒。又有一种,子白,莹澈如水晶者,味亦甘,谓之水晶石榴。

救饥:采嫩叶煠熟,油盐调食。榴果熟时,摘取食之。不可多食,损人肺[1]又及损齿令黑。

治病:文具《本草·果部》条下。

【注释】

[1] 即肺损,病名。

360. Shiliu [石榴, pomegranate, Punica granatum L.]

Shiliu [石榴, pomegranate, Punica granatum L.] is also named Anshiliu, Danruo and Ruoliu according to *Guang Ya* [《广雅》, *Supplement to Literary Expositor*]. It is said that Zhang Qian, an ambassador of Han Dynasty, brought back the pomegranate species when he came back from the Western region in ancient times. Presently, it is planted everywhere. Its branches are close to the trunk that is not too tall. They grow out of the ground and are easy to be alive when its branches are folded off and cut into the soil. Its leaves are like those of Gouqi [枸杞, barbary wolfberry fruit, Lycium chinense Mill.], but longer, slightly sharp; besides, the leaves are green and slightly reddish, and there are two kinds of flowers, yellow and red. The fruit also has two kinds: The sweet kind can be eaten, and the sour kind can be used as medicine. It is sweet and sour in taste, warm in nature and non-toxic. Another kind (the seeds are white, just like the crystal, and sweet in taste) is called crystal pomegranate.

For famine relief: Collect young leaves, blanch and elutriate them in hot water, and then flavor them with oil and salt. The ripe fruit can be eaten, but do not eat much, otherwise it will cause lung injury[1] and make teeth black.

For disease treatment: See the relevant clause in *Materia Medica · Herbaceous Fruit*.

【Notes】

[1] The name of a disease.

361. 杏 树

本草有杏核人。生晋山川谷,今处处有之。其实有数种,黄而圆者名金杏,熟最早。扁而青黄者名木杏,其子皆入药。又小者名山杏,不堪入药。其树高丈余,叶颇圆,淡绿,颇带红色。叶似木葛叶而光嫩,微尖。开花色红,结实金黄色。核人味甘、苦,性温,冷利,有毒。得火良,恶黄芩、黄耆、葛根,解锡毒,畏蘘

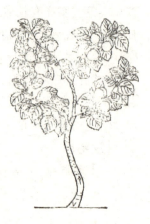

草。杏实味酸,性热。

救饥:采叶煠熟,以水浸渍,作成黄色,换水淘净,油盐调食。其杏黄熟时摘取食。不可多食,令人发热及伤筋骨。

治病:文具《本草·果部》杏核人[1]条下。

【注释】

[1] 现指杏核仁。

361. Xingshu [杏树, apricot tree, Armeniaca vulgaris Lam]

Xingshu [杏树, apricot tree, Armeniaca vulgaris Lam.], also named Xingheren, grows in the valleys where there is flowing water in Mount Jin, and it can be seen everywhere now. There are many kinds of fruits. Jinxing is yellow and round, which becomes ripe as early as possible. Muxing is flat and greenish yellow. The seeds of these two kinds can be used as medicine. Another kind is named Shanxing. It is small, and its seeds can not be used as medicine. The tree is more than one Zhang high; its leaves are quite round, greenish and more reddish. Its leaves are like those of Muge [木葛, muge medicinal, Materia Medica Muge], but relatively bright, soft and tender, and slightly sharp. Its flowers are red, and its fruit is golden yellow. Its kernel is sweet and bitter in taste, warm and cold in nature and toxic. In compatibility, it is averse to Huangqin [黄芩, Radix Scutellariae, Baical Skullcap Root], Gegen [葛根, kudzuvine root, Radix Puerariae] and detoxifies Xi poison, and it is restrained by Rangcao [蘘草, Rhizome of Mioga Ginger, Zingiber mioga Thunb. Rosc.]. Its fruit is sour in taste and hot in nature.

For famine relief: Collect and blanch young leaves, soak and clean them in water, and then flavor them with oil and salt. The ripe fruit when it becomes yellow can be eaten, but do not eat much, otherwise it will make people feel feverish and hurt people's muscles and bones.

For disease treatment: See the clause of Xingheren[1] [杏核人, apricot, Armeniaca vulgaris Lam] in *Materia Medica · Herbaceous Fruit*.

[Notes]

[1] Presently it refers to Xingheren [杏核仁, apricot, Armeniaca vulgaris Lam].

362. 枣 树

本草有大枣,干枣也。一名美枣,一名良枣。生枣出河东平泽及近北州郡,青[1]、晋[2]、绛[3]、蒲州[4]者特佳,江南出者,坚燥少肉。树高一二丈。叶似酸枣叶而大,比皂角叶亦大,尖艄光泽,叶间开青黄色小花,结实种数甚多。《尔雅》云:壶枣,江东呼枣大而锐上者为壶,壶犹瓠也。边,腰枣,一名细腰,又谓辘轳枣。櫅,白枣,即今枣子,白乃熟。遵,羊枣,实小而圆,紫黑色,俗又呼为羊矢枣[5]。洗,大枣,河东猗氏县[6]出大枣,如鸡卵。蹶泄,苦枣,云子味苦。晳,无实枣,云不著子者。还味,稔枣,云还味,短味也。又有水菱枣、御枣,

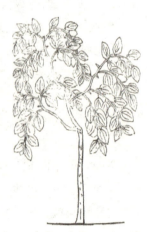

即扑落苏也。又有牙枣。皆味甘美。其余不能尽别其名。大枣味甘,性平,无毒。杀乌头毒。牙齿有病人切忌食。生枣味甘、辛。多食令人寒热腹胀,羸瘦人不可食。蒸煮食,补肠胃,肥中益气。不宜合葱食。

救饥:采嫩叶煤熟,水浸作成黄色,淘净,油盐调食。其枣红熟时摘取食之。其结生硬未红时,煮食亦可。

治病:文具《本草·果部》大枣条下。

【注释】

[1] 古代州名,见《图经本草》。

[2] 古代州名,见《图经本草》。

[3] 古代州名,见《图经本草》。

[4] 见孟诜《食疗本草》。

[5] 即软枣,见本书第356软枣条。

[6] 古代县名,见《图经本草》。

362. Zaoshu [枣树, jujube tree, Ziziphus jujuba Mill.]

Zaoshu [枣树, jujube tree, Ziziphus jujuba Mill.], also named Dazao, Ganzao, Meizao and Liangzao, is produced from the flat wetlands of the east of the river and some counties in the north, especially those produced in Qingzhou[1],

Jinzhou[2], Jiangzhou[3] and Puzhou[4] are of good quality; whereas, those growing in the south of Yangtze River are hard and dried, with less flesh. The tree is 1~2 Zhang high. Its leaves, sharp and shiny, are like those of Suanzao [酸枣, wild jujube, Ziziphus jujuba Mill. var. spinosa (Bunge) Hu ex H. F. Chow], but bigger than the latter and soap pods. The greenish yellow flowers grow in the middle of leaves. There are many kinds of fruits.

According to *Er Ya* [《尔雅》, *Literary Expositor*], Huzao is named after its shape by people in Jiangdong, because this kind is sharp on the top and big in the bottom, just like a jug. Yaozao, thin in the middle, is also named Luluzao. Baizao refers to the current jujube that is familiar to people, and this kind of jujube becomes white when it is ripe. The fruit of Yangzao is small and round, dark purple. So it is also named Yangshizao[5]. Dazao, mainly growing in Yishi County[6] of Hedong, is as big as an egg. Kuzao is named after its taste, which is bitter. Wushizao refers to the kind that does not have fruit. Renzao means this kind of jujube is lacking taste. Here are also many other kinds, such as Shuilingzao, Yuzao (Puluosu) and Yazao. They are all sweet and tasty. Many other kinds can not be identified by their names.

It is sweet in taste, neutral in nature and non-toxic. In compatibility, it suppresses the toxicity of Wutou [乌头, common Monkshood Mother Root, Aconitum carmichaeli Debx.]. People who have teeth problems are not suitable to eat it. It is sweet and pungent in taste. Excessive consumption can make people suffer from deficiency of Yang or abdominal swelling. Those who are feeble or thin are not allowed to eat it. Steaming can treat the deficiency of the intestines and stomach. Do not eat with scallion.

For famine relief: Collect and blanch young leaves, soak and clean them in water, and flavor them with oil and salt. The ripe fruit is edible after becoming red. When the fruit is not ripe yet, it can be cooked.

For disease treatment: See the clause of Dazao [大枣, jujube, Ziziphus jujuba Mill.] in *Materia Medica · Herbaceous Fruit*.

【Notes】

[1] The name of an ancient county. See *Tu Jing Ben Cao* [《图经本草》, *Illustrated Classics of Materia Medica*].

〔2〕The name of an ancient county. See *Tu Jing Ben Cao*〔《图经本草》, Illustrated Classics of Materia Medica〕.

〔3〕The name of an ancient county. See *Tu Jing Ben Cao*〔《图经本草》, Illustrated Classics of Materia Medica〕.

〔4〕The name of an ancient county. See *Shi Liao Ben Cao*〔《食疗本草》, Materia Medica for Dietotherapy〕.

〔5〕Another name for Ruanzao〔软枣, diospyros lotust, Diospyros lotus L.〕. See the 356th clause of this book.

〔6〕The name of an ancient county. See *Tu Jing Ben Cao*〔《图经本草》, Illustrated Classic of Materia Medica〕.

363. 桃 树

本草有桃核人。生太山川谷,河南、陕西出者尤大而美,今处处有之。树高丈余。叶状似柳叶而阔大,又多纹脉。开花红色,结实品类甚多。其油桃光小,金桃色深黄,昆仑桃肉深紫红色。又有饼子桃、面桃、鹰嘴桃、雁过红桃、冻桃之类,名多不能尽载。山中有一种桃,正是《月令》中桃始华者,谓山桃不堪食啖,但中入药。桃核人味苦、甘,性平,无毒。

救饥:采嫩叶煤熟,水浸作成黄色,换水淘净,油盐调食。桃实熟软时,摘取食之。其结硬未熟时,亦可煮食。或切作片,晒干为糁,收藏备用。

治病:文具《本草·果部》桃核人条下。

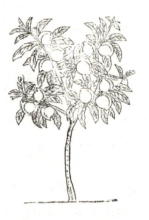

363. Taoshu〔桃树, peach tree, Amygdalus persica L.〕

Taoshu〔桃树, peach tree, Amygdalus persica L.〕, also named Taoheren, grows in the valleys where there is flowing water in Mount Tai. Those produced in Henan Province and Shaanxi Province are especially large and delicious, and they are distributed everywhere. The tree is more than one Zhang high; its leaves are like those of the willow tree, but wider and bigger, with more veins. Its flowers are red, and there are many kinds of fruits. Nectarine is shiny and small, the color of the golden peach is dark yellow, and the flesh of Kunlun peach is dark purple. There are also Bingzitao, Miantao, Yingzuitao, Yanguo Hongtao, Dongtao and many other varieties. It could not be recorded one by one. There is one kind of peaches growing in the mountains and wilderness, and it is called Shantao [山桃, amygdalus davidiana, Amygdalus davidiana (Carri.) de Vos ex L. Henry], which is flowering earliest, with its origin dating back to the record of "The Monthly Order", the sixth chapter in *The Book of Rites*. It is not edible, but it is suitable for being used as medicine. The peach kernel is bitter and sweet in taste, neutral in nature and non-toxic.

For famine relief: Collect and blanch young leaves, soak and clean them in water, and flavor them with oil and salt. The ripe fruit is edible after becoming soft. When the fruit is not ripe yet, it can be cooked, or cut into pieces, dried for food, and stored for future.

For disease treatment: See the clause of Hetaoren [桃核人, peach kernel, Amygdalus persica L.] in *Materia Medica · Herbaceous Fruit*.

新增

New Supplements

364. 沙果子树

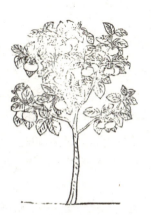

一名花红。南北皆有，今中牟岗野中亦有之，人家园圃亦多栽种。树高丈余。叶似樱桃叶而色深绿；又似急藨子[1]叶而大。开粉红花，似桃花瓣，微长不尖。结实似李而甚大，味甘、微酸。

救饥：摘取红熟果食之。嫩叶亦可爆熟，油盐调食。

【注释】

[1] 吉利子的别名。见本书第306吉利子树条。

364. Shaguozi Shu［沙果子树, crab apple, Malus asiatica Nakai］

Shaguozi Shu［沙果子树, crab apple, Malus asiatica Nakai］, growing in the north and south, is also named Huahong. Presently it can be seen in the wilderness of hills in Zhongmu, and it is planted in the gardens of commn people. The tree is more than one Zhang high. Its leaves are like those of Yingtao［樱桃, cherry, Cerasus pseudocerasus］, but dark green, and like those of Jimeizi[1]［急蘼子, root of Bilobed Grewia, Radix grewiae bilobae］, but larger. Its petals of pinkish red flowers are like those of peach, but longer and not sharp. Its fruit is like that of Lizi［李子, plum, Prunus salicina Lindl.］, but larger than the latter. It is sweet and slightly sour in taste.

For famine relief: Collect ripe fruit, or blanch and elutriate young leaves in hot water, and then flavor them with oil and salt.

【Notes】

［1］Another name of Jilizi. See the 306th clause of this book.

根可食

《本草》原有

Root Edible

Original Ones

365. 芋 苗

本草一名土芝，俗名芋头。生田野中，今处处有之，人家多栽种。叶似小荷[1]叶而偏长不圆，近蒂边皆有一剜儿。根状如鸡弹大，皮色茶褐，其中白色，味辛，性平，有小毒。叶冷，无毒。

救饥：《本草》芋有六种，青芋细长，毒多，初煮须要灰汁，换水煮熟乃堪食。白芋、真芋、连禅芋、紫芋毒少，蒸煮食之。又宜冷食，疗热，止渴。野芋大毒，不堪食也。

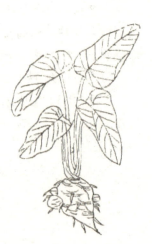

治病：文具《本草·果部》条下。

【注释】

［1］见本书第367莲藕条。

365. Yumiao［芋苗, taro roots, Colocasia esculenta（L.）Schoot］

Yumiao［芋苗, taro roots, Colocasia esculenta（L.）Schoot］, also named Tuzhi and Yutou, growing in the fields, can be seen everywhere presently. Its leaves are like the small lotus[1] leaves, especially long but not round. The leaves have a cornice on one side of the petiole. Its roots, namely taro roots, are as big as eggs. Its bark is dark brown with white flesh. It is pungent in taste, neutral in nature and mildly toxic. Its leaves are cold in nature and mildly toxic.

For famine relief：There are six varieties of Yu［芋, sweet potato/taro roots, Colocasia esculenta（L.）Schoot］in the materia medica. Qingyu, slender and long, has toxicity. The first time it must be cooked with the plant ash juice, and then change water to cook it again. Another four varieties, including Baiyu, Zhenyu, Lianchanyu and Ziyu, which have mild toxicity, are edible after steaming. They are also suitable to heal and quench thirst as the cold food, but Yeyu is not edible because of its strong toxicity.

For disease treatment：See the relevant clause in *Materia Medica · Herbaceous Fruit*.

【Notes】

［1］See the 367th clause of this book.

366. 铁葧脐

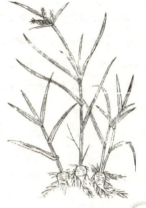

本草名乌芋，又名茨茨，一名藉姑、一名水萍、一名槎牙，亦名茨菰，又名燕尾草，《尔雅》谓之芍。有二种：根黑、皮厚、肉硬白者谓之猪葧脐；皮薄、色淡紫、肉软者谓之羊葧脐。生水田中。叶似莎草而厚肥，梢又长窄。叶间生葶，其葶三棱，梢头开花酱褐色。根即葧脐，味苦、甘，性微寒。

救饥:采根煮熟食,制作粉,食之厚人肠胃,不饥。服丹石人尤宜食,解丹石毒[1]。孕妇不可食。

治病:文具《本草·果部》乌芋条下。

【注释】

[1] 证名。其证头眩耳鸣,发热困笃,恐惧不安。多为服丹药和诸石后产生的副作用。

366. Tieboqi［铁葧脐, water-chestnuts, Bolboschoenus yagara (Ohwi) Y. C. Yang et M. Zhan］

Tieboqi［铁葧脐, water-chestnuts, Bolboschoenus yagara (Ohwi) Y. C. Yang et M. Zhan］is also named Wuyu, Fuci, Jigu, Shuiping, Zhaya, Cigu, Yanweicao and Shao according to *Er Ya*［《尔雅》, *Literary Expositor*］. There are two varieties of Tieboqi. One is called Zhuboqi, which has black roots and thick peels with white and hard flesh. The other is called Yangboqi, which is thin peels with light purple and soft flesh. It grows in the paddy fields, and its leaves are like those of Shacao［莎草, cyperus rotundus, Cyperus rotundus L.］, but thicker, long and narrow in the leaf tip. Its triquetrous scapes grow out of leaves, and brown flowers are among its tip. Its roots are Boqi［葧荠, Chinese water-chestnut, Bolboschoenus yagara (Ohwi) Y. C. Yang et M. Zhan］, which are bitter and sweet in taste and slightly cold in nature.

For famine relief: Pick and cook roots or make them into powder. People will not feel hungry after eating the roots, especially for people who take Danshi, which refers to mineral-contained Chinese medicine, represented by cinnabar with strong toxicity. They can detoxify Danshi[1]. The pregnant women can not eat them.

For disease treatment: See the relevant clause of Wuyu［乌芋, water-chestnuts, Bolboschoenus yagara (Ohwi) Y. C. Yang et M. Zhan］in *Materia Medica · Herbaceous Fruit*.

[Notes]

[1] The name of a syndrome. The main symptom is that people will feel dizzy and tinnitus, fever and sleepy, full of fear, which is caused by the side effect of taking Dan and other medicine.

根及实皆可食

*《本草》原有

Root and Fruit Edible
Original Ones

367. 莲　藕

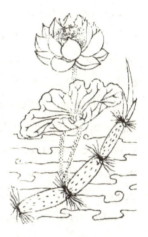

本草有藕实,一名水芝丹,一名莲。生汝南池泽,今处处有之,生水中。其叶名荷,圆径尺余。其花世谓之莲花,色有红白二种。花中结实,谓之莲房,俗名莲蓬。其莲青皮里白,子为的,即莲子也。的中青心为薏。其的至秋,表皮色黑而沉水。就蓬中干者,谓之石莲。其根谓之藕。《尔雅》云:"荷,芙蕖。其茎茄,其叶蕸,其本蔤。"云是茎下白蒻在泥中,藕节间初生萌芽也。"其华菡萏,其实莲,其根藕,其中的,的中薏。"是也。芙蕖其总名,别名芙蓉。又云,其花未发为菡萏,已发为芙蓉。莲实、茎味甘,性平、寒,无毒。

救饥:采藕煤熟食、生食皆可。莲子蒸食,或生食亦可。又可休粮,仙家贮石莲子、干藕经千年者,食之至妙。又以实磨为面食,或屑为米,加粟煮饭食,皆可。

治病:文具《本草·果部》藕实条下。

367. Lian'ou [莲藕, lotus root, Nelumbo nucifera Gaertn.]

Lian'ou [莲藕, lotus root, Nelumbo nucifera Gaertn.], also named Oushi, Shuizhidan and Lian, grows in the ponds and lakes of Runan. Presently it is commonly distributed everywhere and grows underwater. Its leaves are called He, lotus, about more than one Chi in diameter. Its flowers are called Lianhua and the lotus flowers are red or white. The centre of heart is its fruit, which is named Lianfang or lotus seedpod. Its seed peels are green, and the flesh inside is white. The fruit of its seeds is Lianzi, and the green part in the centre of its seeds is named Yi (germ). In autumn, the lotus seed skin turns black and sinks into water. The lotus seeds that are dried in the lotus are called Shilian. The root of the lotus is called Ou. According to the record in *Er Ya* [《尔雅》, *Literary Expositor*], this plant is described that "It is lotus. Its petioles are called eggplants, its leaves are called a dragonfly, and its rhizome underwater is called Lian'ou.", which refers to the germination between the scorpions that is buried in the mud under the petioles. Its flowers are called lotus blooms, its fruit is called lotus, and its root is called lotus root. The seeds in the fruit are called lotus seeds, and the central part of the lotus seeds is called Yi (germ). Fuqu, the general name of this plant, is also called Furong. It is also said that the flowers which are ready to bloom are called Handan, and those which are in bloom are called Furong. Its fruit and roots are sweet in taste, neutral and cold in nature and non-toxic.

For famine relief: Roots can be eaten or cooked. So can its seeds. People may stop eating grain food, but eat the stone lotus seeds and dried lotus roots which are stored in the room where people worship the god, and even after thousands of years, it is still very delicious. Or the lotus is ground into flour or powder to make the congee with millets.

For disease treatment: See the clause of Oushi [藕实, lotus root, *Nelumbo nucifera* Gaertn.] in *Materia Medica · Herbaceous Fruit*.

368. 鸡头实

一名芡,一名雁喙实,幽人谓之雁头。出雷泽,今处处有之,生泽中。叶大如荷而皱,背紫有刺,俗谓鸡头盘,花下结实,形类鸡头,故以名之。中有子,如皂荚子大,艾褐色,其近根茎萩嫩者名蒻,人采以为菜茹。实味甘,性平,无毒。

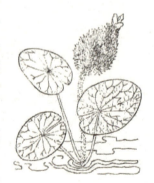

救饥:采嫩根茎煤食。实熟采实,剥人食之。蒸过,烈日晒之,其皮即开,春去皮,捣人为粉,蒸煤作饼,皆可食。多食不益脾胃气,兼难消化。生食动风、冷气,与小儿食不能长大,故驻年耳。

治病:文具《本草·果部》条下。

368. Jitoushi [鸡头实, euryale ferox, Euryale ferox Salisb.]

Jitoushi [鸡头实, euryale ferox, Euryale ferox Salisb.], also named Qian, Yanhuishi and Yantou by the people in Youzhou, once grew in the northeast of Leizhe, but it can be commonly seen everywhere presently and grows in the ponds and lakes. Its leaves are as big as the lotus leaves, but rugose. It is purple at the back of leaves with thorns, so it is also called Jitoupan. Its fruit grows under the flowers, and the ovary is inflated, which is shaped like a chicken head, so it is named after Jitoushi. There are brown seeds in the fruit, as big as the seeds of soap pods. Its young petioles near the roots are called Weigeng, which can be edible as a kind of vegetables. Its fruit is sweet in taste, neutral in nature and non-toxic.

For famine relief: Collect young leaves, blanch and elutriate them in hot water. Collect the ripe fruit, and peel out the kernel. Dry them in the sunshine after steaming, and the seed coat will split open; remove the peels and grind the kernel into powder; and then steam, blanch and cook them to make pancakes. It is not beneficial for the qi of spleen, stomach and digestion if eating them too much. It will lead to wind stiring and syndrome caused by cold. Children will remain young after eating them, so it is thought to protect people from dying early and prolong people's life-span.

For disease treatment: See the relevant clause in *Materia Medica · Herbaceous Fruit*.

菜 部

叶可食

* 《本草》原有

Herbaceous Vegetable
Leaf Edible
Original Ones

369. 芸薹菜

今处处有。叶似菠菜叶,比菠菜叶两傍多两叉。开黄花,结角似蔓菁角。有子如小芥子大。味辛,性温,无毒。经冬根不死,辟蠹。

救饥:采苗叶煠熟,水浸,淘洗净,油盐调食。

治病:文具《本草·菜部》条下。

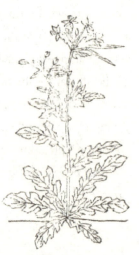

369. Yuntaicai〔芸薹菜, brassica campestris, Brassica campestris L. var. campestris〕

Yuntaicai〔芸薹菜, brassica campestris, Brassica campestris L. var. campestris〕can be seen everywhere presently. Its leaves are like those of Bocai〔菠菜, spinach, Spinacia oleracea L.〕. There are two bifurcations on each side of the leaf compared with the spinach leaf. Its flowers are yellow, and its fruit is like the silique of Manjing〔蔓菁, turnip, Brassica rapa Linn.〕. Its seeds are as small as those of the mustard. It is pungent in taste, warm in nature and non-toxic. Its roots will be in good condition even in winter and also keep the moth away.

For famine relief: Collect young seedlings and leaves, soak and clean them in fresh water, and then flavor them with oil and salt.

For disease treatment: See the relevant clause in *Materia Medica · Herbaceous Vegetable*.

370. 苋 菜

本草有苋实,一名马苋,一名莫实,细苋亦同,一名人苋,幽蓟间人讹呼为人杏菜。生淮阳川泽及田中,今处处有之。苗高一二尺。茎有线楞。叶如小蓝叶而大,有赤白二色。家者茂盛而大,野者细小,叶薄。味甘,性寒,无毒。不可与鳖肉同食,生鳖瘕。

救饥:采苗叶煠熟,水淘洗净,油盐调食。晒干煠食尤佳。

治病:文具《本草·菜部》条下。

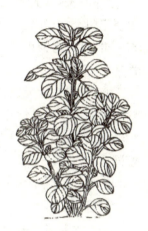

370. Xiancai〔苋菜, amaranth, Amaranthus tricolor〕

Xiancai〔苋菜, amaranth, Amaranthus tricolor〕is also named Xianshi, Maxian, Moshi, Xixian and Renxian. The people in Youji called it Renxingcai by mistake. Growing near the marshes or lakes in Huaiyang or in the fields, it can be seen everywhere presently. Its plants are 1~2 Chi high with string-angulate stems. Its leaves are like those of Xiaolan〔小蓝, vanda coerulescens, Vanda coerulescens Griff.〕but relatively bigger than the latter. There are red or white leaves. Those planted at home are big, but those planted in the wilderness are small and its leaves are thin. It is sweet in taste, cold in nature and non-toxic. Do not eat it with turtle meat, or it may cause Biejia, a syndrome of abdominal mass, or it will lead to stomachache.

For famine relief: Collect young seedlings and leaves, blanch and elutriate them in fresh water, and then flavor them with oil and salt. Especially, it is delicious to blanch after drying them.

For disease treatment: See the relevant clause in *Materia Medica · Herbaceous Vegetable*.

371. 苦苣菜

《本草》云即野苣也,又名䉺苣,俗名天精菜。旧不著所出州土,今处处有之。苗搨地生,其叶光者似黄花苗[1]叶;叶花者似山苦荬[2]叶,茎叶中皆有白汁,味苦,性平,一云性寒。

救饥:采苗叶煠熟,用水浸去苦味,淘洗净,油盐调食。生亦可食。虽性冷,甚益人,久食轻身、少睡,调十二经脉,利五脏。不可与血同食,作痔疾。一云不可与蜜同食。

治病:文具《本草·菜部》条下。

【注释】

[1] 即孛孛丁菜,见本书第 399 孛孛丁菜条。

[2] 见本书第 394 山苦荬条。

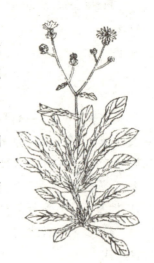

371. Kujucai〔苦苣菜, common sowthistle herb, Sonchus wightianus DC.〕

Kujucai〔苦苣菜, common sowthistle herb, Sonchus wightianus DC.〕, also named Yeju, Bianju and Tianjingcai with no record about its origin in ancient times, can be seen everywhere presently. Its plants creep on the ground. Its lustrous leaves are like those of Huanghuamiao[1]〔黄花苗, dandelion, Taraxacum mongolicum Hand.-Mazz〕, its incised leaves are like those of Shankumai[2]〔山苦荬, paraixeris denticulata, Paraixeris denticulata (Houtt.) Nakai〕, and there is white sauce in its stems and leaves. It is bitter in taste and neutral in nature. It is also said to be cold in nature.

For famine relief: Collect young leaves and seedlings, blanch them and remove the bitterness by elutriating them in water, and then flavor them with oil and salt. The raw leaves and seedlings are edible, which is beneficial, although they are cold in nature. Long-time eating will make people feel their body lighter and more energetic. It also regulates twelve meridians and benefits five-zang organs. It may lead to haemorrhoids when eaten with blood. It is also said that it can not be eaten together with honey.

For disease treatment: See the relevant clause in *Materia Medica · Herbaceous Vegetable*.

【Notes】

［1］See the 399th clause of this book.

［2］See the 394th clause of this book.

372. 马齿苋菜

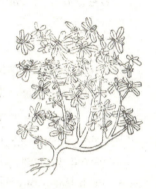

又名五行草。旧不著所出州土,今处处有之。以其叶青、梗赤、花黄、根白、子黑,故名五行草耳。味甘、性寒、滑。

救饥:采苗叶,先以水焯过,晒干,煠熟,油盐调食。

治病:文具《本草·菜部》条下。

372. Machixian Cai ［马齿苋菜, purslane herb, Portulaca oleracea L.］

Machixian Cai ［马齿苋菜, purslane herb, Portulaca oleracea L.］, also named Wuxingcao with no record about its place of origin in ancient times, can be found everywhere presently. It is named after Wuxingcao because of its green leaves, red stalks, yellow flowers, white roots and black seeds. It is sweet in taste and cold in nature, and has the drastic effect so as to cause diarrhea.

For famine relief: Collect and blanch young leaves and seedlings, and then dry them in the sunshine before elutriating, and flavor them with oil and salt.

For disease treatment: See the relevant clause in *Materia Medica · Herbaceous Vegetable*.

373. 苦荬菜

俗名老鹳菜。所在有之,生田野中。人家园圃种者为家苦荬,脚叶似白菜小叶,抪茎而生,稍叶似鸦嘴形。每叶间分叉,攛葶如穿叶状,梢间开黄花。味微苦,性冷,无毒。

救饥:采苗叶煤熟,以水浸洗淘净,油盐调食。出蚕蛾时,切不可取㧅,令蛾子赤烂,蚕妇忌食。

治病:文具《本草·菜部》条下。

373. Kumaicai［苦荬菜, field sowthistle herb, Ixeridium sonchifolium（Maxim.）Shih］

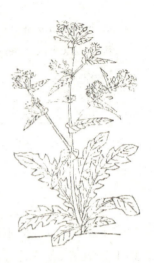

Kumaicai［苦荬菜, field sowthistle herb, Ixeridium sonchifolium（Maxim.）Shih］, also named Laoguancai, growing in the fields, can be found everywhere presently. Those cultivated in the common people's gardens are called Jiakumai. Its basal leaves are like those of Chinese cabbage, clasping with its stems. The shape of its leaves in the stems is like that of raven's bake. Each leaf is bifurcate, and the scapes look like the shape of crossing leaves. Its flowers between branches are yellow. It is slightly bitter in taste, cold in nature and non-toxic.

For famine relief: Collect and blanch leaves and seedlings, soak them in water and make them clean, and then flavor them with oil and salt. It can not be picked when the silkworm becomes the moth, because it will make the moth turn red and die. The silkworm women should abstain from eating them.

For disease treatment: See the relevant clause in *Materia Medica · Herbaceous Vegetable*.

374. 莙荙菜

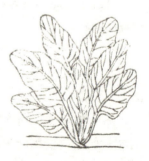

所在有之,人家园中多种。苗叶搨地生,叶类白菜而短,叶茎亦窄,叶头稍团,形状似糜匙样,味咸,性平、寒,微毒。

救饥:采苗叶煤熟,以水浸,洗净,油盐调食。不可多食,动气、破腹。

治病:文具《本草·菜部》条下。

374. Jundacai [莙荙菜, spinach beet, Beta vulgaris L. var. Cicla L.]

Jundacai [莙荙菜, spinach beet, Beta vulgaris L. var. Cicla L.], widely found everywhere presently, is planted in the common people's gardens. Its seedlings and leaves droop on the ground. Its leaves are like those of Baicai, but slightly short. Its stripes are narrow. The top of its leaves is slightly round, and its shape is like a scoop. It is salty in taste, neutral and cold in nature and non-toxic.

For famine relief: Collect and blanch leaves and seedlings, soak them in water and make them clean, and then flavor with oil and salt. It may do harm to spleen qi, or cause diarrhea if eating too much.

For disease treatment: See the relevant clause in *Materia Medica · Herbaceous Vegetable*.

375. 邪 蒿

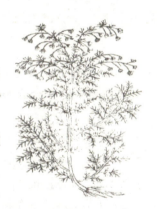

生田园中,今处处有之。苗高尺余,似青蒿,细软。叶又似胡萝卜叶,微细而多花叉,茎叶稠密。梢间开小碎瓣黄花。苗叶味辛,性温、平,无毒。

救饥:采苗叶煠熟,水浸,淘净,油盐调食。生食微动风气,作羹食良。不可同胡荽食,令人汗臭气。

治病:文具《本草·菜部》条下。

375. Xiehao [邪蒿, artemisia carvifolia, Artemisia carvifolia var. schochii (Mattf.) Pamp.]

Xiehao [邪蒿, artemisia carvifolia, Artemisia carvifolia var. schochii (Mattf.) Pamp.], growing in the fields and gardens, can be seen everywhere presently. Its plants are over one Chi high, like Qinghao [青蒿, sweet wormwood herb, Artemisia carvifolia], very slender and soft. Its leaves, which are split, are like those of carrots, but a little slender than the latter. The leaves in stems are dense, and yellow flowers bloom in twigs. Its petals are small. Its seedlings and leaves are pungent in taste, warm and neutral in nature and non-toxic.

For famine relief: Collect and blanch young leaves and seedlings, soak and clean them in water, and then flavor them with oil and salt or steam. It is better for them to be cooked as thick soup than eaten, resulting in deficiency of spleen qi. It is not allowed to eat with Husui [胡荽, coriander herb with root, Herba Coriandri Sativi cum Radice], because it will produce foul smell due to perspiration.

For disease treatment: See the clauses in *Materia Medica · Herbaceous Vegetable*.

376. 茼 蒿

处处有之，人家园圃中多种。苗高一二尺。叶类胡萝卜叶而肥大。开黄花，似菊花。味辛，性平。

救饥：采苗叶煤熟，水浸，淘净，油盐调食。不可多食，动风气，熏人心，令人气满。

治病：文具《本草·菜部》条下。

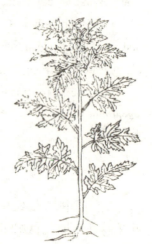

376. Tonghao [茼蒿, garland chrysanthemum, Glebionis coronaria (L.) Cass. Ex Spach]

Tonghao [茼蒿, garland chrysanthemum, Glebionis coronaria (L.) Cass. Ex Spach] can be seen everywhere presently, and especially it is widely planted in the courtyards of common people. Its plants are 1~2 Chi high, and its leaves are like those of carrots, but much stronger and lager than the latter. Its yellow flowers are like chrysanthemum. It is pungent in taste and neutral in nature.

For famine relief: Collect and blanch leaves and seedlings, soak them in water and make them clean, and flavor them with oil and salt. Do not eat them too much, or it will cause the deficiency of qi, and make people feel suffocated.

For disease treatment: See the relevant clause in *Materia Medica · Herbaceous Vegetable*.

377. 冬葵菜

本草冬葵子,是秋种葵,覆养经冬,至春结子,故谓冬葵子。生少室山,今处处有之。苗高二三尺。茎及花、叶似蜀葵而差小。子及根俱味甘,性寒,无毒。黄芩为之使。根解蜀椒毒。叶味甘,性滑利。为百菜主,其心伤人。

救饥:采叶煠熟,水浸,淘净,油盐调食。服丹石人尤宜食。天行病后食之,顿丧明。热食亦令人热闷动风。

治病:文具《本草·菜部》条下。

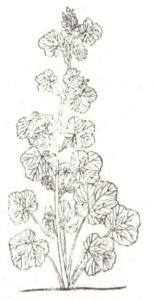

377. Dongkuicai [冬葵菜, malva verticillata, Malva verticillata L. var. Crispa L.]

Dongkuicai [冬葵菜, malva verticillata, Malva verticillata L. var. Crispa L.], also named Dongkuizi, is a kind of mallows planted in the autumn, cultivated in the whole winter, so it is also called Dongkuizi. It grew in Mount Shaoshi, and it can be seen everywhere presently. Its plants are 2~3 Chi high. Its stems, flowers and leaves are like those of Shukui [蜀葵, althaea rosea, Althaea rosea (Linn.) Cavan.], but a bit smaller than the latter. Both its seeds and roots are sweet in taste, cold in nature and non-toxic. In compatibility, Huangqin [黄芩, radix Scutellariae, Baical Skullcap Root] is its assistance. Its roots can detoxify Shujiao [蜀椒, Sichuan pepper, Zanthoxylum bungeanum Maxim.]. It is sweet in taste and has the drastic effect so as to cause diarrhea. It is regarded as one of chief vegetables of many kinds, but its central part will do harm to people.

For famine relief: Collect and blanch leaves and seedlings, soak them in water and make them clean, and flavor them with oil and salt. It is beneficial for people who take cinnabar and stone, and those who recover from epidemic diseases will be blind as soon as they eat them. People will feel stuffy if it is heated to eat.

For disease treatment: See the relevant clause in *Materia Medica · Herbaceous Vegetable*.

378. 蓼芽菜

本草有蓼实。生雷泽川泽,今处处有之。叶似小蓝叶微尖;又似水荭叶而短小,色微带红。茎微赤。梢间出穗,开花赤色。茎叶味辛,性温。

救饥:采苗叶煠熟,换水浸去辣气,淘净,油盐调食。

治病:文具《本草·菜部》蓼实条下。

378. Liaoyacai [蓼芽菜, polygonum hydropiper, Polygonum hydropiper L.]

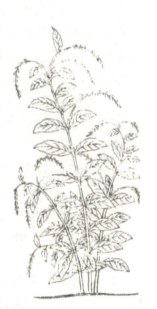

Liaoyacai [蓼芽菜, polygonum hydropiper, Polygonum hydropiper L.], also named Liaoshi, growing near the lakes or marshes in Leize, can be seen everywhere presently. Its leaves are like those of Xiaolan [小蓝, vanda coerulescens, Vanda coerulescens Griff.], but a little sharper than the latter, and like those of Shuihong [水荭, polygonum hydropiper, Polygonum hydropiper L.], shorter and smaller. Its leaves are green and slightly red, and its stems are slightly red. Its spica in the stem is red. Both its stems and leaves are pungent in taste and warm in nature.

For famine relief: Collect and blanch young leaves and seedlings, change water to remove pungent taste, and then flavor them with oil and salt.

For disease treatment: See the clause of Liaoshi [蓼实, polygonum hydropiper, Polygonum hydropiper L.] in *Materia Medica · Herbaceous Vegetable*.

379. 苜 蓿

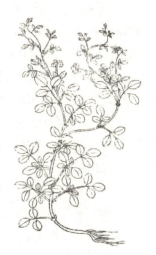

出陕西，今处处有之。苗高尺余。细茎，分叉而生。叶似锦鸡儿花叶，微长；又似豌豆叶，颇小，每三叶攒生一处。梢间开紫花，结弯角儿，中有子如黍米大，腰子样。味苦，性平，无毒。一云微甘、淡，一云性凉。根寒。

救饥：苗叶嫩时，采取煤食。江南人不甚食，多食利大小肠。

治病：文具《本草·菜部》条下。

379. Muxu［苜蓿, medicago sativa, Medicago sativa L.］

Muxu［苜蓿, medicago sativa, Medicago sativa L.］ grew in Shaanxi Province, and it can be seen everywhere presently. Its plants are over one Chi high with thin stems and twigs. Its leaves are like those of Jinji'er［锦鸡儿, caragana, Caragana sinica (Buchoz) Rehd.］, but a little longer, and like those of peas, but quite small. They are the trifoliate and compound leaves. There are purple flowers in twigs. Its seeds in the curved horn are as small as those of millets, and its shape is like kidney. It is bitter in taste, neutral in nature and non-toxic. It is also said to be slightly sweet or light in taste, and cool in nature. Its roots are cold in nature.

For famine relief: Collect and blanch young leaves and seedlings. It is not popular among people in the south of the Yangtze River, but it is beneficial for large and small intestines.

For disease treatment: See the relevant clause in *Materia Medica · Herbaceous Vegetable*.

380. 薄 荷

一名鸡苏。旧不著所出州土，今处处有之。茎方。叶似荏子[1]叶，小颇细长；又似香菜[2]叶而大。开细碎黪白花。其根经冬不死，至春发苗。味辛、苦，性温,无毒。一云性平。东平[3]龙脑岗[4]者尤佳。又有胡薄荷,与此相类,但味少甘为别,生江浙间,彼人多作茶饮,俗呼为新罗薄荷。又有南薄荷,其叶微小。

救饥:采苗叶煠熟,换水浸去辣味,油盐调食。与薤作齑食相宜,煎豉汤、暖酒和饮、煎茶并宜。新病瘥人勿食,令人虚汗不止。猫食之即醉,物相感尔。

治病:文具《本草·菜部》条下。

【注释】

[1] 见本书第411 荏子条。
[2] 见本书第383 香菜条。
[3] 古代州名。
[4] 古代地名。

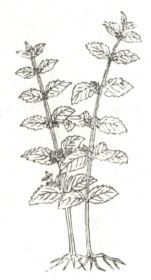

380. Bohe [薄荷, field-mint, Mentha canadensis L.]

Bohe [薄荷, field-mint, Mentha canadensis L.] is also named Jisu, but there was no record of its place of origin in ancient times, and presently it is cultivated everywhere. Its stems are squarish. Its leaves are like those of Renzi[1] [荏子, perilla frutescens, Perilla frutescens (L.) Britt.], but a little smaller, thinner and longer. Its leaves are also like those of Xiangcai[2] [香菜, coriander herb with root, Ocimum basilicum L.], but relatively larger than the latter. Its flowers are small and dark white. Its roots will not be withered in the whole winter. When the spring comes, it will come to a bud. It is pungent and bitter in taste, warm in nature and non-toxic. It is also said that it is neutral in nature. Among all the species, the quality of it which is growing Longnaogang[3] of Dongping[4] is better than that of other places. Hubohe is similar to Bohe, just different from its taste. Hubohe is not sweet and grows in Jiangsu and Zhejiang Province, where people drink them as tea. So it is also called Xinluo Bohe. Another kind is called Nanbohe, and its leaves are a little smaller.

For famine relief: Collect and blanch young leaves and seedlings. Soak them in water to remove the pungency, and then flavor them with oil and salt. It is also suitable to make seasonings with Allium baker. Boil them to make bean curd soup or drink with warm wine tea. The people who recover after illness should not eat, otherwise it will make people sweat. When a cat eats mint, it will immediately get drunk.

For disease treatment: See the relevant clause in *Materia Medica · Herbaceous Vegetable*.

【Notes】

[1] See the 411th clause of this book.

[2] See the 383th clause of this book.

[3] The name of an ancient place.

[4] The name of an ancient county.

381. 荆 芥

本草名假苏,一名鼠蓂、一名姜芥。生汉中川泽,及岳州、归德州,今处处有之。茎方窊面。叶似独扫叶而狭小,淡黄绿色。结小穗,有细小黑子,锐圆。多野生,以香气似苏,故名假苏。味辛,性温,无毒。

救饥:采嫩苗叶煠熟,水浸去邪气,油盐调食。初生香辛可咂,人取作生菜腌食。

治病:文具《本草·菜部》假苏条下。

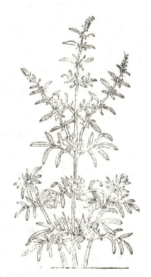

381. Jingjie〔荆芥, schizonepeta herba, Nepeta tenuifolia Benth.〕

Jingjie〔荆芥, schizonepeta herba, Nepeta tenuifolia Benth.〕, also named Jiasu, Shuming and Jiangjie, grows near the lakes or marshes in Hanzhong, Yuezhou and Guidezhou. Now it is distributed everywhere. There are concaves on the squarish stems. Its leaves are like those of Dusao〔独扫, kochia, Kochiae Fructus〕, but relatively narrow, small and yellowish green. Small black seeds, which are sharp and round, are placed on its spikelets. It is mostly planted in the wild. Because its aroma is like Suzi〔苏子, perilla seed, Fructus Perillae〕, it is also named Jiasu. It is pungent in taste, warm in nature and non-toxic.

For famine relief: Collect young leaves and seedlings, blanch and soak them in water to remove the strange taste, and then flavor them with oil and salt. Newborn Jingjie is pungent and can be used for making pickles.

For disease treatment: See the clause of Jiasu [假苏, schizonepeta tenuifolia, Nepeta tenuifolia Benth.] in *Materia Medica · Herbaceous Vegetable*.

382. 水　蕲

俗作芹菜，一名水英。出南海池泽，今水边多有之。根茎离地二三寸，分生茎叉，其茎方，窊面四楞。对生叶，似痢见菜叶而阔短，边有大锯齿；又似薄荷叶而短。开白花，似蛇床子花。味甘，性平，无毒。又云大寒。春、秋二时，龙带精入芹菜中，人遇食之，作蛟龙病。

救饥：发英时采之，煠熟食。芹有两种，秋芹取根，白色，赤芹取茎叶，并堪食。又有渣芹，可为生菜食之。

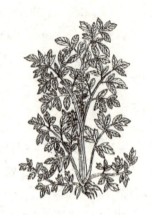

382. Shuiqin [水蕲, cress, Oenanthe javanica (Blume) DC.]

Shuiqin [水蕲, cress, Oenanthe javanica (Blume) DC.], also named Qincai or Shuiying, is produced in the ponds or lakes of South China Sea. Now it mostly grows near the water. Its roots and stems are 2~3 Cun high off the ground. Its split stems are squarish and tetragonal with caves on the surface. Its opposite leaves are like those of Lijiancai [痢见菜, copperleaf herb, Acalypha australis L.], but slightly wide and short with large serrations at the fringe. It is also like that of Bohe [薄荷, field-mint, Mentha canadensis L.], but shorter than the latter. Its white flowers are like those of Shechuangzi [蛇床子, chidium Fruit, Fructus Cnidii Common]. It is sweet in taste, neutral in nature and non-toxic. It is also said to be cold in nature. In the spring and autumn, once men eat this kind of celery, which is flavored with Daijing [带精, Daijing medicinal, Materia Medica Daijing], it will decrease their semen volumes.

For famine relief: Collect and blanch them after flowering. There are two kinds of celery: One is called Qiuqin, and the other is Chiqin. Collect the roots of the former one, and its roots are white. Collect the stems and leaves of the latter one. Another kind is Zhaqin [渣芹, Zhaqin medicinal, Materia Medica Zhaqin], and it can be eaten directly.

新增
New Supplements

383. 香 菜

生伊洛间[1],人家园圃种之。苗高一尺许。茎方,窊面四棱,茎色紫。稔叶似薄荷叶微小,边有细锯齿,亦有细毛。梢头开花作穗,花淡藕褐色。味辛香,性温。

救饥:采苗叶煠熟,油盐调食。

【注释】

[1] 古代地区名,指伊水和洛水间的区域。即今河南洛河,黄河支流。

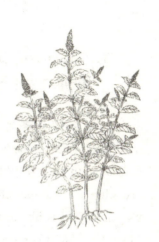

383. Xiangcai [香菜, coriander herb with root, Ocimum basilicum L.]

Xiangcai [香菜, coriander herb with root, Ocimum basilicum L.] grew in the area of Luo River[1], and it is more cultivated in the courtyards of common people. Its plants are one Chi high. The stems with some caves on the surface are squarish, tetragonal and purple. Its serrulation-fringed leaves are like those of mint, with short fuzz, a little smaller. Its flowers, which are spicate and light pinkish purple, bloom on the top of branches. It is pungent in taste and warm in nature.

For famine relief: Collect young leaves and seedlings, blanch and elutriate them in hot water, and then flavor them with oil and salt.

[Notes]

[1] The name of an ancient place. It is presently located in the areas between Luo River and Yi River, here it refers to Luo River, the branch of the Yellow

River, in Henan Province.

384. 银条菜

所在人家园圃多种。苗叶皆似莴苣,细长,色颇青白。撺葶高二尺许,开四瓣淡黄花。结蒴似荞麦蒴而圆,中有小子如油子大,淡黄色。其叶味微苦,性凉。

救饥:采苗叶煠熟,水浸,淘净,油盐调食。生揉亦可食。

384. Yintiaocai [银条菜, rorippa globosa, Rorippa globosa (Turcz.) Hayek]

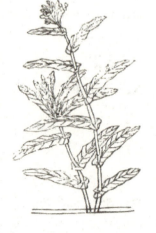

Yintiaocai [银条菜, rorippa globosa, Rorippa globosa (Turcz.) Hayek] is mostly cultivated in the courtyards of common people, and its seedlings and leaves are similar to those of Woju [莴苣, lettuce, Lactuca sativa Linn.], slender, green and white. The scapes are about two Chi high, and four yellowish flowers are in bloom. Its fruit is like that of Qiaomai [荞麦, buckwheat, Fagopyrum esculentum Moench.], but it is round. There are yellowish seeds in the fruit, as big as Youzi. The leaves are slightly bitter in taste and cold in nature.

For famine relief: Collect young leaves and seedlings, blanch and elutriate them in water, and then flavor them with oil and salt. It can be eaten after rubbing.

385. 后庭花

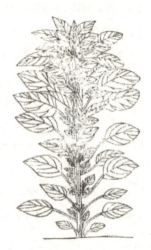

一名雁来红。人家园圃多种之。叶似人苋叶,其叶中心红色,又有黄色相间,亦有通身红色者,亦有紫色者。茎叶间结实,比苋实微大。其叶众叶攒聚,状如花朵,其色娇红可爱,故以名之。味甜、微涩,性凉。

救饥:采苗叶煠熟,水浸淘净,油盐调食。晒干煠食尤佳。

385. Houtinghua〔后庭花, amaranthus, Amaranthus tricolor L.〕

Houtinghua〔后庭花, amaranthus, Amaranthus tricolor L.〕, also named Yanlaihong, is cultivated in the gardens of common people. Its leaves are like those of Renxian〔人苋, acalypha australis, Acalypha australis L.〕. The center of the leaves is red, and some are yellow, red or purple. Its fruit grows in the middle of stems and leaves, which is slightly larger than Xian〔苋, amarantus mangostanus, Amaranthus tricolor L.〕. It is called Yanlaihong because its leaves grow together, just like flowers, red and lovely. Its leaves are sweet and a bit astringent in taste; besides, it is cold in nature.

For famine relief: Collect young leaves and seedlings, blanch and elutriate them in water, and then flavor them with oil and salt. It is especially delicious to blanch them after drying.

386. 火焰菜

人家园圃多种。苗叶俱似菠菜,但叶稍微红,形如火焰。结子亦如菠菜子。苗叶味甜,性微冷。

救饥:采苗叶煠熟,水淘洗净,油盐调食。

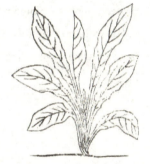

386. Huoyancai〔火焰菜, beta vulgaris, Beta vulgaris L.〕

Huoyancai〔火焰菜, beta vulgarist, Beta vulgaris L.〕is mainly cultivated in the courtyards of common people. Its leaves are like those of spinach, but the leaves on the top are reddish. Its shape is like the flame, and its seeds are like those of spinach. Its leaves are sweet in taste, and a bit cold in nature.

For famine relief: Collect young leaves and seedlings, blanch and elutriate them in water, and then flavor them with oil and salt.

387. 山 葱

一名隔葱,又名鹿耳葱。生辉县太行山山野中。叶似玉簪叶微团,叶中撺葶,似蒜葶,甚长而涩。稍头结膏葖,似葱膏葖微小,开白花,结子黑色。苗味辣。

救饥:采苗叶煠熟,油盐调食。生腌食亦可。

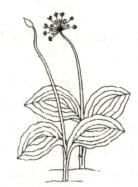

387. Shancong [山葱, scallion, Allium victorialis L.]

Shancong [山葱, scallion, Allium victorialis L.], also named Gecong and Lu'ercong, grows in the wilderness of Mount Taihang in Huixian County. Its leaves are like those of Yuzan [玉簪, hosta, Hosta plantaginea (Lam.) Aschers.], but a bit round. Its scapes are like those of Suan [蒜, garlic, Allium sativum L.], very long and rough. The follicles, growing on the tip, just like those of scallion, are a little smaller; its flowers are white, and its seeds are black. Its seedlings are pungent in taste.

For famine relief: Collect young leaves and seedlings, blanch and elutriate them in water, and then flavor them with oil and salt. It is also used for making pickles.

388. 背 韭

生辉县太行山山野中。叶颇似韭叶而甚宽大。根似葱根,味辣。

救饥:采苗叶煠熟,油盐调食。生腌食亦可。

388. Beijiu [背韭, allium paepalanthoides, Allium paepalanthoides Airy-Shaw]

Beijiu [背韭, allium paepalanthoides, Allium paepalanthoides Airy-Shaw] grows in the mountains and fields of Mount Taihang in Huixian County. Its leaves are like those of Jiucai [韭菜, Chinese chive, Allium tuberosum], but very wide and large. Its roots are like those of Cong [葱, scallion, Allium fistulosum L.]. It is pungent in taste.

For famine relief: Collect young leaves and seedlings, blanch and elutriate them in water, and then flavor them with oil and salt. It is also used for making pickles.

389. 水芥菜

水边多生。苗高尺许。叶似家芥菜叶,极小,色微淡绿,叶多花叉。茎叉亦细,开小黄花。结细短小角儿。叶味微辛。

救饥:采苗叶煠熟,水浸去辣气,淘洗过,油盐调食。

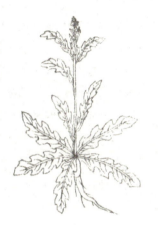

389. Shuijiecai [水芥菜, rorippa palustris, Rorippa palustris (L.) Bess.]

Shuijiecai [水芥菜, rorippa palustris, Rorippa palustris (L.) Bess.] grows by the water. Its seedlings are about one Chi high. Its leaves are like those of Jiecai [芥菜, mustard, brassica juncea (L.) Czern. et Coss.], small and light green. There are many divergences at the fringe of leaves. Its branches in stems are very thin. Its flowers are yellow, and its pointed fruit is small and short. Its leaves are slightly pungent in taste.

For famine relief: Collect young leaves and seedlings, blanch and elutriate them in water, and then flavor them with oil and salt.

390. 遏蓝菜

生田野中下湿地。苗初揭地生。叶似初生菠菜叶而小,其头颇团。叶间撺葶分叉,上结荚儿,似榆钱状而小。其叶味辛香、微酸,性微温。

救饥:采苗叶煠熟,水浸取酸辣味,复用水淘净,作齑,油盐调食。

390. Elancai [遏蓝菜, boor's mustard herb, Thlaspi arvense L.]

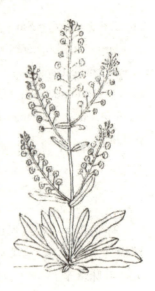

Elancai [遏蓝菜, boor's mustard herb, Thlaspi arvense L.] grows in the fields of lowland or damp places. Its seedlings creep on the ground. Its leaves are like those of Bocai [菠菜, spinach, Spinacia oleracea L.], but very small. The top leaves are round. Its scapes are in the leaves, and the pods, growing in the twigs, are like those of Yuqian [榆钱, the fruit of elm, Ulmus pumila L.], but a little smaller. Its leaves are pungent and a bit sour in taste. It is warm in nature.

For famine relief: Collect young leaves and seedlings, blanch and soak them to remove the sourness and pungency, mince them after elutriating, and then flavor them with oil and salt.

391. 牛耳朵菜

一名野芥菜。生田野中。苗高一二尺。苗茎似莴苣色，叶似牛耳朵形而小。叶间分撺葶叉，开白花。结子如粟粒大。叶味微苦辣。

救饥：采苗叶淘洗净，煠熟，油盐调食。

391. Niu'erduo Cai [牛耳朵菜, chirita eburnea, Brassica rapa L. var. Olefera DC.]

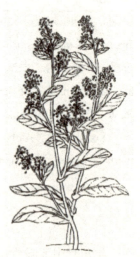

Niu'erduo Cai [牛耳朵菜, chirita eburnea, Brassica rapa L. var. Olefera DC.], also named Yejiecai, grows in the fields. Its plants are 1～2 Chi high. Its stems are like those of Woju [莴苣, lettuce, Lactuca sativa Linn.]. Its leaves are like the ears of cows, but a little smaller. Its scapes grow out of the leaves with white flowers. Its fruit is as small as millets. Its leaves are slightly bitter and pungent in taste.

For famine relief: Collect young leaves and seedlings, blanch and elutriate them in water, and then flavor them with oil and salt.

392. 山白菜

生辉县山野中。苗叶颇似家白菜，而叶茎细长。其叶尖艄，边有锯齿叉；又似莙荙菜叶而尖瘦，亦小。味甜、微苦。

救饥：采苗叶煤熟，水淘净，油盐调食。

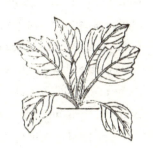

392. Shanbaicai [山白菜, aster, Aster tataricus L. f.]

Shanbaicai [山白菜, aster, Aster tataricus L. f.] grows in the mountains and fields of Huixian County. Its leaves are like those of Baicai [白菜, Chinese cabbage, Brassica rapa pekinensis], and its petioles are slender and long. Its leaf apex with some serration at the fringe is narrow, and also like that of Jundacai [莙荙菜, spinach beet, Beta vulgaris L.], but very sharp, thin and small. It is sweet and slightly bitter in taste.

For famine relief: Collect young leaves and seedlings, blanch and elutriate them in water, and then flavor them with oil and salt.

393. 山宜菜

又名山苦菜。生新郑县山野中。苗初揭地生。叶似薄荷叶而大，叶根两傍有叉，背白；又似青荚儿菜叶，亦大。味苦。

救饥：采苗叶煤熟，油盐调食。

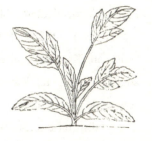

393. Shanyicai [山宜菜, lactuca raddeana, Lactuca raddeana Maxim.]

Shanyicai [山宜菜, lactuca raddeana, Lactuca raddeana Maxim.], also named Shankucai, grows in the mountains and fields of Xinzheng County. Its seedlings initially creep on the ground. Its leaves are like those of Bohe [薄荷, field-mint, Mentha canadensis L.], but slightly big. With the bifurcation on both sides of the base of leaves, the back of leaves is white. Its leaves are also like those of Qingjia'er Cai [青荚儿菜, heterophyllous patrinia, Patrinia heterophylla Bunge]. It is bitter in taste.

For famine relief: Collect young leaves and seedlings, blanch and elutriate them in water, and then flavor them with oil and salt.

394. 山苦荬

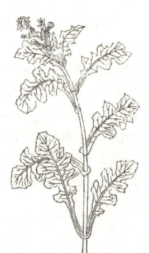

生新郑县山野中。苗高二尺余。茎似莴苣葶而节稠。其叶甚花,有三五尖叉,似花苦苣叶,甚大。开淡棠褐花,表微红。味苦。

救饥:采嫩苗叶煠熟,水淘去苦味,油盐调食。

394. Shankumai [山苦荬, field sowthistle herb, Paraixeris denticulata (Houtt.) Nakai]

Shankumai [山苦荬, field sowthistle herb, Paraixeris denticulata (Houtt.) Nakai] grows in the mountains and fields of Xinzheng County. Its plants are over two Chi high. Its stems are like the scapes of Woju [莴苣, lettuce, Lactuca sativa Linn.], but slightly dense. Its leaves are split, like those of Huakuju [花苦苣, common sowthistle herb, Sonchus wightianus DC.], very large. Its flowers are light brown, and reddish on the top. It is bitter in taste.

For famine relief: Collect young leaves and seedlings, blanch and elutriate them in water to remove the bitterness, and then flavor them with oil and salt.

395. 南芥菜

人家园圃中亦种之。苗初揭地生，后擎葶叉。叶似芥菜叶，但小而有毛涩。茎叶梢头开淡黄花，结小尖角儿。叶味辛辣。

救饥：采苗叶煤熟，水浸淘去涩味，油盐调食。生焯过，腌食亦可。

395. Nanjiecai [南芥菜, nanjiecai medicinal, Cruciferae]

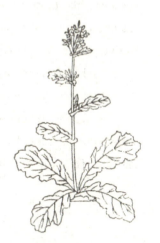

Nanjiecai [南芥菜, nanjiecai medicinal, Cruciferae] is often cultivated in the courtyards of common people. Its plants initially creep on the ground, and then its scapes appear. Its leaves are like those of Jiecai [芥菜, mustard, Brassica juncea (L.) Czern. et Coss.], but smaller and strigillose. Its yellowish flowers bloom on the top of stems, with small pointed fruit. Its leaves are pungent in taste.

For famine relief: Collect young leaves and seedlings, blanch and elutriate them in water, and then flavor them with oil and salt. It is also used for making pickles.

396. 山莴苣

生密县山野间。苗叶揭地生。叶似莴苣叶而小；又似苦苣叶而却宽大，叶脚花叉颇少，叶头微尖，边有细锯齿。叶间擎葶，开淡黄花。苗叶味微苦。

救饥：采苗叶煤熟，水浸淘去苦味，油盐调食。生揉亦可食。

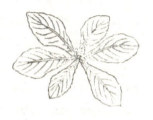

396. Shanwoju [山莴苣, herb of Indian Lettuce, Lactuca indica L.]

Shanwoju [山莴苣, herb of Indian Lettuce, Lactuca indica L.] grows in the mountains and wilderness of Mixian County. Its plants creep on the ground. Its leaves are like those of Woju 〔莴苣, lettuce, Lactuca sativa Linn.〕, but a little smaller, and also like those of Kuju 〔苦苣, endive, Cichorium endivia L.〕, but relatively wide and large. There are a few lobes in the base, but its apexes which are fringed with serration are slightly sharp. The scapes grow out of leaves. Its flowers are light yellow. Its seedlings and leaves are slightly bitter in taste.

For famine relief: Collect young leaves and seedlings, blanch them and remove the bitterness by elutriating them in water, and then flavor them with oil and salt. They can also be eaten after rubbing.

397. 黄鹌菜

生密县山谷中。苗初搨地生。叶似初生山莴苣叶而小,叶脚边微有花叉;又似字字丁叶而头颇团。叶中撺生葶叉,高五六寸许。开小黄花,结小细子,黄茶褐色。叶味甜。

救饥:采苗叶煤熟,换水淘净,油盐调食。

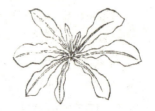

397. Huang'ancai 〔黄鹌菜, herb of Japanese Youngia, Youngia japonica (L.) DC.〕

Huang'ancai 〔黄鹌菜, herb of Japanese Youngia, Youngia japonica (L.) DC.〕 grows in the valleys of Mixian County. Initially, its seedlings creep on the ground. Its leaves are like those of new Shanwoju 〔山莴苣, herb of Indian Lettuce, Lactuca indica L.〕, but slightly small with some lobes in the base of leaves. It is also like that of Beibeiding 〔字字丁, dandelion, Taraxacum mongolicum Hand.-Mazz.〕 with round apexes. Its scapes, which have some twigs, grow out of leaves, about 5~6 Cun high. Its flowers are yellow and the seeds, being small and thin, are yellow and brown. Its leaves are sweet in taste.

For famine relief: Collect young leaves and seedlings, blanch and elutriate them in water, and then flavor them with oil and salt.

398. 燕儿菜

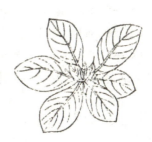

生密县山涧边。苗叶塌地生。叶似匙头样,颇长;又似牛耳朵菜叶而小,微涩;又似山莴苣叶亦小,颇硬而头微团,味苦。

救饥:采苗叶煤熟,换水浸淘净,油盐调食。

398. Yan'ercai [燕儿菜, herb of Hygrometric Boea, Boea hygrometrica (Bunge) R. Brown]

Yan'ercai [燕儿菜, herb of Hygrometric Boea, Boea hygrometrica (Bunge) R. Brown] grows in the valleys of Mixian County. Both its seedlings and leaves creep on the ground. Its leaves are like those of Shitoucai [匙头菜, violet, Violae Formosanae Herba], but very long, and like those of Niu'erduo Cai [牛耳朵菜, Chirita eburnea, Brassica rapa L. var. Olefera DC.], but small and rough. It is also like that of Shanwoju [山莴苣, Herb of Indian Lettuce, Lactuca indica L.], small and hard in texture, and it is round on the top of leaves and bitter in taste.

For famine relief: Collect and blanch young plants and leaves, soak them in fresh water, wash and clean them, and then flavor them with oil and salt.

399. 孛孛丁菜

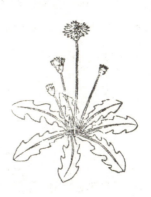

又名黄花苗。生田野中。苗初塌地生。叶似苦苣叶微短小。叶丛中间撺葶,梢头开黄花。茎叶折之皆有白汁。叶微苦。

救饥:采苗叶煤熟,油盐调食。

399. Beibeiding Cai [孛孛丁菜, dandelion, Taraxacum mongolicum Hand.-Mazz.]

Beibeiding Cai [孛孛丁菜, dandelion, Taraxacum mongolicum Hand.-Mazz.], also named Huanghuamiao, grows in the fields. Initially, its seedlings creep on the ground. Its leaves are like those of Kuju [苦苣, endive, Sonchus oleraceus L.], but relatively small. Its scapes grow out of leaves, and its flowers on the top are yellow. When the stems and leaves are broken, the white juice will flow out. Its leaves are slightly bitter in taste.

For famine relief: Collect young leaves and seedlings, blanch and soak them in fresh water, and flavor them with oil and salt.

400. 柴 韭

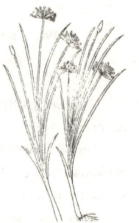

生荒野中。苗叶形状如韭,但叶圆细而瘦。叶中撺葶开花,如韭花状,粉紫色。苗叶味辛。

救饥:采苗叶煠熟,水浸淘净,油盐调食。生腌食亦可。

400. Chaijiu [柴韭, allium, Allium tenuissimum L.]

Chaijiu [柴韭, allium, Allium tenuissimum L.] grows in the wilderness. Its plants are like Jiu [韭, Chinese chives, Allium tuberosum L.], but its leaves are round and slender. Its scapes growing out of leaves are just like Jiuhua [韭花, flower of Chinese chives, Allium tuberosum L.], pinkish purple. Both its seedlings and leaves are pungent in taste.

For famine relief: Collect young leaves and seedlings, blanch and elutriate them in water, and then flavor them with oil and salt. It is also used for making pickles.

401. 野 韭

生荒野中。形状如韭,苗叶极细、弱。叶圆,比柴韭又细小。叶中撺葶,开小粉紫花,似韭花状。苗叶味辛。

救饥:采苗叶煠熟,油盐调食。生腌食亦可。

401. Yejiu [野韭, allium, Allium tenuissimum L.]

Yejiu [野韭, allium, Allium tenuissimum L.] grows in the wilderness. Its shape is like Jiu [韭, Chinese chives, Allium tuberosum], and both its seedlings and leaves are slender and tender. Compared with the leaves of Chaijiu, its leaves are round and smaller. Its scapes growing out of leaves are just like those of Jiuhua [韭花, flower of Chinese chives, Allium tuberosum], pinkish purple. Both its seedlings and leaves are pungent in taste.

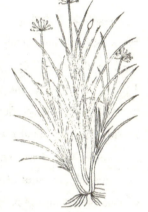

For famine relief: Collect young leaves and seedlings, blanch and elutriate them in water, and then flavor them with oil and salt. It is also used for making pickles.

根可食

新增

Root Edible

New Supplements

402. 甘露儿

人家园圃中多栽。叶似地瓜儿叶甚阔,多有毛涩。其叶对节生,色微淡绿;又似薄荷叶,亦宽而皱。开红紫花。其根呼为甘露儿,形如小指,而纹节甚稠,皮色黲白,味甘。

救饥:采根洗净,煤熟,油盐调食。生腌食亦可。

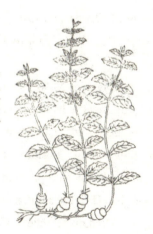

402. Ganlu'er [甘露儿, Chinese artichoke Stachys sieboldii Miq., Stachys sieboldii Miq.]

Ganlu'er [甘露儿, Chinese artichoke Stachys sieboldii Miq., Stachys sieboldii Miq.] is cultivated in the gardens of common people. Its leaves, with some hair, are like those of Digua'er [地瓜儿, wayaka yambean root, Lycopus lucidus Turcz.], very wide and rough. Its opposite leaves are light green, and also like those of Bohe [薄荷, field-mint, Mentha canadensis L.], with some rugose edges. Its flowers are reddish purple. Its roots are called Ganlu'er, and its shape is like the little finger with dense knots. Its stem bark is dark white. It is sweet in taste.

For famine relief: Collect and blanch roots, and flavor them with oil and salt, or make them into pickles.

403. 地瓜儿苗

生田野中。苗高二尺余。茎方四楞。叶似薄荷叶，微长大；又似泽兰叶，㧒茎而生。根名地瓜，形类甘露儿，更长，味甘。

救饥：掘根洗净，煤熟，油盐调食。生腌食亦可。

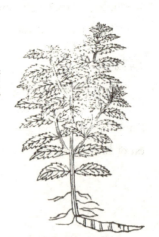

403. Digua'er Miao [地瓜儿苗, lycopus lucidus, Lycopus lucidus Turcz.]

Digua'er Miao [地瓜儿苗, lycopus lucidus, Lycopus lucidus Turcz.] grows in the fields. Its plants are over two Chi high. The squarish stems are tetragonal. Its leaves are like those of Bohe [薄荷, field-mint, Mentha canadensis L.], slightly long. Besides, it is like that of Zelan [泽兰, hirsute shiny bugleweed herb, Herba Lycopi] and scatters on the stems. Its rhizome is called Digua, which is shaped like Ganlu'er, but longer than the latter. It is sweet in taste.

For famine relief: Collect and wash and clean its tubers, blanch and flavor them with oil and salt, or make them into pickles.

根叶皆可食

《本草》原有

Root and Leaf Edible
Original Ones

404. 泽 蒜

又名小蒜。生田野中,今处处有之。生山中者名 藠。苗似细韭。叶中心撺葶,开淡粉紫花。根似蒜而 甚小,味辛,性温,有小毒。又云热,有毒。

救饥:采苗根作羹,或生腌,或煠熟,油盐调,皆可食。

治病:文具《本草·菜部》小蒜条下。

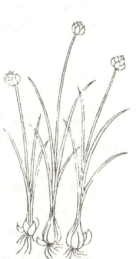

404. Zesuan [泽蒜, allium macrostemon, Allium macrostemon Bunge]

Zesuan [泽蒜, allium macrostemon, Allium macrostemon Bunge], also named Xiaosuan, grows in the fields. Presently it can be seen everywhere, and those which grow in the mountains are called Li. Its plants are like those of Xijiu [细韭, Chinese chive, Allium tenuissimum L.]. Its scapes grow out of leaves. Its flowers are pinkish purple. Its bulbs are like Suan [蒜, garlic, Allium sativum L.], but very small, pungent in taste and warm in nature, mildly toxic. It is also said to be hot in nature and toxic.

For famine relief: Collect seedlings and bulbs to make thick soup, or wash bulbs clean, blanch and flavor them with oil and salt, or make them into pickles.

For disease treatment: See the clause of Xiaosuan [小蒜, allium macrostemon, Allium macrostemon Bunge] in *Materia Medica · Herbaceous Vegetables*.

New Supplements

405. 楼子葱

人家园圃中多栽。苗叶根茎俱似葱。其叶梢头又生小葱四五枝,叠生三四层,故名楼子葱。不结子,但掐下小葱,栽之便活。味甘、辣,性温。

救饥:采苗茎连根,择去细须,煠熟,油盐调食。生亦可食。

治病:与《本草·菜部》下葱同用。

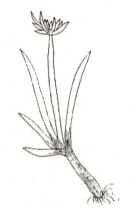

405. Louzicong [楼子葱, allium cepa, Allium cepa L. var. prolife rum (Moench) Regel]

Louzicong [楼子葱, allium cepa, Allium cepa L. var. prolife rum (Moench) Regel] is cultivated in the gardens of common people. Its leaves and rhizomes are like those of Cong [葱, scallion, Allium victorialis L.], four or five shallots grow out of its tip of inflorescences and stacked three or four layers, so it is called Louzicong. Without bearing seeds, it begins to grow after its being cultivated scallion. It is sweet and pungent in taste, and warm in nature.

For famine relief: Collect seedlings and roots, pick fine whiskers to blanch, and then flavor them with oil and salt. It can be eaten directly.

For disease treatment: See the clause of Cong [葱, scallion, Allium victorialis L.] in *Materia Medica · Herbaceous Vegetable*.

406. 薙 韭

一名石韭。生辉县太行山山野中。叶似蒜叶而颇窄狭;又似肥韭叶微阔。花似韭花颇大。根似韭根甚粗,味辣。

救饥:采苗叶煠熟,油盐调食。生亦可食。冬月采取根煠食。

406. Xiejiu [薤韭, Chinese chive, Allium hookeri]

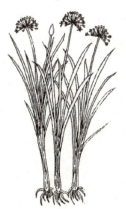

Xiejiu [薤韭, Chinese chive, Allium hookeri], also named Shijiu, grows in the mountains and fields of Mount Taihang in Huixian County. Its leaves are like those of Suan [蒜, garlic, Allium macrostemon Bunge.], but very narrow; besides, it is like that of Jiu [韭, Chinese chives, Allium tuberosum], succulent and slightly wide. Its flowers are like those of Jiu [韭, Chinese chives, Allium tuberosum], very large. Its bulbs and fibrous roots are like those of Jiu [韭, Chinese chives, Allium tuberosum], strong and pungent in taste.

For famine relief: Collect and blanch young leaves and seedlings, blanch and elutriate them in hot water, and then flavor them with oil and salt, or eat them directly. Its bulbs and fibrous roots can be eaten by blanching and elutriating them in winter.

407. 水萝卜

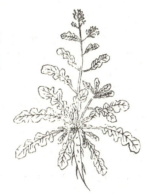

生田野下湿地中。苗初揭地生。叶似荠菜形而厚大,锯齿尖花叶;又似水芥叶,亦厚大。后分茎叉,稍间开淡黄花,结小角儿。根如白菜根而大,味甘、辣。

救饥:采根及叶煤熟,油盐调食。生亦可食。

407. Shuiluobo [水萝卜, summer radish, Brassicaceae]

Shuiluobo [水萝卜, summer radish, Brassicaceae] grows in the fields, where the terrain is low and humid. Its plants initially creep on the ground. Its leaves are like those of Jicai [荠菜, shepherd's purse, Capsella Bursa-pastoris Herba], but thick and large, with serrated lobes at the edge, and they are like those of Shuijiecai [水芥菜, rorippa palustris, Rorippa palustris (L.) Bess.], but thicker and larger than the latter. Its yellowish flowers grow out of twigs in the stalk fork, with small fruit. Its roots are like those of Chinese cabbage, but relatively large. It is sweet and pungent in taste.

For famine relief: Collect and blanch young leaves and roots, blanch and elutriate them in hot water, and then flavor them with oil and salt, or eat them directly.

408. 野蔓菁

生辉县栲栳圈山谷中。苗叶似家蔓菁叶而薄小，其叶头尖艄，叶脚花叉甚多。叶间撺出枝叉，上开黄花。结小角，其子黑色。根似白菜根颇大。苗、叶、根味微苦。

救饥：采苗叶煠熟，水浸淘净，油盐调食。或采根，换水煮去苦味，食之亦可。

408. Yemanjing [野蔓菁, wild turnip, Brassica rapa Linn.]

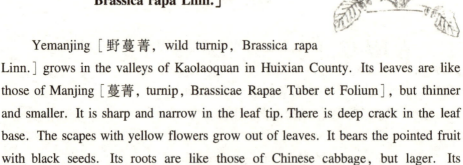

Yemanjing [野蔓菁, wild turnip, Brassica rapa Linn.] grows in the valleys of Kaolaoquan in Huixian County. Its leaves are like those of Manjing [蔓菁, turnip, Brassicae Rapae Tuber et Folium], but thinner and smaller. It is sharp and narrow in the leaf tip. There is deep crack in the leaf base. The scapes with yellow flowers grow out of leaves. It bears the pointed fruit with black seeds. Its roots are like those of Chinese cabbage, but lager. Its seedlings, leaves and roots are slightly bitter in taste.

For famine relief: Collect and blanch young leaves and seedlings, blanch and soak them by filtration with water, and then flavor them with oil and salt. Or cook roots to remove the bitterness.

叶及实皆可食

✱ **《本草》原有**

Leaf and Fruit Edible
Original Ones

409. 荠　菜

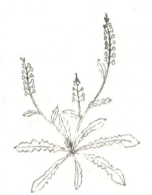

生平泽中,今处处有之。苗搨地生,作锯齿叶。三四月出薹,分生茎叉。梢上开小白花。结实小,似菥蓂子。苗叶味甘,性温,无毒。其实亦呼菥蓂子。其子味甘,性平。患气人食之动冷疾。不可与面同食,令人背闷。服丹石人不可食。

救饥:采子,用水调搅,良久成块,或作烧饼,或煮粥食,味甚粘滑。叶煤作菜食,或煮作羹,皆可。

治病:文具《本草·菜部》条下。

409. Jicai [荠菜, shepherd's purse, Capsella bursa-pastoris (L.) Medic.]

Jicai [荠菜, shepherd's purse, Capsella bursa-pastoris (L.) Medic.] was recorded in ancient times that it grew up in a flat, grassy wetland. Presently it can be seen everywhere. Its plants creep on the ground with serration lobes. In March and April, its scapes, with some twigs, grow out of leaves. Its white flowers are on the twigs. Its seeds are like those of Ximi [菥蓂, thlaspi arvense, Thlaspi arvense L.]. Both its leaves and seedlings are sweet in taste, warm in nature and non-toxic. Its fruit is also called Ximi [菥蓂, thlaspi arvense, Thlaspi arvense L.], its seeds are sweet in taste and neutral in nature, and people who have syndrome of qi will get diseases owing to cold. It will make people stuffy when eaten with noodles. People who take cinnabar and stone can't eat it either.

For famine relief: Collect young seeds, mix them with water and stir for a long time or make pancakes or congee. Blanch leaves to make dishes or soup.

For disease treatment: See the relevant clause in *Materia Medica · Herbaceous Vegetable*.

410. 紫　苏

一名桂荏。又有数种,有勺苏、鱼苏、山苏。出简州[1]及无为军[2],今处处有之。苗高二尺许。茎方。叶似苏子叶,微小。茎叶背面皆紫色,而气甚香。开粉红花。结小蒴,其子状如黍颗。味辛,性温。又云味微辛、甘。子无毒。

救饥:采叶煠食,煮饮亦可。子研汁、煮粥,食之皆好。叶可生食,与鱼作羹,味佳。

治病:文具《本草·菜部》苏子条下。

【注释】

[1] 古代州名,辖境相当今四川简阳市及金堂县部分地区。

[2] 古代军名,见《图经本草》药图。

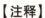

410. Zisu〔紫苏, perilla frutescens, Perilla frutescens (L.) Britt.〕

Zisu〔紫苏, perilla frutescens, Perilla frutescens (L.) Britt.〕is also named Guiren, with many varieties, including Shaosu, Yusu and Shansu. It was recorded that it was produced in Jianzhou[1] and the areas controlled by Wuwei Army[2]. Presently it can be seen everywhere. Its seedlings are about two Chi high, and its stems are squarish. Its leaves are like those of Suzi〔苏子, perilla seeds, Perilla frutescens (L.) Britt.〕, but slightly small. The back of its stems and leaves are purple with fragrant smell. Its flowers are pinkish purple. With small pods, its seeds are shaped like broomcorn millets. It is pungent in taste and warm in nature. It is also said to be slightly pungent and sweet in taste, and its seeds are non-toxic.

For famine relief: Collect leaves, blanch them, and drink them after boiling. Its seeds are ground into juice or made into congee, and then flavor them with oil and salt. It is tasty to eat leaves or make soup with fish.

For disease treatment: See the clause of Suzi〔苏子, perilla seeds, Perilla frutescens (L.) Britt.] in *Materia Medica · Herbaceous Vegetable*.

【Notes】

[1] The name of an ancient prefecture. Presently, it refers to Jianyang City, Sichuan Province.

[2] The name of an ancient army. See the picture in *Tu Jing Ben Cao* [《图经本草》, *Illustrated Classics of Materia Medica*].

411. 荏 子[1]

所在有之，生园圃中。苗高一二尺。茎方。叶似薄荷叶，极肥大。开淡紫花。结穗似紫苏穗，其子如黍粒。其枝茎对节生。东人呼为蘇，以其"蘇"字但除禾边故也。味辛，性温，无毒。

救饥：采嫩苗叶煤熟，油盐调食。子可炒食。又研之杂米作粥，甚肥美。亦可笮油用。

治病：文具《本草·菜部》条下。

【注释】

[1] 与本书第 410 条紫苏是同一种。

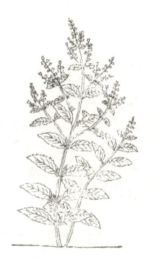

411. Renzi[1] [荏子, perilla frutescens, Perilla frutescens (L.) Britt.]

Renzi [荏子, perilla frutescens, Perilla frutescens (L.) Britt.], distributed in all areas, grows in the gardens. Its plants are 1~2 Chi high, with squarish stems. Its leaves are like those of Bohe [薄荷, field-mint, Mentha canadensis L.], strong and big. Its flowers are light purple. Its spicas are like those of Zisu [紫苏, perilla frutescens, Perilla frutescens (L.) Britt. Var.], and its nutlets are like those of broomcorn millets. Its branches are opposite on the knot. People in the eastern region of Shanxi Province call it "Yu", which is from part of Chinese character 蘇 (Su). It is pungent in taste, warm in nature and non-toxic.

For famine relief: Collect young leaves and seedlings, blanch and elutriate them in hot water, and then flavor them with oil and salt. It is delicious to cook seeds or make congee with rice. It can also be used for oil extraction.

For disease treatment: See the relevant clause in *Materia Medica · Herbaceous Vegetable*.

【Notes】

[1] It is considered to be the same kind as the 410th clause of this book.

新增
New Supplements

412. 灰 菜

生田野中,处处有之。苗高二三尺。茎有紫红线楞。叶有灰葧。结青子,成穗者甘,散穗者微苦。性暖。生墙下、树下者不可用。

救饥:采苗叶煠熟,水浸淘净,去灰气,油盐调食。晒干煠食尤佳。穗成熟时,采子捣为米,磨面作饼蒸食,皆可。

412. Huicai [灰菜, chenopodium album, Chenopodium album L.]

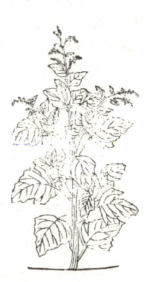

Huicai [灰菜, chenopodium album, Chenopodium album L.], growing in the fields, is distributed everywhere presently. Its plants are 2~3 Chi high with purple and red arris on the stems. There is grey cystic hair on the leaves. Its fruit is green, the spicate plants are sweet in taste, and the inflorescence-dispersed plants are slightly bitter in taste. It is warm in nature, and those growing under the wall or trees are not edible.

For famine relief: Collect and blanch young leaves, soak them in fresh water and remove the smell of the grey cystic hair, and flavor them with oil and salt. It is especially delicious after drying. When the tassel is ripe, grind the seeds into flour, make into pancakes and steam for food.

413. 丁香茄儿

亦名天茄儿。延蔓而生。人家园篱边多种。茎紫多刺,藤长丈余。叶似牵牛叶,甚大而无花叉;又似初生嫩苘[1]叶却小。开粉紫边紫色心筒子花,状如牵牛花样。结小茄,如丁香样而大。有子如白牵牛子,亦大。味微苦。

救饥:采茄儿煠食,或腌作菜食。嫩叶亦可煠熟,油盐调食。

【注释】

[1] 苘麻。见本书第191苘子条。

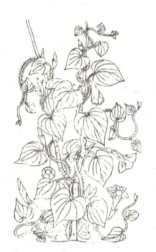

413. Dingxiang Qie'er [丁香茄儿, calonyction muricatum, Calonyction muricatum (L.) G. Don]

Dingxiang Qie'er [丁香茄儿, calonyction muricatum, Calonyction muricatum (L.) G. Don], also named Tianqie'er, is planted on the fence side of common people's gardens with its vines creeping along the ground. Its stems with thorniness is purple, and its vines are more than one Zhang long. Its leaves are like those of Qianniu [牵牛, Morning glory, Pharbitis nil (L.) Choisy], very big with no lobes, and also like those of Qingma[1] [苘麻, abutilon, Abutilon theophrasti Medicus], but smaller. Its flowers are cylindrical with the purple edge and center. It is shaped like the flowers of the Morning Glory, with small eggplant-shaped fruit, which is like the shape of a lilac, but larger. Its seeds are like those of Baiqianniu [白牵牛, pharbitidis, semen, Cissus repens Lamk.], but bigger. It is bitter in taste.

For famine relief: Collect and blanch the eggplant-shaped fruit or pickle them for food. Or collect and blanch young leaves, and then flavor them with oil and salt.

【Notes】

[1] See the 191th clause of this book.

根及实皆可食

❋ 《本草》原有

Root and Fruit Edible

Original Ones

414. 山 药

本草名薯蓣,一名山芋,一名诸薯,一名修脆,一名儿草,秦楚名玉延,郑越名土藷。出明州、滁州,生嵩山山谷,今处处有之。春生苗,蔓延篱援。茎紫色。叶青,有三尖角,似千叶狗儿秧叶而光泽。开白花。结实如皂荚子大。其根皮色黪黄,中则白色。人家园圃种者,肥大如手臂,味美。怀孟间产者,入药最佳。味甘,性温、平,无毒。紫芝为之使,恶甘遂。

救饥:掘取根,蒸食甚美。或火烧熟食,或煮食,皆可。其实亦可煮食。

治病:文具《本草·草部》薯蓣条下。

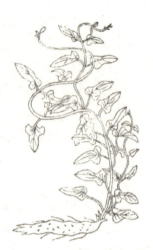

414. Shanyao〔山药, common yam rhizome, Dioscorea polystachya Turcz.〕

Shanyao〔山药, common yam rhizome, Dioscorea polystachya Turcz.〕, also named Shuyu, Shanyu, Zhuyu, Xiucui and Ercao, was called Yuyan in the regions of Qin and Chu, and Tushu in the regions of Zheng and Yue in ancient China. It grows in Mingzhou, Chuzhou and in the valleys of Mount Song. Presently, it can be seen everywhere. Its seedlings grow in spring, and its plants creep on the fence. Its stems are purple. Its leaves are green, with three pointed fruit, just like those of wrapped peonies, but lustrous. Its flowers are white. Its fruit is as small as the seeds of soap pods. The bark of its rhizome is dark yellow with white flesh. The kind of Shanyao, which is planted in the gardens of common people, is as strong as an arm and delicious. Those that grow in Huaizhou and

Mengzhou are appropriate to be used as medicine. It is sweet in taste, neutral in nature and non-toxic. In compatibility, Zizhi [紫芝, Chinese ganoderma, Ganoderma Sinensis] is its assistance, and it is averse to Gansui [甘遂, gansui root, Radix Euphorbiae Kansui].

For famine relief: It is delicious to steam or cook the stem tubers. Its fruit (bulbil) is also edible after cooking.

For disease treatment: See the relevant clause of Shuyu [薯蓣, common yam rhizome, Dioscorea polystachya Turcz.] in *Materia Medica · Herbaceous Vegetable*.